# Pharmacology
## *for the*
# Dental Hygienist
## *For Students and Practitioners*

*O love that wilt not let me go, I rest my weary soul in thee;*
*I give thee back the life I owe, that in thine ocean depths its flow may richer, fuller be.*

GEORGE MATHESON, 1842-1906

# Pharmacology
## *for the*
# Dental Hygienist
### *For Students and Practitioners*

FRED F. COWAN, B.S. (Pharm.), Ph.D.

*Professor of Pharmacology*
*Chairman, Department of Pharmacology*
*School of Dentistry*
*University of Oregon Health Sciences Center*
*Portland, Oregon*

## *Lea & Febiger*     *Philadelphia ·*

**Library of Congress Cataloging in Publication Data**
Cowan, Fred F.
  Pharmacology for the dental hygienist.

  Bibliography
  Includes index.
  1. Dental pharmacology.  2. Dental hygiene.
I. Title.
RK701.C68                    615'.1'0246176                    77-17477
ISBN 0-8121-0626-1

Published in Great Britain by Henry Kimpton Publishers, London
Printed in the United States of America
Print number 3 2

*To the glory of God*
*and to my loving family,*
*Phyllis, Caroline, and Kirk*

# PREFACE

My primary reason for writing this text is to provide students and practitioners of dental hygiene with their own accurate, up-to-date, unembellished study guide to information regarding the drugs of specific interest and concern to them. Secondly, I want to establish a higher level of understanding between the dental hygiene profession and pharmacology by demonstrating the specific relationships between our two disciplines. Thirdly, I believe that there is a current need for such a text. This is not to say that the *Pharmacology for the Dental Hygienist* by Kutscher and his associates, published in 1967, is completely out-of-date. There will always be a need for the enormous amount of such clinical detail regarding drug use in dentistry.

The present textbook is more oriented toward the basic science aspects of pharmacology with just the appropriate amount of clinical dental hygiene application to keep the student making necessary correlations. It is hoped that the text supports the principles and the specifics of the American Dental Hygiene Association's curriculum essentials as they have been modified over recent years.

It is, of course, difficult to know where to begin in acknowledging individuals for assistance in the preparation of this book. Before I do so I must explain that, in reality, I look upon myself as an arranger of pharmacological information; I did not compose the original music nor write the original lyrics; what I have done is pick and choose from a large, ever-growing body of knowledge that I thought most appropriate at the time. I know there are areas of pharmacology that should be included in future editions, and I am expecting every reader to offer suggestions for what should be added and what should be deleted. As an arranger, then, each thought found herein probably can be accredited to someone else, for my own present understanding of pharmacology is the summation of what all my teachers, colleagues, and students have taught me.

I am specifically grateful to my colleague and fellow arranger, Samuel E. Taylor, Ph.D., who has contributed the material on the adrenergic stimulants and blocking agents, as well as the following complete chapters: Characteristics of Drug Action, Vitamins, Drugs in the Treatment of Cardiovascular Disorders, and Drugs in the Treatment of Endocrinological Disorders. In addition, he has given continuous encouragement and valuable advice on many other sections. Surely, he is my friend.

Writing words on paper is only a small part of the preparation of a textbook, even one as narrow in scope as this; however, having the manuscript typed in a presentable, accurate form takes manipulative skills as well as dedication to the smallest detail. I am grateful to Colleen M. Gooding who has typed this textbook not just once but countless times. Surely, she is an artist.

Lastly, I can state honestly that I am even grateful to Martin C. Dallago, my editor at Lea & Febiger, who originally convinced me to undertake this task and who has since waited so patiently for so long. Surely, he is a saint.

Portland, Oregon                                    Fred F. Cowan

# CONTENTS

PART  *I*

# ORIENTATION AND GENERAL PRINCIPLES

# 1

# THE ROLE OF PHARMACOLOGY IN DENTAL HYGIENE

Pharmacology is the science that deals with all facets of drugs, especially the action of drugs on living tissue. Since a drug is usually defined as any chemical substance that affects living tissue, pharmacology is a broad discipline. More commonly a drug is considered as any chemical substance, with the exception of food, that is used as an aid in the diagnosis, treatment, or prevention of disease or to control or improve any physiological or pathological condition.

Although a course in pharmacology is included in most dental hygiene educational programs, it has been difficult to find what the role of pharmacology is or should be in dental hygiene. In many instances the pharmacology courses in dental hygiene education appear to be general, selected surveys of a variety of drug groups with or without special emphasis on the drugs particularly used in dentistry. It would seem if pharmacology is important enough to include in the dental hygiene curriculum there should be some attempt to agree upon what it is doing there and to orient it strongly toward that pharmacology necessary for the competent practice of dental hygiene.

It will no doubt come as a surprise to many pharmacologists, but today's dental hygienists do utilize a small number of drugs as adjuncts to the procedures they perform. These selected agents are administered under the supervision of a dentist, and the kinds of drugs that the dental hygienist may give to the patient are spelled out in the practice acts of each state. Even at this time, because of the rapid evolution of the dental hygiene profession, there is wide variation from state to state regarding what drugs, if any, may be used by the dental hygienist. Changes will continue to come in terms of what drugs may be used, how the drugs may be administered, and the degree of actual supervision required by the dentist. Based upon this background several roles of pharmacology in dental hygiene are offered for discussion.

It could be argued quite validly that the dental hygienist must know the pertinent pharmacology of at least those drugs that are utilized as adjuncts to the dental hygiene procedures and are administered by the dental hygienist. On the other hand, what pharmacology would be considered essential if the dental hygienist does not make the final decision whether a particular drug should be used in a particular patient, or even what dose should be administered? In most instances the supervising dentist must make the final decision concerning a drug's use, how much to give, and how it must be taken.

This pharmacologist does not accept the dental hygiene profession as an overeducated group of "go-fors." To be realistic the dental hygienist may most likely be the dental health team member who first recognizes the dental patient's need for a particular drug. The dental hygienist would then verify this need with the dentist who, with the dental hygienist, would make the final decision as to which drug, the dose, and route of administration. In other words, the dental hygienist must be aware of the specific indications for which these drugs are used. Furthermore, the dental hygienist must know what effects the drug may be expected to produce as well as any precautions to be observed in the drug's use.

If this general philosophy is acceptable, then the specific pharmacological information for dental hygienists to learn and know regarding those drugs they will be using as adjuncts to their procedures may be outlined. This approach has the added advantage of allowing to be identified all that other pharmacology dental hygienists should not be required to learn. Therefore, one of pharmacology's roles in dental hygiene is to supply the appropriate and selective information about the specific drugs the dental hygienist will be using as adjuncts to their procedures.

Pharmacology has another role to play in the life of a competent dental hygienist. Even if the dental hygienist finds no need to administer or to recommend any drug to a particular patient, the hygienist would still need an adequate background in pharmacology to handle properly the drug information regarding each dental patient. An important part of patient pretreatment evaluation is the accurate recording of the patient's personal, medical, and dental history which includes a number of inquiries about drugs. Some of these questions would include, but not be limited to the following: Is the patient taking any drugs (both prescription drugs and over-the-counter drugs) currently or within the past month? If so, what are the names of the drugs? Has the patient experienced allergic or any unusual effects to any drug, in particular any of the drugs the patient may be required to encounter during dental hygiene or dental treatment? Does the patient now have, or has the patient ever had, any one of a number of disorders or diseases which require special drug administration (e.g., chemoprophylaxis) before dental hygiene or dental procedures can be carried out?

Once the dental hygienist has obtained this critical drug information from each patient, then it must be evaluated and translated into how it may or may not alter the planned course of dental or dental hygiene treatment for the patient. It is this translation process that requires a definite understanding of pharmacology.

Another role of pharmacology in dental hygiene is to guide the dental hygienist toward the most reliable sources of drug information. The dental hygienist is a busy professional involved in a special aspect of public health. Like colleagues in medicine, dentistry, and nursing, the dental hygienist will need to know how and where to find accurate, up-to-date information regarding drugs used in dental hygiene, drugs used in dentistry, and drugs dental patients are taking when they seek your services.

As an important and active member of the health team in the dental office, it is only natural, desirable, and to be expected that the dental hygienist have some degree of general understanding of all aspects of the care of dental patients. The dentist uses drugs in the treatment of oral diseases and as adjuncts to the dental procedures performed. Although the dental hygienist will not be administering many of these drugs, it is necessary that the dental hygienist have a general understanding regarding at least the types of situations for which the drugs are indicated in dentistry, what effects they will produce in the patient that will indicate the drug is giving the desired response, as well as what precautions should be observed in employing any drug used in the dental office. By being the second person in the office who knows this information, the dental hygienist can aid immeasurably in the general safety of the patient. Unusual drug-induced effects can be noted and immediately conveyed to the dentist. Moreover, an active and effective role in the handling of the dental office emergencies can be assumed by the dental hygienist.

As the dental hygiene profession continues to grow and take on new and broader responsibilities, it seems only inevitable that the future will require the dental hygienist to possess a deeper understanding of pharmacology.

# 2

## CHARACTERISTICS OF DRUG ACTION

Pharmacology is a truly integrative science, borrowing heavily from such disciplines as physiology, biochemistry, and other biological sciences, and as such has become one of the most complex and all-encompassing of the basic medical or dental sciences. Some of the specialties of pharmacology are defined in Table 2.1

Although pharmacology may be said to have had its beginnings with early man's observations of the effects of herbs and plant extracts on himself and other animals, pharmacology as a science could not begin until hundreds of years later when chemists began to improve their techniques for the extraction and purification of active principles from plants. This was a necessary precursor to the advancement of pharmacology, since any conclusions about how drugs work must be based on knowledge of exactly what substance and how much of this substance is being administered. Only then can hypotheses be developed that may be tested by reproducible experimentation.

Historically, physiology has contributed the most to the science of pharmacology, and most of the early pharmacologists were originally trained in physiology. Of these men, Rudolf Buchheim is usually credited with establishing the first "modern" laboratory of pharmacology.[1] As modern technology advances, allowing scientists to study the action of drugs at the cellular and molecular levels, biochemical and molecular pharmacology are areas of increasing research interests. Much as been learned in the past decade or so about the biochemical fate of many drugs within the body. However, many intriguing questions remain to be answered: How is the drug's initial contact with a particular cell translated into changes within the intracellular physicochemical

## Table 2.1. Specialties of Pharmacology

| | Definitions |
|---|---|
| Biochemical pharmacology | the metabolism and other biochemical aspects of drugs |
| Clinical pharmacology | the study of the effects of drugs in man |
| Descriptive pharmacology | the consideration of the qualitative effects of drugs |
| Molecular pharmacology | a study of drug effects at the molecular level |
| Pharmacodynamics | the study of the biochemical and physiological effects of drugs and their mechanisms of action |
| Pharmacogenetics | the interrelationships between drug effects and the genetic makeup of the responding individual |
| Pharmacognosy | the study of the botanical sources and properties of naturally occurring drugs |
| Pharmacokinetics | the absorption, distribution, biotransformation, and excretion of drugs |
| Pharmacotherapeutics | the art and science of using drugs in the prevention, diagnosis, and treatment of disease |
| Pharmacy | the art and science of preparing and dispensing of drugs as medicines |
| Posology | the study of the general subject of dosage |
| Toxicology | the study of the adverse effects of drugs; the science of poisons |

environment which eventually lead to the characteristic drug effect? How do variations in an individual's genetic composition affect his response to a given drug? Can more specific drugs be developed for the treatment of cancer and for suppression of the immune and inflammatory responses?

Of more immediate concern to the dentist and the dental hygienist is the application of present and future pharmacological knowledge to the safer and more effective use of drugs in their patients. A thorough understanding of the general principles of drug action to be discussed in this chapter is the foundation upon which this goal may be accomplished. Such an understanding not only is important for the proper administration and monitoring of drugs by the practitioner, but also is imperative for any mature understanding of the possible interactions between drugs administered by the practitioner and other drugs the patient may be taking, either self-administered or under medical supervision.

The first medical uses of drugs by man were based strictly on empiricism, that is, the use of a drug in particular situation based only upon the dictates of past experience without any sound knowledge of what the drug was doing. Some drugs are still used empirically in both medicine and dentistry because they "work"; they alleviate illness, or at least its manifestations, but what the drug is actually doing to cause these improvements (its mechanism of action) is not known. However, with our present understanding of pharmacology, as meager as it may be, the use of drugs should be based on a rational approach whenever possible. The rational use of drugs includes an understanding of how the drug acts, what effects it has on normal physiological and biochemical processes of the body (both desirable and undesirable), and then using this knowledge to produce safely the desired effect. Paramount to rational therapeutics is the concept of the therapeutic end point. A drug should never be administered to a patient unless the practitioner has a clear understanding of the appropriate type and intensity of therapeutic effect the drug is to produce, as well as how to determine when this point has been reached.

## DRUG RECEPTORS

Probably everyone has at one time or another taken an aspirin to relieve the pain of mild headache. Within a brief time after taking the aspirin, the headache pain usually disappears. Few people, however, stop to wonder how the aspirin brings this about. Similarly, most people have comfortably undergone potentially painful dental treatment while under local anesthesia. By injecting a solution containing a local anesthetic into the patient's oral tissues the dentist can perform traumatic procedures with the patient feeling little, if any, pain. How does the local anesthetic produce this effect? If one drank the local anesthetic solution, it would not relieve headache pain; nor would injection of an aspirin solution into the oral tissues produce local anesthesia. What is it then that makes aspirin, with its characteristic headache-relieving properties, an analgesic, and the local anesthetic, with its characteristic ability to produce profound absence of local pain, a local anesthetic?

The answer to this question lies in the chemical sturcture of the drug itself, as well as in the physicochemical composition of the body's biological systems. All drugs have their own individualized chemical structures, just as each person has his own unique set of fingerprints. Knowledge of the drug's chemical structure alone, however, is not enough to predict the type of characteristic pharmacological response a drug will produce. Only when aspirin and a local anesthetic are introduced into a patient under the proper conditions does a difference become apparent. These two drugs require the presence of a viable biological system in order to express their biological activity.

This is an obvious point, but take this analysis a step further and ask, What elements in the two drugs and the biological system combine to produce the characteristic pharmacological effect? The biochemical reactions involved in cellular respiration and metabolism are exceedingly complex, but when these complex reactions are broken down to their basic components they all involve the reaction of the one molecule with another molecule. Drug molecules are also capable of reacting with molecules of an organism and in this way causing some change in the cell's chemical environment.

The idea that drugs had to combine with components of living cells in order to produce an effect was proposed by J. N. Langley in the late 1800's.[2] After studying the effects of atropine and pilocarpine on salivary flow, he suggested that the two substances must combine with some component of the nerve endings or salivary gland cells to form compounds and that the formation of these compounds was related in some way to their chemical affinities for these two substances. Paul Ehrlich, the father of chemotherapy, extended this concept and applied the term "receptive substances" to chemical groups of the "protoplasmic molecule" which gave a biological response by combining with complementary groups of natural or foreign molecules.[3] This concept of binding of complementary groups is similar to that proposed by the chemist, Emil Fisher, with respect to the interaction of enzymes with their respective substrates. In noting the relatively high degree of specificity of enzymes, he concluded that the enzyme and its substrate must fit together like a "lock and key" through complementary structures.[4]

The work of these men contributed to the acceptance of the idea that drugs produce their pharmacological and toxicological effects by chemically interacting with biological tissue, but it remained for A.J. Clark (1933) to suggest how much of the total cell surface was actually involved in this drug-tissue interaction.[5] Through a series of involved calculations, he estimated that if an isolated organ was exposed to a concentration of acetylcholine sufficient to produce an effect, the amount of acetylcholine actually bound to the organ would cover less than 1% of the total cell surface area. This led to the concept of a highly specialized and localized area of the cell surface which acts as a receptor for a specific drug. Clark concluded that drugs occupy certain specific receptors on the cell surface, and that these specific receptors only comprise a small fraction of the total cell surface. The theory of a drug combining with a specialized receptor has great importance in explaining, to a limited degree, how minute quantities of drug can produce such profound effects in a patient.

Since these earliest formulations of the drug-receptor concept, pharmacologists have identified many types of receptors with respect to which drugs will or will not combine with a specific receptor, the kinetics of the binding, and the final outcome of the drug-receptor interaction. Drug receptors appear to be macromolecules located either on the cell membrane or within the cell itself. By virtue of their large size, receptor molecules are not homogeneous with respect to the distribution of their electrochemical forces. Some areas of the molecule may be electropositive, while others may be electronegative. Some areas may be hydrophilic, others hydrophobic. This heterogeneity within the receptor molecule determines the pattern of electrochemical forces being exerted outwardly in the immediate vicinity of the receptor.

The drug molecule, which has its own pattern of electrochemical forces, is in constant, random motion due to its thermal energy. When the drug molecule approaches close enough to the receptor that the attractive forces between them become great enough to overcome the random motion of the drug molecule, the drug binds to the receptor.

Most drug-receptor interactions consist of weak chemical bonds such as ionic bonds, hydrogen bonds, hydrophobic bonds, and Van der Walls forces. The energy involved in the formation of these types of bonds is very low. Consequently they are easily formed and easily broken, and almost as soon as the drug binds to its receptor, it disengages and another drug molecule takes its place. This reversibility accounts in part for the relatively short duration of action of most clinically useful drugs. A few drug-receptor interactions are formed of strong covalent bonds that require significant amounts of energy to make and break. Drugs that bind to their receptors by these types of bonds do not disassociate readily, and that particular receptor is unavailable for further combination for a significant period of time.

AFFINITY. Regardless of the type of bond formed, there are at least two potential components of initial drug-receptor interaction. The first step is the actual coupling of the drug to the receptor. The tendency for this coupling to occur is defined as the affinity of the drug for its receptor; one drug is said to have a greater affinity than another if it binds more readily to the receptor. The affinity that a drug has for its receptor is related to its potency as illustrated in Figure 2.1.

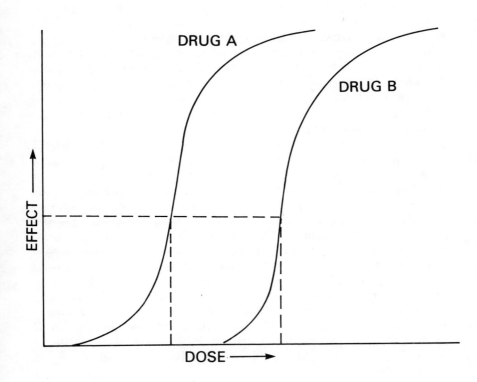

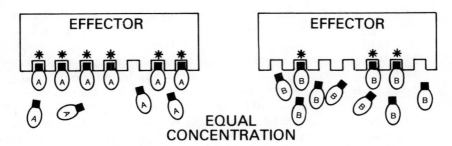

**Figure 2.1** Relationship between drug affinity for its receptor and potency. This figure diagrammatically illustrates that when equal concentrations of two drugs are in equilibrium with the same receptor population (square indentions), the drug with the greater affinity (drug A) will undergo a greater number of effective bindings (*) at any given instant. Thus, a lower concentration of drug A will be required to produce the same level of pharmacological effect.

In this example two drugs, A and B, both have affinity for the same pharmacological receptor, interaction with which results in the same pharmacological response. If drug A has a greater affinity for the receptor than drug B, and if the same number of molecules of the two drugs is in equilibrium with the receptors, then it follows that more molecules of drug A than of drug B will be bound to the receptors at any given time. This concept is illustrated diagrammatically in Figure 2.1. Since it appears that the magnitude of the pharmacological response is in some way dependent on the number of drug-receptor interactions, the receptor will be expressed outwardly as requiring a smaller dose of drug A than drug B to produce the same level of pharmacological response, and drug A is said to be more potent than drug B.

INTRINSIC ACTIVITY. The actual coupling or binding of the drug to the receptor is not all that is involved in drug-receptor interaction. Some drugs have more ability than others to "stimulate" the receptor once the drug has bound to it. The ability of a drug to stimulate the receptor and thus produce an effect is termed its intrinsic activity or efficacy. Intrinsic activity cannot be measured directly and must be expressed in relation to some standard drug, that is, some drug known to be capable of producing the maximal effect. A drug that is capable of binding to a receptor, stimulating it, and thus producing a characteristic effect is called an agonist. If such a drug possesses full intrinsic activity and is capable of producing the maximum effect possible, it is called a full agonist. If a drug does not possess full intrinsic activity and therefore cannot produce the same degree of maximum effect, it is called a partial agonist. As one would suspect from the nature of intrinsic activity, these are relative terms.

Some drugs have the ability to bind to the receptor (thus they have affinity), but have no intrinsic activity. If such a drug binds to the receptor, it interferes with the binding of the agonist, since, obviously, the agonist cannot occupy the receptor at the same time another drug is occupying it. With a given number of the receptors occupied by the second drug, fewer of the receptors can be occupied by the agonist, and the second drug antagonizes the action of the agonist. Such drugs are called competitive antagonists or competitive blocking agents, since they are competing for the same receptor as the agonist.

It is also possible for a second drug to bind with a site which is separate from the agonist's receptor, but which influences the agonist-receptor interaction. When this second drug binds to its site, it evidently distorts the agonist's receptor in such a way that the agonist fails to bind properly and cannot express its full intrinsic activity. This type of antagonism is called noncompetitive antagonism, since the two drugs are not competing for the same receptor. The end result is the same, that is, less effect for a given dose of agonist in the presence of the antagonist as compared with the effect caused by the same dose in the absence of the antagonist. The concepts of potency, intrinsic activity, and antagonism will be discussed in greater detail below.

PHARMACOLOGICAL ACTION. Pharmacologists have learned a great deal about the kinetics of drug-receptor binding, but until recently little was known about what happens between the time when the drug binds to the receptor and when an observable effect is produced. Presumably, the interaction of a drug with its receptor triggers an initial physicochemical change in the receptor's immediate environment. This change leads to some initial event termed the pharmacological action. An example of drug action might be a change in the membrane permeability to calcium. Such an action might then initiate one or more pharmacological effects, for example, smooth muscle contraction. In the last decade or so, significant progress has been made toward identifying the various components in the chain of events linking drug-receptor binding to the final pharmacological effect. It is now known that many drugs and hormones, such as epinephrine, produce some of their effects by activating an enzyme, adenyl cyclase. This enzyme catalyzes the conversion of adenosine triphosphate (ATP) to adenosine-3',5'-monophosphate (cyclic AMP). The cyclic AMP thus formed acts as a "second messenger" to cause other changes in the cellular and subcellular physicochemical environment. For example, the stimulation of salivary secretion by 5-hydroxytryptamine (5-HT) is mediated, in part, through activation of adenyl cyclase.[6] Interactions of 5-HT with its receptor on the basal side of the salivary secretory cell leads to activation of adenyl cyclase. The resultant increase in cyclic AMP appears to stimulate transport of cations at the apical surface of the cell through a yet undefined mechanism. Many other questions remain to be answered, including the mechanism whereby the binding of drug to receptor is transformed into activation of adenyl cyclase. In addition, undoubtedly still other "second" and possibly even "third" and "fourth" messengers are involved in other drug effects. These are areas of intense research activity at the present time.

PROPERTIES OF RECEPTORS. Much of what little is known about the actual chemical structures of pharmacological receptors has been derived indirectly. Comparison of the kinetics of drug-receptor interaction with that of enzyme-substrate reactions has led to the conclusion that receptors must have many properties in common with enzymes. It is generally agreed that receptors are macromolecules and that, like enzymes, their steric or three-dimensional structure is vital to their activity. Steric structure deals not with which atoms make up a given molecule, but rather with how the various groups of atoms are arranged in space and how the molecule coils around itself. Present evidence indicates that when a substrate binds to an enzyme it causes physicochemical changes in the enzyme molecule which than allow more binding to occur. In other words, the substrate "induces a better fit" between itself and the enzyme. This is in contrast to the old idea of the enzyme as a rigid template into which the substrate must fit. This additional binding then causes a steric realignment of the entire molecule. It should be noted that this makes an attractive hypothesis for explaining the coupling of drug-receptor binding (affinity) to the pharmacological action. The ability of a drug to induce secondary changes in the receptor molecule after initial binding would be an expression of its intrinsic activity. These secondary changes might then cause steric realignment of the entire receptor molecule with resultant changes in surrounding molecules, i.e., activation of adenyl cyclase or some other pharmacological action.

One way to examine indirectly the chemical structure of a receptor is by considering a complementary fit between a structurally known drug and the hypothetical receptor. Figure 2.2 very simply illustrates what is meant by a complementary fit between a drug and its receptor. L-epinephrine is the pharmacologically active form of epinephrine while its optical isomer, D-epinephrine, is inactive. In this figure it is assumed that for effective interaction to take place, the drug must bind to three areas on the molecule: (1) a point on the receptor that binds the aromatic portion of epinephrine, (2) a point that binds the hydroxyl group on the beta carbon, and (3) a point that binds the methylamine group. Although the structure of L-epinephrine fulfills these prerequisites, the steric configuration of D-epinephrine is such that there is no way for the molecule to align itself so that all three groups are in proper position to bind simultaneously. By changing the drug molecule in various ways and then noting how these changes affect the drug's activity, the groups necessary for the particular activity being investigated can be determined. Studies of this type are called structure-activity-relationship (SAR) studies. The practical importance of studies of this type is that in many cases they have provided the knowledge necessary for "tailor-making" new drugs. It should be emphasized that receptors vary with respect to rigidity, i.e., how readily a drug can "induce a better fit." The more rigid the receptor, the more specific will be the relationship between the structure of the drug and its activity.

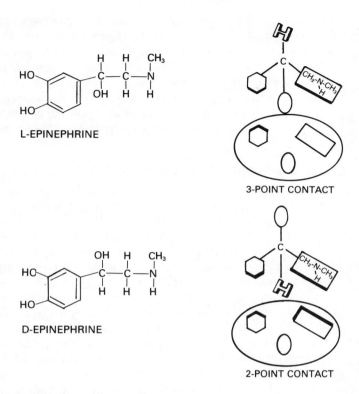

**Figure 2.2** Complementary fit between drug and receptor. L-epinephrine fits into the three essential parts of the receptor, but D-epinephrine can fit into only two parts at any one time. (Redrawn from Csaky, 1969.[4])

In addition to the fact that more than one drug may interact with the same receptor, it is also true that one drug may interact with more than one type of receptor. Not only can some drugs interact with more than one type of pharmacological receptor, but also some drugs bind to chemical components of various tissues, such as hydroxyapatite of bone and plasma protein. Binding sites that do not elicit any pharmacological response when a drug binds to them are called acceptors to distinguish them from those molecules that are capable of eliciting a pharmacological response, i.e., pharmacological receptors. Finally, it should be noted that not all drugs produce their pharmacological effects by interacting with pharmacological receptors. Some drugs cause profound changes by virtue of their physical presence only and are called nonspecific drugs. The anesthetic gases are examples of nonspecific drugs; they cause loss of consciousness without interacting (as far as is known) with receptors in the central nervous system.

Therefore, specific drugs do react with specialized drug receptors, and this interaction depends on the chemical structure of both drug and receptor. Basically, then, it is this specificity between drug and receptor that makes aspirin, an analgesic and the local anesthetic, a local anesthetic. The specificity is not so great, however, that a drug can bind with only one type of receptor. Drugs can, and do, react with more than one type of receptor, and one of the fundamental axioms of pharmacology is that no drug has only one action.

## QUANTITATIVE ASPECTS OF DRUG ACTION

The most obvious comparison that can be made between two drugs is with respect to the qualitative effect produced by the drugs, that is, both drugs produce the same type of effect. Within the same qualitative class, drugs are further classified on the basis of their quantitative relationships. The quantitative aspects of drug action are important experimentally and clinically. To the pharmacologist, careful measurement of the alterations caused by drugs under carefully defined conditions is the cornerstone for the analytical investigation of the mechanisms by which drugs produce their effects. Conversely, similar studies lead to the discovery of new information which emerges when the response of living tissue to drugs whose mechanisms of action are known is carefully measured.

Although the dentist and dental hygienist are not directly concerned with these types of studies, nevertheless, an understanding of the knowledge gained from such studies is essential to the rational clinical use of drugs. The quantitative aspects of drug action can be considered from several perspectives, including the following: How does the intensity of the drug effect change as the dose is changed? How does the intensity of effect change with time? How is the desired level of therapeutic effect related to dose, or more specifically, how should the practitioner arrive at the proper dose of a drug for a particular patient? How are the adverse effects and therapeutic effects of a drug related with respect to dose? What should the practitioner expect regarding the variability of response of the patient population? These questions cannot be precisely answered for a given drug in a given patient, but the general principles of drug action, if understood and applied clinically, can guide the practitioner's safe use of drugs in patients.

For anyone who administers or prescribes drugs, an appreciation of the variability of one's patient population is essential. The magnitude of the response of a patient to a given dose of a drug is determined by several factors. Two of these, the affinity and intrinsic activity, are properties of the drug and receptor molecules and contribute little to patient variability. The magnitude of effect is also modified by the responsiveness of the target cell or tissue itself and the effectiveness of both cellular and systemic reflexes in modifying the changes induced by the drug. These latter factors are all in a state of dynamic equilibrium and are subject to wide variation. In addition, many processes acting upon a drug once it enters the body can influence the concentration of drug in equilibrium with its pharmacological receptors. Consequently, all of these factors combine to contribute to much of the variation seen when drugs are administered to a group of patients. The term *biological variation* connotes the sum total of all the sources of variation that combine to cause one biological unit to vary from another and is most often manifest as differences in the quantitative aspects of drug action as opposed to qualitative differences (although these too can exist).

GRADED DOSE-RESPONSE CURVE. The relationship between dose and effect can be perceived from two different perspectives. In one of these, the relationship between dose and change in magnitude of effect is of primary importance. This relationship is based upon one of the most fundamental principles of pharmacology, i.e., the magnitude of drug effect is some function of the dose administered, and is most easily visualized by means of a graded dose-response curve as illustrated in Figure 2.3. The term *graded* refers to that characteristic of an effect which begins at some low level and increases through progressive stages until it reaches some higher level. The lowest dose of a drug that will produce a measurable response is called the threshold dose. This dose is of greater theoretical than practical interest. As the dose of drug administered is increased further, the response continues to increase in some gradual and smooth fashion, usually at a fairly rapid rate of change. As the dose is increased still further, the rate of change of the response decreases and a point is reached above which further increases in dose cause no change in response. This plateau is called the ceiling or maximum effect. The graded dose-response curve may take many forms, but is usually some type of hyperbolic relationships when the dose is plotted on an arithmetic scale (Figure 2.3A). More commonly, for analytical convenience, a mathematical transformation of the dose axis is made by plotting the logarithm of the dose (Figure 2.3B).

The graded dose-response curve is a convenient expression of three important characteristics of a given drug for the conditions under which the dose-response curve was obtained: (1) The position of graded dose-response curve along the dose axis is a measure

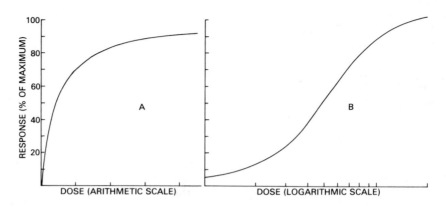

**Figure 2.3**   Graded dose-response curves. A, Arithmetic scale. B, Logarithmic scale.

of the drug's potency, i.e., how much of the drug it takes to produce a certain intensity of response. (2) Knowledge of the complete dose-response curve is the only reliable way of determining the maximum effect that the drug will produce under the defined conditions. The maximum effect is sometimes referred to as the efficacy of the drug. (3) The rate of change of response intensity as the dose is increased is given by the slope of the graded dose-response curve. These three characteristics are illustrated in Figure 2.4 in which graded dose-response curves of three hypothetical drugs, all producing the same pharmacological effect, are shown. In this example, drug A is more potent than drug B, and drug C is the least potent. The maximum effect, or efficacy, of a drug is of greater clinical interest, however, especially with respect to the therapeutic effect, since the practitioner would usually like the drug to produce as great a therapeutic effect as possible (for example, the level of pain relief). In Figure 2.4, drugs A and B have equal efficacy, whereas drug C has significantly less efficacy than the other two drugs. The clinical significance of the slope of the graded dose-response curve can be seen by noting the difference between the doses of drug B required to produce two levels of effect (indicated by points X and Y) as compared to that of drug C. If point X represents some desired level of therapeutic effect (for example, sedation) and point Y represents a level of effect which, in this case, is undesired (for example, hypnosis), then it should be apparent that the practitioner has a much narrower dose range in which to maintain the desired effect without progressing to the undesired level of response with drug B because of the steeper slope of its graded dose-response curve.

The graded dose-response curve for a drug is usually constructed from pooled data obtained from several individuals. Such curves then give some measure of the variability of the dose-response relationship for that representative sample. This variability is usually expressed on the graded dose-response curve as the variation around the mean level of response produced by a given dose of the drug, as indicated by the brackets on the dose-response curve for drug A in Figure 2.4. The dose of a drug required to cause a given level of response in a group of patients also varies. This type of variability is best examined by means of the quantal or "all-or-none" dose-response curve.

QUANTAL DOSE-RESPONSE CURVE. When the dose-response relationship is examined with respect to the frequency with which a specified dose of a drug produces a defined, "all-or-none" response, a quantal dose-response curve can be constructed. In the usual clinical situation, the practitioner administers a specified dose of drug which he expects to produce some effect, or some level of effect, established by his therapeutic end point. Any deviation from this point, either above or below, can be considered as failure of the drug in producing the desired response (in the idealized case). The desired therapeutic effect can then be considered as all-or-none, i.e., it either does or does not occur. Similarly, toxic or adverse effects can be treated as all-or-none effects.

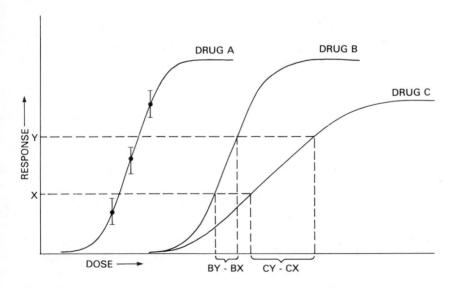

**Figure 2.4**   Potency, efficacy, and variation in graded dose-response curves.

If the minimal effective doses required to produce a certain effect in a group of patients is plotted against the number of people responding at a particular dose, a "normal" or bell-shaped distribution will be approached. There will be some central dose around which the sample of patients tends to cluster as illustrated in Figure 2.5. The most commonly used estimate of this central tendency is the arithmetic mean. About 95% of the patients will fall within the range indicated by the shaded area in Figure 2.5 (± two standard deviations of the mean dose) and thus the great majority of patients will usually fall within a fairly narrow dosage range which elicits the response being measured. The other patients, however, may require a noticeably different dose from the majority of patients. A few of these will require a significantly smaller dose than the mean dose in order to respond with the particular effect being observed, i.e., they are hyperreactive to the drug; others will require a significantly higher dose than the majority in order to elicit the required response, i.e., they are hyporeactive to the drug. This type of examination provides the best illustration of the variability of a patient population with respect to the dose-response relationship, and it should be readily apparent that in some patients it may be necessary to adjust the dose of a drug either up or down from the average dose in order to elicit the appropriate level of effect.

The "normally" distributed variation in reactivity of individuals with respect to dose may also be expressed as an integrated or accumulative quantal dose-response curve as illustrated in Figure 2.6. If the frequency of response at any given dose is expressed as the percentage of the total number of individuals, rather than simply the number of individuals responding to a minimally effective dose as in Figure 2.5, then at the lower doses only a small percentage of individuals will respond. As the dose is progressively increased, a

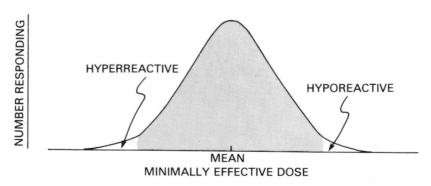

**Figure 2.5** Normal distribution.

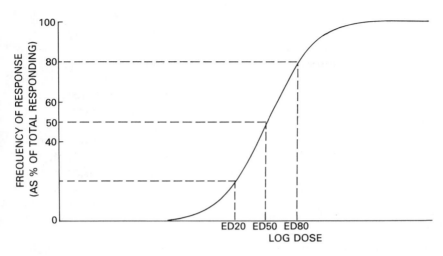

**Figure 2.6**  Quantal dose-response curve.

greater percentage of the total group will be recruited until a dose is reached to which all individuals of the group will be responsive.

This type of representation has several analytical advantages over the bell-shaped distribution of responses to minimally effective doses. The central portion of the S-shaped curve is usually fairly linear, and the linearity can be extended further by mathematical transformations of both the dose and the frequency of response. This linear portion can then be used for comparing one drug to another, as well as two effects of the same drug. Thus, this type of curve can be used to compare the potencies of two drugs in causing a given effect, since it shows the dose at which a specified percentage of individuals will respond to each of the drugs. There is a standardized way of referring to the dose of a drug which will produce a given response in a specified percentage of individuals (Figure 2.6). The smallest dose causing the given pharmacological effect in 50% of the individuals of a sample is called the ED50 (effective dose in 50% of the sample). Similar designations can be used to refer to doses causing other percentages of response, e.g., ED20, ED80.

The most important use of the quantal dose-response curve is in comparing the relative safety of one drug to that of another. The determination of the relative safety of a drug is based upon the fact that every drug has at least two quantal dose-response curves. It has one (or more) characterizing the therapeutic effect (or effects) and one (or more) characterizing its toxic effect (or effects). Relative safety refers to the dose of the drug required to produce the desired therapeutic effect relative to the dose of the drug required to produce toxic or lethal effects. More simply stated, the relative safety refers to how close the toxic effect curve is located to the curve for the therapeutic effect on the dose axis.

THERAPEUTIC INDEX. Several indices have been developed for referring to relative safety in an attempt to devise a more quantitative way of indicating the degree of separation between the therapeutic effects and the toxic or lethal effects of a drug. The oldest of these is the therapeutic index which, contrary to the implications of the name itself, is not an index of the therapeutic value of the drug. The therapeutic index is merely an approximate statement of the relative safety of the drug expressed as the ratio of the lethal or toxic dose to the therapeutic dose as illustrated in Figure 2.7. The therapeutic index is usually calculated at the 50% level of response since this has the greatest statistical accuracy, in which case the LD50, the minimum dose causing death in 50% of the individuals in a sample, divided by the ED50 would give the therapeutic index. For example, the therapeutic index for drug A in Figure 2.7 would be calculated as follows: the ED50 taken from the integrated quantal dose-response curve for the therapeutic effect is 2, while the LD50 taken from the integrated quantal dose-response curve for lethality is 21. The therapeutic index for drug A is, therefore, 10.5 (21 divided by 2). Similarly, the therapeutic index for drug B is 5.5. Based on these values alone, drug A appears to have greater relative safety than drug B.

The therapeutic index calculated in this way, however, has several disadvantages. For instance, the therapeutic index gives no information of the slopes of the quantal dose-response curves or the degree of overlap of their extremes. This can be a distinct disadvantage as illustrated in Figure 2.7. In the usual clinical situation, one would like to produce the therapeutic effect in all patients without producing toxic or lethal effects in any. With this in mind, it is apparent that drug A, because of the flat slope of its quantal dose-response curve, is actually less safe than drug B, since the dose of drug A causing the therapeutic effect in 99% of the individuals of a sample would also be expected to produce death in 15%. Another index, the certain safety factor, has been proposed to remedy this deficiency. The certain safety factor is actually a special case of the therapeutic index which is calculated by dividing the LD1 by the ED99 as illustrated for drug B in Figure 2.7. (It should be noted that the certain safety factor for drug A is less than 1.) A certain safety factor greater than 1, therefore, indicates that the dose of a drug causing the therapeutic effect in 99% of the individuals in a sample would be expected to be smaller than the

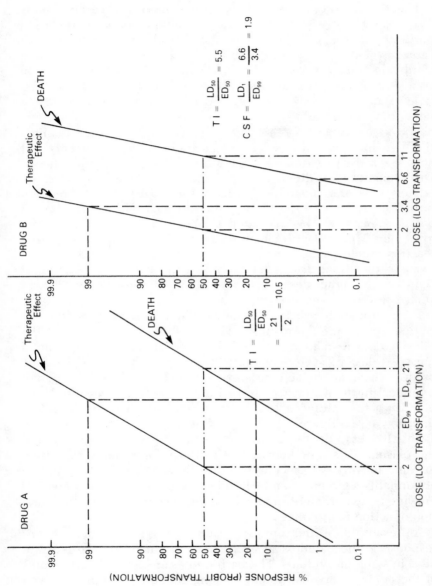

**Figure 2.7** Therapeutic index (TI) and certain safety factor (CSF), (Redrawn from Goldstein, Aronow, and Kalman, 1974.[7])

dose causing death in 1%, and that, generally, the greater the certain safety factor, the more the therapeutic dose has to be raised before toxic effects or death are to be expected.

The therapeutic index and its special case, the certain safety factor, can be accurately determined in laboratory animals during the initial phases of drug testing. Very rarely, however, are such values available for a drug as determined in humans. More commonly, the relatively safety of a drug in humans is extrapolated from animal data and less complete clinical data and is usually referred to in relative terms such as "one drug having a greater margin of safety than another."

UNDESIRABLE RESPONSES. Patient variation with respect to undesirable responses to drugs is seen in a variety of forms; usually, but not always, the variation takes the form of dose-related phenomena. Drug toxicity and idiosyncrasy are the two most important dose-related types of undesirable effects of drugs. Toxic effects are often further extensions of the therapeutic effect to undesirable levels, but they may also be unrelated to the therapeutic effect. Drug idiosyncrasy is a term used to describe a unique or unexpected drug reaction. Such reactions may be expressed either as extreme reactivity to the usual drug effects seen in the normal population at significantly higher doses or as unique qualitative effects not seen at any dose in the normal population.

Present evidence indicates many of the former types of idiosyncratic response are the results of genetic abnormalities, such as the idiosyncratic response seen in a few individuals to the skeletal muscle relaxant, succinylcholine. Low doses of succinylcholine produce skeletal muscle relaxation which is of short duration (minutes) in the majority of individuals receiving this drug. However, in a few individuals relaxation is of much longer duration (hours) at comparable doses. Succinylcholine is usually metabolized rapidly by an enzyme, pseudocholinesterase, found in the plasma. It is now known that in those individuals exhibiting extreme sensitivity to succinylcholine, there is a genetically linked abnormality of their pseudocholinesterase. Because this atypical enzyme is less efficient in metabolizing succinylcholine, the duration of action is prolonged.[7]

An example of the unique qualitative type of idiosyncratic response is the paradoxical excitement produced by the barbiturates in some individuals. The barbiturates are general depressants of the central nervous system causing sedation, sleep, and even general anesthesia in high doses. In some individuals, especially those on the extremes of the age spectrum, these same agents produce overt signs of excitation of the central nervous system instead of depression. The mechanism of this reaction is not completely understood.

Another important type of undesirable response to drugs, allergic hypersensitivity, is unrelated to the dose administered. Drugs vary with respect to their potential for producing allergic reactions. The antibiotic, penicillin, the local anesthetics, and even aspirin, all of which are used frequently by the dental practitioner, although low in total incidence, still cause allergic reactions in a large enough percentage of the population to cause concern. Allergic reactions to drugs can range in severity from a mild skin rash to severe, even fatal anaphylactic shock.

The major difference between the toxic response, the idiosyncratic response, and the allergic response can be summarized as follows:

(1) *Relationship to Dose.* Both the toxic and idiosyncratic responses are dose related, i.e., the intensity of the response increases as the dose is increased. The severity of the allergic reaction, on the other hand, is unrelated to dose; a small dose potentially may produce as severe a reaction as a large dose. For this reason, it is extremely important to avoid administration of any drug to which a patient has a known or suspected hypersensitivity, even in small doses. This rule applies equally to drugs similar in chemical structure to the offending drug.

(2) *Incidence among Drugs.* All drugs have the potential to produce toxic effects if the dose is increased to sufficient levels. Only a few drugs cause idiosyncratic and allergic responses, and even these drugs do not cause them in all patients.

(3) *Necessity of Prior Exposure.* Toxic and idiosyncratic responses are similar in that prior exposure to the drug is unnecessary for these responses to occur. In contrast, prior exposure to a drug is essential before it can elicit an allergic reaction.

(4) *Mechanism of Response.* Toxic and idiosyncratic responses are similar in that both are the result of drug-receptor interaction, and the effect is antagonized by specific antagonists at the receptor. The allergic response is the result of the antigen-antibody reaction. The antibody is specific, but the effects of the reaction are due to the release of mediators of the immunological response and, therefore, have no relation to the drug producing the effect. The antagonists which are used to counteract these undesirable effects also have no relation to the drug's pharmacological effect; rather they are drugs which tend to counteract the immunological responses, agents such as antihistamines, epinephrine and antiinflammatory steroids.

TIME-EFFECT RELATIONSHIP. The relationship between dose

and response is not the only quantitative aspect of drug action; the relationship between time and response is also important. A complete discussion of this relationship is beyond the scope of this text, and the interested reader is referred to more complete discussions in the references listed in the bibliography. Nevertheless, Figure 2.8 illustrates some elementary concepts and terminology for this relationship with respect to a single administration of a drug. After initial administration of a drug, there is a period of time before any perceptible effect of the drug is observed in the patient. The period from the time of administration, $T_0$, to the first observable effect, $T_1$, is called the drug's onset of action and is denoted by the letter A. The effect then increases with time up to a maximum point, termed the peak effect, after which the effect begins to subside. The period from the time of administration, $T_0$, to the time of peak effect, $T_2$, is called the time to peak effect and is denoted by the letter B in Figure 2.8. As the drug effect begins to subside, there is a significant period of time over which the effect of the drug can be

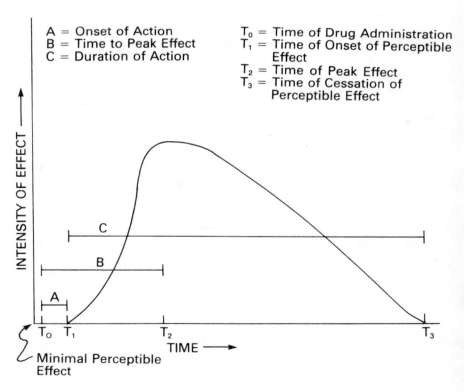

Figure 2.8  Drug response-time relationships.

observed. Finally, however, the drug effects will no longer be seen. The period from the time of onset, $T_1$, to the time of cessation of perceptible effect, $T_3$, is called the duration of action of the drug and is denoted by letter C in Figure 2.8.

The above parameters are the net result of many processes acting simultaneously; each influences the other. General statements can be made, nevertheless, regarding which of these processes are most important for each parameter. The time of onset is determined primarily by the rate and degree of absorption. The duration of action is affected primarily by the rate of inactivation and excretion of the drug, although compensatory reflexes and continued absorption modify the duration of action. The peak effect is primarily related to the rate of distribution of the drug to its site of action. Generally, the peak effect will be reached when the drug is in contact with the greatest number of reactive cells.

In addition to the factors mentioned above, the time of onset, the time of peak effect, and the duration of action of a drug are all dependent upon the dose administered. In general, the larger the dose which is administered the shorter will be the time of onset, the shorter will be the time of peak effect, and the longer will be the duration of action.

One of the most important clinical uses of these time-effect relationships is in the formulation of dosage schedules for a particular drug. When a drug is administered in multiple doses over a period of time the dosage schedule must be constructed in such a way as to avoid giving more drug than has been eliminated during the period since the last dose. Failure to do this may lead to build up of blood and tissue levels of the drug which will produce toxic effects. This type of toxicity, i.e., toxicity resulting from accumulation of drug over a long period of time, is called cumulative toxicity.

## ABSORPTION, DISTRIBUTION, BIOTRANSFORMATION, AND EXCRETION

In this section some of the things that happen to the drug once it has been administered to a patient will be presented. In other words, what are the effects of the normal biochemical and physiological processes of the body on the drug which has been administered? These processes both cause and modify the absorption of the drug, its distribution throughout the body, its metabolism (or biotransformation), and its excretion from the body.

An overview of factors influencing the concentration of a drug at its site of action is shown in Figure 2.9. After a drug has been introduced into a patient's body, either by topical administration,

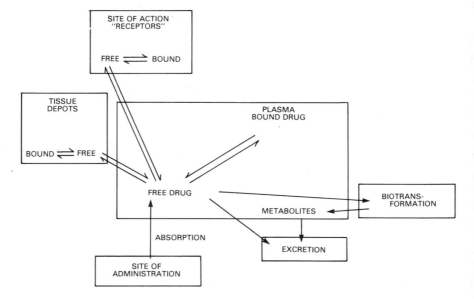

**Figure 2.9** Overview of influencing factors on drug at site of action. (Adapted and redrawn from Fingl and Woodbury, 1975.[16])

oral administration, or injection, the drug is then absorbed to varying degrees into the systemic circulation.

As the drug is absorbed, it enters the blood which transports it throughout the body. In the blood the drug can exist either in a free form or bound to plasma protein. These two forms of the drug, free and bound, exist in equilibrium with each other. Molecules of the drug thus constantly go back and forth between the two forms. This fact is important, since only the free form of the drug can diffuse out of the blood and become distributed in other tissues of the body, including the drug's site of action.

As the drug becomes distributed to its site of action, an equilibrium is established with its pharmacological receptor depending on the drug's concentration in the immediate vicinity (biophase) of the receptor. The drug, while in equilibrium with its receptor, is also in equilibrium with the free form in the plasma; thus, drug molecules constantly go back and forth between the site of action and the plasma.

In a similar way the free form of the drug is also distributed to other tissues of the body, some of which act as storage depots of the drug. Here too the drug can exist in free or bound form. The free form equilibrates with that which is bound to components of the tissue. Again the free form of the drug is in equilibrium with the free drug in the plasma so that here, too, the drug molecules constantly go back and forth between the plasma and tissue depots.

Figure 2.9 also illustrates how the action of a drug is terminated. A portion of the free drug is usually metabolized, or undergoes biotransformation, to an inactive form. These metabolites, as well as the free drug itself, can then be excreted from the body. As the drug is eliminated from the body, either by biotransformation or excretion, the concentration of free drug in the plasma falls, and new equilibria are established between the amount of drug bound to plasma protein, the amount that may be stored in tissue depots, and the amount of drug in equilibrium with its pharmacological receptor. Consequently the level of pharmacological response will begin to fall as the active drug is cleared from the body by these two processes, biotransformation and excretion, acting either alone or in combination.

The absorption, distribution, biotransformation, and excretion of drugs, as well as the processes that modify them, form the basis for evaluating the proper drug, dosage, and route of administration for a patient based on both that particular patient's physical history and the purpose for which the drug is given.

### Drug Passage through Biological Membranes

In all of the travels of a drug molecule around the body, it has to cross biological membranes. These biological membranes can act as significant barriers to the passage of drugs throughout the body. Figure 2.10 illustrates diagrammatically one of the more widely accepted concepts of the structure of the cell membrane. According to this concept, the cell membrane is a bimolecular layer of lipid bounded on both sides by a layer of protein. The membrane is thought to be about 100 angstroms in thickness. Scattered throughout the membrane are water-filled pores of from 4 to 40 angstroms in diameter which provide some continuity between the extracellular and intracellular fluids. The functional significance of this particular type of structure is that the lipoid nature of the membrane influences the passage of drugs through it. Since drugs generally must be soluble in the lipid phase of the membrane in order to pass through, lipid-soluble drugs will pass through the membrane, but lipid-insoluble drugs are barred from passage. Thus, the chemical structure of the drug influences, primarily through its lipid solubility, the rate and extent to which a drug will cross the lipoid cell membrane.

There are several different processes by which drugs can cross the membranes of the body. The most important of these with

**CELL MEMBRANE**

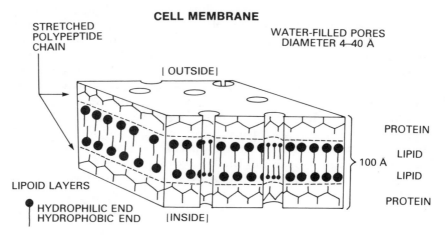

STRETCHED
POLYPEPTIDE
CHAIN

WATER-FILLED PORES
DIAMETER 4–40 Å

| OUTSIDE|

PROTEIN

LIPID
100 Å
LIPID

LIPOID LAYERS

PROTEIN

● HYDROPHILIC END
| HYDROPHOBIC END      |INSIDE|

**Figure 2.10**   Cell membrane.

respect to the movement of the vast majority of drugs is passive diffusion. Simple diffusion results in the movement of a solute from an area of higher concentration to one of lower concentration, i.e., diffusion down a concentration gradient. The energy that drives the diffusion of a solute down its concentration gradient is derived from the inherent thermal activity of the drug molecules themselves; no outside energy source is required. In any solution, solute particles are in constant random motion. As drug molecules move around because of their thermal energy, some molecules, if they are lipid soluble, will enter the membrane. Some of these molecules will move back out, while others will move on through to the other side. The greater concentration of molecules on the outside of the membrane increases the probability of two molecules colliding; therefore, the tendency is to move into an area of lower concentration where there is less probability of collision.

If the drug is a nonelectrolyte, its ability to cross biological membranes generally is dependent entirely upon its solubility. A lipid-soluble drug should be able to pass through the membrane and establish an equilibrium across the membrane. A drug which is not lipid soluble will be barred from passing through the membrane. In this way, diffusion and lipid solubility can lead to the selective distribution of a nonelectrolyte depending upon that particular drug's chemical structure which in turn determines its lipid solubility. A lipid-soluble drug will be distributed on both sides of the membrane, whereas a lipid-insoluble drug will be barred from entering the membrane and thus be contained outside the cell.

Drugs that are organic electrolytes present a more complex problem with respect to their ability to cross biological membranes. Organic electrolytes are drugs which have the ability to ionize or become charged. The ionized form of the drug is more polar than its nonionized form and, therefore, is less lipid and more water soluble. The nonionized form of the drug, for all practical purposes, is a nonelectrolyte, and its ability to pass through the cell membrane is governed by the same properties, i.e., its lipid solubility as determined by its chemical structure.

The water-filled pores that are distributed throughout the cell membrane form a communication between the extracellular and intracellular media through which some drugs may pass independent of their lipid solubility. Such passsage depends primarily on their molecular size and in some cases also on the electrical charge of the molecule. As has been mentioned, the caliber of these pores is about 4 to 40 angstroms in diameter. In general, most drugs whose molecular weights are less than 200 will pass through the membrane, whereas those drugs with molecular weight greater than 200 will not. This is only a general rule, and a great deal depends on the charge of the molecule and its three-dimensional structure. If there is a hydrostatic pressure or some other type of driving force across the membrane, water will flow through the pores, and a drug, if it is small enough, will follow the bulk flow of water through the membrane. An example of this type of passage is the glomerular filtration of drugs and other solutes from the plasma into the tubular fluid by filtration through pores in the glomerular cells of the kidney.

Carrier facilitated processes are another major class of processes by which drugs may cross biological membranes. These types of processes derive their name from the fact that there appears to be some chemical compound inside the membrane which combines with the drug on the outside and carries it through the membrane to the other side where the drug is released. Carrier facilitated processes are characterized by the following attributes: (1) Since the carrier is some chemical substance, there is a certain degree of structural specificity for the particular drug being transported. This results in selective transport of a particular drug dependent upon its chemical structure. (2) There is usually enough nonspecificity in drug binding to a given carrier molecule, however, to allow competition for this carrier molecule between similar chemical types. This results in competitive inhibition of transport between two drugs of similar chemical structure. (3) Since a finite quantity of carrier is available at any one time, carrier facilitated transport can become saturated if the concentration of drug is high enough to bind all available carrier molecules. The result of saturability of carrier facilitated transport mechanisms is that transport of a drug will increase as the concentration of the drug is increased up to the point where the carrier mechanism is saturated and then transport of the drug will level off and continue at some steady-state level independent of the concentration of transported drug.

The most important of the carrier facilitated types of transport processes is active transport. In addition to the three general characteristics of all carrier mediated processes, active transport has two additional features. First of all, the solute crosses the membrane against a concentration or electrochemical gradient. Secondly, active transport processes require an external source of energy. Active transport processes play an important role in the transfer of drugs throughout the body, especially in the kidney and intestine.

Facilitated diffusion is another type of carrier facilitated process, but of less importance than active transport in the transport of drugs throughout the body. It has all of the general characteristics of carrier facilitated transport. Its main distinguishing feature is that transport of a drug by this mechanism moves down a concentration gradient as the name implies. Carrier facilitated diffusion is usually more efficient or may occur at a greater rate than would be expected from simple diffusion alone.

### Factors Affecting Absorption of Drugs

Regardless of the process by which a drug passes through the cell membrane, it first must be dissolved in the aqueous fluids bathing the cells. For this reason, a drug must have some degree of both lipid and water solubility—water solubility to get it to the cell and lipid solubility to get it through the cell membrane. In general, the greater the water solubility, the faster the rate of absorption. The form in which a drug is administered can, therefore, affect its rate of absorption. For example, the rate and degree of absorption of a drug administered in solid form is influenced by the rate and degree of disintegration and dissolution of the solid drug. Similarly, the chemical form of an administered drug is another modifying factor. This is taken advantage of by the dental practitioner in his use of the corticosteroids. These drugs are often applied topically for the local treatment of inflammatory lesions of the oral mucosa. In such situations the practitioner wants the drug to remain at the site of administration and a water-insoluble form of the corticosteroid is used to retard absorption into the systemic circulation. In the emergency treatment of adrenal insufficiency, however, these same types of steroids are injected in a water-souble form to enhance their rapid distribution throughout the body.

Several other factors modify the rate of absorption: (1) Drug concentration at the site of absorption—in general, the greater the concentration, the faster will be the rate of absorption. (2) Circulation to the site of absorption—the greater the blood flow, the faster the rate of absorption. The dental hygienist takes advantage of this factor when a vasoconstrictor, such as epinephrine, is included in the local anesthetic solution. Epinephrine acts to constrict the blood vessels and decrease the blood flow in the area into which the local anesthetic solution has been injected. This slows absorption of the local anesthetic, keeping it at its site of action. (3) Area of absorptive surface—the greater the area to which the drug is exposed, the faster the rate of absorption.

### Factors Affecting the Distribution of Drugs.

After absorption into the systemic circulation, the primary factor determining the passive distribution of a drug is its lipid solubility Several factors influence the amount of lipid-soluble drug available for passive diffusion across the cell membrane. One such factor is the tendency of some drugs to bind to various macromolecules of body tissues.

BINDING TO MACROMOLECULE. The bonds formed between drug and macromolecule are usually weak in nature and result in reversible binding. This reversible binding of drugs to various intracellular and extracellular substances influences the length of time a drug remains in the body. Without these storage pools many drugs would be metabolized and excreted so rapidly that they would have little time in which to exert their pharmacological action. Binding also plays an important role in determining the pattern of distribution of drugs.

Selective distribution as a result of binding to macromolecules is illustrated in Figure 2.11. In this example, two compartments are separated by a semipermeable membrane. The characteristics of this hypothetical system are such that 90% of the total amount of a certain drug is bound to macromolecules on the right side of the membrane, and on the left side, 50% of the total amount is bound. Only the unbound drug is free to diffuse across the membrane, since macromolecules normally do not cross cell membranes. If the drug is originally placed in the right compartment, it will be distributed according to its binding characteristics, i.e., 10% free and 90% bound. The free form of the drug will then diffuse down its concentration gradient to the left side, limited only by its lipid solubility. As the free drug diffuses out of the right compartment, it is simultaneously replaced by molecules from the bound pool, still maintaining the 10% free to 90% bound ratio. As free drug enters

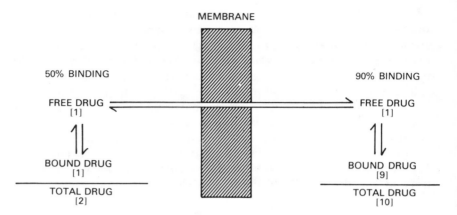

MEMBRANE

50% BINDING

FREE DRUG
[1]

BOUND DRUG
[1]

TOTAL DRUG
[2]

90% BINDING

FREE DRUG
[1]

BOUND DRUG
[9]

TOTAL DRUG
[10]

**Figure 2.11** Selective distribution: effect of protein binding. (Redrawn from Schanker, 1971.[17])

the left compartment, it is distributed according to the 50% free to 50% bound ratio. This maintains the concentration "sink" until equilibrium has been reached. Since the free drug diffuses across the membrane in both directions, at equilibrium the concentration of free drug will be the same on both sides of the membrane. If the percentages are converted into relative concentrations, with the concentration of free drug assigned a value of 1, Figure 2.11 illustrates that this difference in the degree of binding results in a fivefold concentration difference between the two sides of the membrane.

Selective distribution resulting from drug binding can have an important clinical significance. For example, the tetracyclines are antibiotics that have an affinity for some of the components of developing bone and bonelike structures (including the teeth). This leads to the selective distribution of these agents in the developing teeth of the fetus and young children. Consequently, these antibiotics are contraindicated during pregnancy and in young children, since their use in such patients has led to permanent discoloration of the teeth.[8]

COMPETITION FOR ACCEPTOR SITES. Of the macromolecules to which drugs may become bound, the plasma proteins are by far the most important. If a drug is significantly bound to plasma protein, then the dose required to produce a given magnitude of effect (i.e., to produce the required concentration of free drug in equilibrium with its pharmacological receptors) must include, in addition, enough drug to occupy the binding sites on the plasma protein.

Two drugs with similar chemical structures may have an affinity for the same sites on the protein molecule and will compete for these acceptor sites. For this reason, administration of a second drug having a higher affinity for the same binding sites as the drug already being taken by a patient will cause displacement of the original drug from its acceptor sites, increasing the blood level of its free form. The resultant increase in concentration of free drug in equilibrium with its pharmacological receptors will increase the pharmacological effects, possibly causing toxic effects.

An example of this phenomenon is found in the oral hypoglycemic agent, chlorpropamide, which is significantly bound to plasma protein. This agent lowers the blood sugar of diabetics by stimulating the secretion of insulin by the pancreas. Aspirin competes with chlorpropamide for its binding sites so that administration of aspirin to a patient taking chloropropamide displaces the hypoglycemic agent from the plasma protein. The resultant increase in free, pharmacologically active drug increases pancreatic insulin secretion which, in turn, causes a further fall in blood sugar and increases the possibility of hypoglycemic shock.

HYDROGEN CONCENTRATION. The hydrogen concentration is another factor affecting the passive transfer of drugs across the cell membrane. Many drugs are either weak acids or weak bases. As a result, their ionization is affected by the pH of the surrounding solution, i.e., the pH determines the relative concentrations of ionized and nonionized drug. Acidic drugs ionize according to the following chemical equation.

$$HR \rightleftharpoons H^+ + R^-$$

The nonionized form of the drug, which is in effect a nonelectrolyte, will diffuse across the membrane, depending upon its lipid solubility. On the other hand, the ionized form of the drug, which is much less lipid soluble, will not diffuse across. From the above equation it can be seen that if the pH is decreased (i.e., the hydrogen ion concentration is increased), then by the laws of mass action the equation will shift toward the nonionized form of the drug, increasing its passage through the cell membrane. If on the other hand, the pH is raised, (i.e., the hydrogen ion concentration is decreased), the chemical equation will shift toward the ionized form of the drug, and passage through the cell membrane will be suppressed.

Basic drugs ionize according to the following chemical equation:

$$RNH_3 + H^+ \rightleftharpoons RNH_4^+$$

In this instance a decrease in pH will shift the equation toward the ionized state, decreasing the drug's passage through the cell membrane. An increase in pH will cause dissociation toward the nonionized state, increasing the drug's passage through the membrane.

An acid can be defined as any drug that will give up a hydrogen ion; a base can be defined as any drug that will accept a hydrogen ion. Examination of the above equation for the ionization of a basic drug shows that the ionized form of the drug ($RNH_4^+$) is actually an acid, since it dissociates, giving up a hydrogen ion; it is called the conjugate acid of the base. Application of the law of mass action to the above chemical equation for the dissociation of the conjugate acid of a basic drug results in the following relationship:

$$\frac{[H^+][RNH_3]}{[RNH_4^+]} = K$$

where the brackets indicate the concentration of the respective elements at equilibrium and K is the equilibrium constant. Taking the logarithm of both sides of the equation and rearranging,

$$-\log[H^+] = -\log K + \log\frac{[RNH_3]}{[RNH_4^+]}$$

By definition, $-\log[H^+]$ is equal to the pH. Similarly, $-\log K$ can be given the designation of $pK_a$; so by substitution the final equation is

$$pH = pK_a + \log\frac{[RNH_3]}{[RNH_4^+]} \qquad \text{(Equation 1)}$$

This equation is one form of the familiar Henderson-Hasselbalch equation.

A similar equation can be derived from the chemical equation for the ionization of an acid drug with the following result:

$$pH = pK_a + \log\frac{[R^-]}{[HR]} \qquad \text{(Equation 2)}$$

It should be noted that these two equations, (1) and (2), are similar except that the ratio of nonionized to ionized drug is inversely related. In both these equations, the $pK_a$ is a constant characteristic of a given drug which is determined by its structure and is equal to the pH at which the drug is 50% ionized. Derived in the above manner, the $pK_a$ is a convenient index for comparing the ionization of both acidic and basic drugs. For example, drugs with $pK_a$ values less than 7 are usually acids ($pK_a$ of aspirin = 3.5), and drugs with $pK_a$ values greater than 7 are usually basic drugs ($pK_a$ of local anesthetic, lidocaine = 7.86). Decreasing the pH below the $pK_a$ of an acidic drug (equation 2) means that over 50% of the drug will be in the nonionized form; decreasing the pH below the $pK_a$ of a basic drug (equation 1) means that over 50% of the drug will be in the ionized form. Conversely, increasing the pH above the $pK_a$ of an acidic drug means that over 50% of the drug will be in the ionized form; increasing the pH above the $pK_a$ of a basic drug means that over 50% of the drug will be in the nonionized form.

Through its influence on lipid solubility, a difference in pH across a semipermeable membrane can lead to selective distribution of a drug in a manner analogous to a difference in binding. Figure 2.12 illustrates this phenomenon for an acidic drug having a $pK_a$ of 4.4. In this example two compartments are separated by a semipermeable membrane: the right compartment represents the gastric juice with a pH of 1.4; the left compartment represents the plasma with a pH of 7.4. If the drug is placed in the right compartment, it will ionize according to the pH and its $pK_a$ as governed by the Henderson-Hasselbalch equation for a weak acid, as indicated at the bottom of Figure 2.12. For any given amount of the drug, this will result in 1,000 times more nonionized than ionized drug. The nonionized drug will then diffuse down its concentration gradient, limited only by its lipid solubility. As nonionized drug diffuses out of the right compartment, it is simultaneously replaced by molecules from the ionized pool with the 1,000-fold concentration difference between the two forms being maintained. As the nonionized drug enters the left compartment, it ionizes according to the higher pH as indicated, i.e., there will be 1,000 times more ionized than nonionized drug. This maintains the concentration "sink" until equilibrium has been reached. Since the nonionized drug is free to diffuse across the membrane in both directions, at equilibrium the concentration of nonionized drug will be the same on both sides of the membrane. If all concentrations are converted to relative concentrations with the concentration of nonionized drug assigned a value of 1, Figure 2.12 illustrates that this difference in pH results in an approximately 1,000-fold concentration difference between the two sides of the membrane.

From the discussion of the ionization of drugs, it should not be too surprising that acidic drugs are absorbed to a greater extent than basic drugs in the low pH of the gastric fluids. The effects of pH on ionization and absorption of acidic and basic drugs is sometimes

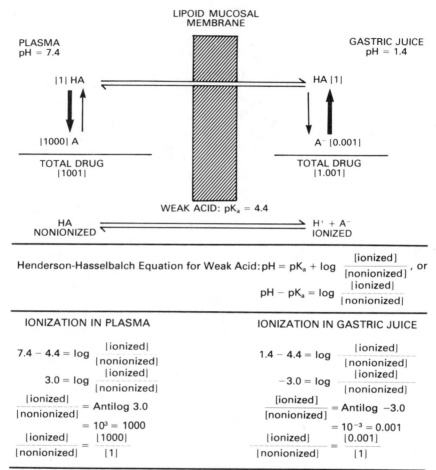

Henderson-Hasselbalch Equation for Weak Acid: $pH = pK_a + \log \dfrac{[ionized]}{[nonionized]}$ , or

$$pH - pK_a = \log \dfrac{[ionized]}{[nonionized]}$$

| IONIZATION IN PLASMA | IONIZATION IN GASTRIC JUICE |
|---|---|

$7.4 - 4.4 = \log \dfrac{[ionized]}{[nonionized]}$

$3.0 = \log \dfrac{[ionized]}{[nonionized]}$

$\dfrac{[ionized]}{[nonionized]} = $ Antilog 3.0

$= 10^3 = 1000$

$\dfrac{[ionized]}{[nonionized]} = \dfrac{[1000]}{[1]}$

$1.4 - 4.4 = \log \dfrac{[ionized]}{[nonionized]}$

$-3.0 = \log \dfrac{[ionized]}{[nonionized]}$

$\dfrac{[ionized]}{[nonionized]} = $ Antilog $-3.0$

$= 10^{-3} = 0.001$

$\dfrac{[ionized]}{[nonionized]} = \dfrac{[0.001]}{[1]}$

NOTE: Drugs that are weak bases are handled in a similar manner, except that the Henderson-Hasselbalch equation for weak bases is employed.

**Figure 2.12**   Selective distribution: effect of pH. (Adapted and redrawn from Fingl and Woodbury, 1975.[16])

taken advantage of by manipulating the stomach pH to increase or decrease the absorption of orally administered drugs. For example, excess use of antacids by a patient can significantly increase stomach pH, decreasing absorption of acidic drugs like penicillin. Hydrogen ion concentration also plays important roles both in the renal excretion of drugs and the pharmacodynamics of the local anesthetics.

DONNAN EQUILIBRIUM. The Donnan equilibrium is another, but less important, process that can influence the passage and distribution of drugs. The Donnan equilibrium results from the presence of a nondiffusible, charged molecule on one side of a semipermeable membrane which tends to retard the diffusion of oppositely charged molecules. In other words, an electrochemical gradient as well as a concentration gradient is established. As a result of this process there may be a higher concentration of solute on one side of the membrane than might be expected from concentration differences alone.

TIME. One of the most important principles of drug distribution is that distribution is a dynamic process. The drug is constantly undergoing change and redistribution. Three major factors determine the distribution of a drug with respect to time.

(1) *Relative Rate of Blood Flow to the Various Tissues.* This is most important immediately after initial drug administration. After absorption into the systemic circulation, the drug will be distributed first to those tissues receiving the greatest portion of the heart's cardiac output. The brain, kidney, and liver have a high rate of blood flow relative to their tissue mass. The skeletal muscle is less well supplied with blood, and fat depots are generally poorly supplied.

(2) *Ability of the Drug to Penetrate a Given Tissue.* Some drugs penetrate all tissue; some drugs are distributed only to the body water and do not enter the fat depots of the body. Other drugs have a higher affinity for fat, resulting in a somewhat selective distribution within the fat depots of the body.

(3) *Immediate Availability of Binding Sites or Concentration Gradient within a Given Tissue.* Since diffusion is one of the primary driving forces for the distribution of the drug, a drug will diffuse rapidly into a tissue (into which it can penetrate) if there is a favorable concentration gradient. As the tissue becomes saturated with the drug, however, diffusion decreases.

The influence of the above factors on the distribution of thiopental is illustrated on Figure 2.13. Thiopental, one of the barbiturates, is a general depressant of the central nervous system with a very short onset and duration of action after a single intravenous injection. Both the quick onset and short duration of action can be explained by the temporal pattern of the drug's distribution. Thiopental is very lipid soluble. As a result, it is widely distributed to all tissues of the body, especially fat.

The rapid onset of action of thiopental is a result of the high rate of blood flow to the brain. After rapid intravenous injection of a single dose, the drug goes, undiluted, to the heart where it is pumped out, still relatively undiluted, as part of the cardiac output. Since a large portion of the cardiac output goes to the brain, thiopental rapidly diffuses down the steep concentration gradient

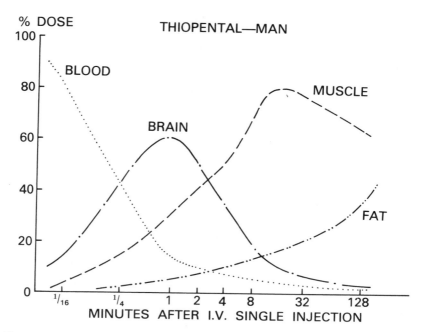

**Figure 2.13** Redistribution of thiopental. (Adapted and redrawn from Price, et al., 1960.[18])

into the brain tissue, quickly reaching therapeutic levels. The drug will continue to diffuse into the brain as long as the blood concentration is greater than that of the brain tissue concentration. From Figure 2.13 it can be seen that because of the above factors, within the first few seconds after injection, most of the total amount of administered drug is in the brain.

As the drug becomes mixed within the total blood volume, thiopental begins to diffuse, first, into the large skeletal muscle mass, and, later, into the fatty tissues of the body. The rate with which diffusion occurs is directly related to the relative blood flow to these areas. As diffusion into skeletal muscle and fat continues, the amount of thiopental in the blood begins to fall. Eventually, the concentration of drug in the blood falls below that in the brain and thiopental begins to diffuse out of the brain back into the blood, resulting in a decrease in its depressant effect on the central nervous system.

As thiopental continues to diffuse out of the brain, and later the skeletal muscle, an adequate blood level is maintained which allows the drug to diffuse down the concentration gradient into the fatty tissue. As a result, the thiopental that was administered eventually finds its way into the fat depots of the body. The total body concentration of thiopental during the first few minutes after the single intravenous injection is for all practical purposes the same as after the initial injection. Thus, the termination of thiopental's action is not due to excretion or biotransformation, but rather a shifting of drug from a high concentration in the brain, which is the site of desired action, to other areas of the body such as muscle and fat.

This is not the case when thiopental is infused intravenously for long periods of time. As administration is continued, the drug continues to diffuse into the skeletal muscle and fatty tissues. Eventually, these tissues become saturated and act as storage depots. When administration is stopped, any drop in blood level results in diffusion of thiopental out of the muscle and fat back into the blood, thus maintaining an effective concentration in the brain. The duration of action of thiopental under these conditions may be measured in hours.

## Biotransformation of Drugs

The biotransformation of drugs is one of the major ways by which the activity of a drug is terminated. Although some drugs are metabolized by enzymes in the plasma, kidney, and other tissues, the liver is the major site of biotransformation of drugs. The pharmacological significance of biotransformation is basically that the metabolite is usually less pharmacologically active than the parent drug. In addition, most drugs, being lipid soluble, are generally readily reabsorbed from the renal tubules back into the blood at normal urinary pH. As a result, their elimination by the kidney tends to be relatively slow. Biotransformation of most drugs results in more polar, water-soluble metabolites which are more readily excreted by the kidney.

Most drugs are metabolized by one, or both, of two general types of chemical reactions. The nonsynthetic reactions do not require an outside utilization of energy by the cell. These include oxidation reactions (e.g., the removal of alkyl groups from the amino group of morphine), reductions (e.g., the addition of two hydrogen atoms to chloral hydrate), and hydrolysis (e.g., the hydrolysis of procaine, an ester, into paraaminobenzoic acid and diethylaminoethanol). The second type of metabolic reaction is the synthetic reaction in which a drug is combined with some naturally occurring chemical moiety. These synthetic (conjugation) reactions require an external energy source.

Biotransformation of drugs by nonsynthetic reactions may result in the activation of an initially inactive or less active drug, a decrease in the original activity of the parent drug in such a way that it still retains a significant amount of pharmacological activity, or complete inactivation of an initially active parent drug. In any case, nonsynthetic biotransformation tends to lead to the formation of polar groups on the parent drug molecule.

In contrast, synthetic biotransformation of drugs almost invariably results in the inactivation of the parent drug through combination with some endogenous substrate (conjugate). In many instances drugs undergo both types of reactions, the nonsynthetic reactions producing a place for attachment of the endogenous substrate by synthetic reaction. Another importance of the increased polarity of the drug metabolite is its positive effect on the excretion of the drug by inhibiting the reabsorption of the drug from the renal tubules.

Of the many biochemical systems in the body that are involved in the metabolism or the biotransformation of drugs, probably the most important is the microsomal drug metabolizing system. This system of enzymes is located primarily in the smooth endoplasmic reticulum of hepatic cells, but similar enzyme systems have also been isolated in cells of other tissues including lung, intestine, and kidney. The microsomal enzyme system of hepatic endoplasmic reticulum appears to be a series of enzymes involved in oxidative, electron-transport processes. Of these, cytochrome P450 appears most important. Through interaction with this enzyme, drugs are oxidized by combination with molecular oxygen. The rate of drug biotransformation is dependent on the amount of drug-cyctochrome P450 complex formed and the rate of its enzymatic reduction.

The activity of the drug metabolizing enzymes of the hepatic endoplasmic reticulum is influenced by various factors such as drugs, sex, and age. In man, a number of drugs inhibit the metabolism of other drugs. For example, ethanol inhibits the metabolism of barbiturates when they are present in the body together. Drugs may also increase their own rate of metabolism or that of other drugs by the process of enzyme induction. Enzyme induction results in increased activity of the microsomal enzyme system, probably in large part owing to the enhanced synthesis of the cytochrome P450 enzyme. Phenobarbital is one drug known to induce the enzymes of the hepatic microsomal system. For example, administration of phenobarbital for two to five days increases the metabolism of hexobarbital (a similar barbiturate), as well as phenytoin, cortisone, and many other drugs.

### Excretion of Drugs

The second major process (which usually occurs in combination with biotransformation) by which drug activity is terminated is the excretion of drugs and their metabolites from the body. The kidney is by far the most important organ for drug excretion, although small amounts of basic and lipid-soluble drugs are excreted in the sweat and saliva. Some drugs are excreted in the milk of lactating mothers, this excretion leading to pharmacological effects in the nursing infant. The excretion of drugs in expired air via the lungs can be a significant route of elimination for the anesthetic gases and volatile liquids, such as diethyl ether, as well as the inhalational sedative, nitrous oxide.

The renal excretion of drugs involves three processes. The first of these is glomerular filtration. As blood passes through the glomerulus, both ionized and nonionized forms of the drug are filtered through the pores of the glomerular cells into the tubules of the nephron. The rate and amount of drug entering the tubular fluid by filtration is primarily dependent upon the glomerular filtration rate but is also influenced by the degree of plasma protein binding. Drug molecules that are bound to plasma protein are not filtered because the protein molecules are too large to pass through the pores of the glomeruli.

The second process is the active tubular secretion and reabsorption of drugs. This occurs primarily in the proximal tubules, although it can occur at other levels of the nephron as well. The active tubular secretion of drugs from the blood into the tubular fluid and the active reabsorption of drugs from the tubular fluid back into the blood are active transport processes. These processes are carrier mediated and have the other characteristics of active transport. They are the same processes that transport naturally occurring anionic and cationic substances across the tubular cells. As a result, competition for the transport carriers exists among various anionic and cationic compounds within respective tubular transport systems. For example, the drug probenecid can competitively inhibit the secretion of penicillin from the blood into the tubular fluid, thus delaying the excretion of penicillin from the body.

A third process that influences the renal excretion of drugs is the passive tubular diffusion of drugs. This can occur in both the proximal and the distal tubules of the nephron. Lipid-soluble drugs may diffuse across the tubular cells in either direction, depending on the concentration gradient and the pH of the blood and the renal tubular fluid. Under normal conditions the concentration gradient for a drug in the distal tubule will be from the urine to the plasma as a result of the increasing concentration of drugs in the distal tubule as water is reabsorbed.

Even though the concentration gradient is most important, the pH of the tubular fluid can have a significant effect on the excretion of weak acids and weak bases. An alkaline urine increases, but an acidic urine decreases the rate of excretion of a weak acid, since lowering the pH of the urine tends to suppress ionization, causing more of the drug to be in the nonionized state which can diffuse through the tubular cells back into the blood. This is sometimes taken advantage of by changing the urinary pH in such a way as to increase the excretion of a drug. For example, an increasing tubular urinary pH will increase the excretion of the weak acid salicylate; this technique has been used in the treatment of salicylate (aspirin) poisoning.

Hydrogen ion concentration has an opposite effect on the excretion of weak bases, since increasing the pH of the tubular fluid shifts the dissociation of a weak base toward the nonionized state, resulting in increased absorption and, hence, decreased excretion. Similarly an acidic urine increases excretion of a weak base.

In addition to renal excretion there is another important mechanism for the excretion of some drugs from the body. This is found in the liver. The liver appears to have several active transport processes for the biliary excretion of many poorly lipid-soluble organic compounds as well as some lipid-soluble substances. By these processes a drug, or its metabolite, may be excreted into the intestine via the bile. Part of it may then be excreted in the feces, but usually a greater portion is reabsorbed into the blood. This cycle of intestinal excretion via the bile followed by reabsorption may then be repeated and is referred to as the enterohepatic cycle. The enterohepatic cycle can cause a significant delay in the elimination of drugs from the body.

## ALTERATION OF DRUG EFFECTS

From the discussion of the absorption, distribution, biotransformation, and excretion of drugs it should be readily apparent that many factors contribute to biological variation and thus may alter drug effects and drug dosages. One such factor is the weight of the individual patient. Weight can vary greatly from one patient to another. As a general rule the greater the body weight, the greater the dose of drug required to produce a given concentration of the drug at the site of action and as a result to produce a given level of pharmacological effect. This is not always true in extreme cases, however, since the average dose that will produce the desired level of pharmacological effect in most individuals is influenced by the amount of active tissue relative to the total body weight. Active tissue can be defined as that tissue which plays a role in metabolizing and actively responding to the drug. Hence, the relative amount of inactive tissue such as bone, edema fluid, and the fat depots of the body may significantly affect drug dosage. For example, a lean well-muscled 200-pound man with a medium bone structure will probably require a higher dose of a drug that is distributed in the total body water than an obese, edematous 200-pound man with a heavy skeleton.

Individuals at the extremes of the age scale, i.e., young children and elderly adults, often are unusually sensitive to drugs. Elderly people may be particularly sensitive to the central nervous system depressant drugs. Both children and the elderly frequently respond to the barbiturates with idiosyncratic "paradoxical excitement." In addition, aging brings about an alteration in the cardiovascular system, the nervous system, the endocrine system, and other tissues in general. Glomerular filtration rate is often decreased in the elderly.

The female patient often reacts more strongly to many drugs and suffers a higher incidence of adverse effects than the male; therefore, a lower dosage is often indicated. The basis for this difference is not completely understood, but it undoubtedly is due in part to the differences in hormonal makeup between males and females. The use of all drugs should be approached with caution in treating the pregnant patient, since many drugs have the potential for causing teratogenic effects with resulting damage to the development of the fetus. The most widely known example of this is the thalidomide tragedy in which women who took the sedative, thalidomide, gave birth to infants in which the development of the limb buds had been retarded by the drug, resulting in babies born with phocomelia.[9]

Obviously, the rate of inactivation and excretion of the drug can modify drug dosage and drug effect. If the function of the organs of inactivation or excretion of a given drug is impaired, then both the intensity and duration of effect of the drug at a particular dose may be greater than desired, and toxic effects may occur. For example, the tetracycline antibiotics are contraindicated in patients with kidney disease, since their serum half-life is 8 to 9 hours in a normal person but is increased to 57 to 108 hours in anuric patients.[10]

Similarly, other pathological conditions of a patient may influence drug dosage and effect. The practitioner may not notice the respiratory depressant effect of morphine at therapeutic doses in the normal patient, but this same dose may produce significant problems in a patient who has chronic pulmonary disease. A patient with hyperthyroidism may tolerate larger doses of morphine than an otherwise normal patient, but may be sensitive to a dose of epinephrine that would not affect the euthyroid patient.

The psychological makeup of the patient may also modify drug dosage and effect. The well-known placebo effect is a good example. The placebo effect is seen most commonly with drugs, such as the analgesic (pain-relieving) drugs, whose effects include a subjective component. A placebo may be defined as a chemical substance that resembles in appearance a pharmacological agent but has no pharmacological activity of its own. To illustrate, consider a clinical trial in which each of a large group of patients is told he is to receive a "pain-reliever" for his toothache. In reality, the patient receives either drug A, a known effective analgesic, or drug B, lactose in a form resembling drug A. If the patients are then asked if the drug they received relieved their pain, a few of the patients who received lactose will report that the drug relieved their pain. These patients are called "placebo reactors."

Every person is genetically unique, but in most individuals these differences in genetic makeup are subtle and contribute only to the normal biological variability of drug effect. In a few individuals, however, there are genetic abnormalities that are responsible for a number of quantitatively and qualitatively identifiable modifications in drug effects. For example, a genetically transmitted abnormality of certain cholinesterase enzymes found in the blood has been identified. These enzymes are involved in the inactivation of certain local anesthetics, notably procaine and tetracaine, as well as the skeletal muscle relaxant, succinycholine. In one study the plasma of 5 of 16 subjects having an atypical cholinesterase enzyme was incapable of hydrolyzing procaine.[11] The decreased inactivation of procaine in these patients could possibly lead to potentiation of its effects and in increase in systemic toxicity.

A final important factor that can modify drug dosage or the selection of a drug that the dental practitioner may want to administer is the presence of other drugs which the patient may be taking either as self-medication or on the order of a physician. This factor is given the general name of drug-drug interaction and will be discussed with each drug group. Drug-drug interactions are becoming more important now as more and more patients with chronic illnesses that are being controlled by powerful drugs are seeking oral health care.

The presence of any of the preceding factors may necessitate adjustment of the usual dosage as stated by the manufacturer or in official publications. Of primary concern to the dental hygienist should be that the proper dose for an individual patient be given which will produce the predetermined therapeutic end point with as few adverse effects as possible. It should be appreciated, however, that any deviation from the recommended dosage should be based upon defensible reasons, since there may be legal responsibilities for any such change.[12]

## ROUTES OF ADMINISTRATION

The routes of administration of drugs can be divided into two broad classes: (1) enteral routes which include those routes in which absorption of the drug takes place through the gastrointestinal tract and (2) parenteral routes in which drugs are absorbed directly into the blood, bypassing the gastrointestinal tract. The choice of the proper route of administration involves several factors, including the physical and chemical properties of the drug, safety versus the desired onset of action, and the convenience and cost to the patient.

### Enteral Routes

The most common of the enteral routes of administration is the oral route in which the drug is swallowed by the patient. This route of administration has several advantages, the most important of which is its safety. Absorption is slow, and if need be, gastric lavage or other measures may be used to remove a portion of an administered dose before it is absorbed. It is also the most convenient route, since the patient can administer the drug himself and does not require the presence of a skilled professional to administer the drug. It is also generally the most economical route.

Many of the disadvantages of the oral route of administration are related to the relatively poor and erratic absorption of drugs from the gastrointestinal tract. For example, many drugs are insoluble in the gastrointestinal fluid; some may react with food substances in the gastrointestinal tract to form nonabsorbable complexes. The digestive enzymes and low pH of the stomach may chemically inactivate many drugs. Other disadvantages of the oral route are the unpleasant taste and irritation associated with many drugs.

Some of these disadvantages can often be avoided by coating the active drug with an enteric coating. An enteric coating is a chemical coating that does not dissolve at the low pH of the stomach. This protects the drug until it passes into the duodenum where it then dissolves at the higher pH of the small intestine. The enteric coating actually serves the dual function of protecting the stomach from the irritant effects of the drug, as well as protecting the drug from destruction by the gastric contents.

In addition to the aforementioned factors, the variable rates of absorption attendant to the oral route are due to physiological factors such as gastrointestinal motility and gastric emptying time. Although the stomach constitutes a significant site of absorption for many acidic and neutral compounds because of the favorable pH, it is the upper small intestine which serves as the major site of absorption of drugs in general. This is true because of the extremely large absorptive surface area of the small intestine. An example of this is seen clinically with the anticholinergic agents that inhibit gastric emptying and therefore may retard the absorption of drugs which rely on the small intestine for their major absorption.[13]

Another type of enteral route of administration is by topical application of the drug to the oral mucosa. The drug is not swallowed but is absorbed from the oral mucosa itself. An example of this route is the sublingual administration of the antianginal agent, nitroglycerin. One chief advantage of this route is that higher initial blood concentrations are reached than with oral administration, since the drug does not pass through the hepatic portal system as it does after absorption from the gastrointestinal tract. This route avoids many of the disadvantages of gastrointestinal tract administration. However, it does have the disadvantages of unpleasant taste, irritation, and, generally, a longer length of time needed for administration.

A third enteral route of administration is through the rectal mucosa. Again, the drug does not pass through the liver after absorption through the rectal mucosa. Drugs are most often administered by this route in the form of suppositories or retention enemas. Rectal administration is useful for unconscious or vomiting patients, or for patients who otherwise cannot take drugs by oral administration. It has the disadvantage of resulting in both irregular and incomplete absorption.

### Parenteral Routes

Of the parenteral routes of administration, administration of drugs to the skin is the most convenient. Drugs are administered topically for local effects in the form of ointments, liniments, lotions, creams, and pastes. Absorption of drugs through the skin generally does not constitute a major route of administration for the systemic effects of drugs, since the epidermal layer serves as an effective lipoid barrier. However, when the epidermal layer has been removed by burns or abrasions, the dermis is freely permeable to most solutes. This has led to the poisoning of burn patients when drugs, such as local anesthetics, were administered topically to large areas.

Absorption of drugs through the intact skin can be enhanced by the following processes: (1) Iontophoresis is a procedure in which galvanic current is applied across the skin. This route is used to aid the passage of ionized drugs across the skin. (2) Inunction is a procedure by which the drug is applied in a chemical vehicle. For example, dimethylsulfoxide aids the passage of drugs through the skin by acting as a solvent.[14] This process has served as a significant mode of accidental poisoning and death. For example, insecticides dissolved in organic solvents can be absorbed significantly through the skin if allowed to remain for a long enough period of time on a large enough area of skin.[15]

The respiratory tract also serves as a route of parenteral administration. Many drugs are absorbed readily through the pulmonary endothelium and mucous membranes of the respiratory tract, gaining rapid access to the systemic circulation. This route is used primarily for the administration of gases and volatile liquids by inhalation, usually for the induction of general anesthesia and inhalational sedation. The absorption of gaseous drugs is regulated by the gas laws of respiratory physiology. Drugs can be administered in nongaseous forms as aerosols, which are air suspensions of liquid or solid particles of minute size. Inhalation, too, serves as a route of accidental poisoning when paints or other volatile agents are inadvertently inhaled.

Drugs can also be administered parenterally by injection. They may be injected underneath the skin (subcutaneously). This route allows rapid absorption of aqueous drug solutions but is limited to nonirritating drugs since subcutaneous injection of some agents may produce inflammation and necrosis. Three major factors affect the rate of absorption of drugs after subcutaneous injection: (1) ease of penetration of the capillary walls, (2) the area in contact with the drug solution, and (3) the rate of blood flow through the area. The rate of absorption can be increased by massage of the area of injection, the application of heat locally, and in some cases the administration of hyaluronidase, an enzyme that breaks down the ground substance of the connective tissue. The rate of absorption can be decreased by local cooling, the use of vasoconstrictors, and by the injection of drug in a repository form. The latter includes implantation of a solid pellet or injection as a suspension in a vehicle, both of which retard absorption.

Another parenteral route of administration is the intramuscular route. Irritating substances that cannot be injected subcutaneously may be injected deeply into skeletal muscle. Aqueous drug solutions are rapidly absorbed, and the same factors influence the rate of absorption after intramuscular injection as after subcutaneous injection. The intramuscular route is used for repository forms of drugs more often than the subcutaneous route.

Drugs may also be injected directly into a vein (intravenous injection). This route provides a method of delivering to the systemic circulation very irritating and hypertonic solutions safely, since the drugs are rapidly diluted by the blood. Among other advantages, intravenous administration avoids all the delays and variables of absorption. Since the distribution to the site of drug action is rapid, intravenous administration is the most useful route for emergency therapy. This route can also allow continuous control of the degree of pharmacological drug action by slow administration (for example, intravenous administration of a sedative in outpatient dentistry). It allows the greatest accuracy in drug dosage. It also allows administration of large volumes of solutions over a long period of time. It has several disadvantages, however. This is the most dangerous route because of the speed of onset of the pharmacological action. An overdose cannot be withdrawn. If a therapeutic dose is given too rapidly, so rapidly that mixing and dilution do not occur, toxicity may result from the initially high concentration. Finally, allergic reactions to drugs are usually most severe if they occur during and/or after intravenous administration. Drugs in suspension or dissolved in oily vehicles or precipitating readily at blood pH should not be injected intravenously.

There are more sophisticated, less commonly used, routes by which drugs may be injected. One is the intra-arterial injection, a route of administration used to achieve high drug concentration in a particular organ or area of the body. This route is used most often for the treatment of localized tumors with antineoplastic agents. Finally, intra-articular injection (injection directly into a joint) of antiinflammatory steroids is used by dental practitioners trained in this specialized technique for treatment of temporomandibular joint arthritis.

## REFERENCES

1. Habermann, E.R.: Rudolf Buchheim and the beginning of pharmacology as a science. Annu. Rev. Pharmacol., *14*:249, 1974.
2. Langley, J.N.: On the physiology of salivary secretion. Part II. On the mutual antagonism of atropin and pilocarpin, having especial reference to their relations with the sub-maxillary gland of the cat. J. Physiol. (Lond.), *1*:339, 1878.
3. Ehrlich, P., and Morgenroth, J.: Studies on haemolysis. *In* Studies in Immunity. 2nd Edition. Edited by P. Ehrlich. New York, John Wiley, 1910.
4. Csaky, T.Z.: Introduction to General Pharmacology. New York, Appleton-Century-Crofts, 1969.
5. Clark, A.J.: General pharmacology. *In* Handb. exp. Pharmak. Vol. 4. Edited by A. Heffter. Berlin, Springer-Verlag, 1937.
6. Berridge, M.J., and Prince, W.T.: The role of cyclic AMP in the control of fluid secretion. *In* Advances in Cyclic Nucleotide Research. Vol. 1. Edited by P. Greengard, R. Paoletti, and G. A. Robison. New York, Raven Press, 1972.
7. Goldstein, A., Aronow, L., and Kalman, S.M. (Eds.): Principles of Drug Action: The Basis of Pharmacology. 2nd Edition. New York, John Wiley, 1974.
8. Council on Dental Therapeutics: Significance of dental changes induced by tetracyclines. J. Am. Dent. Assoc., 68:277, 1964.
9. Taussig, H.B.: The thalidomide syndrome. Sci. Am., *207*:29, 1962.
10. Sanford, J.P.: Guide to Antimicrobial Therapy. Dallas, University of Texas Southwestern Medical School, 1972.

11. Foldes, F.F., Foldes, V.M., Smith, J.C., and Zsigmond, E.K.: The relation between plasma cholinesterase and prolonged apnea caused by succinylcholine. Anesthesiology, 24:208, 1963.
12. Council conference: Notes on the package insert. J. Am. Med. Assoc., 207:1335, 1969.
13. Smyth, D.H.: Alimentary absorption of drugs: physiological considerations. In Absorption and Distribution of Drugs. Edited by T.S. Binns. Baltimore, Williams & Wilkins, 1964.
14. David, N.A.: The pharmacology of dimethylsulfoxide. Annu. Rev. Pharmacol., 12:353, 1972.
15. Wolfe, H.R., Durham, W.F., and Armstrong, J.F.: Exposure of workers to pesticides. Arch. Environ. Health, 14:622, 1967.
16. Fingler, E., and Woodbury, D.M.: General principles. In The Pharmacological Basis of Therapeutics. 5th Edition. Edited by L.S. Goodman and A. Gilman. New York, Macmillan, 1975.
17. Schanker, L.S.: Intimate Study of Drug Action. I. Absorption, distribution, and excretion. In Drill's Pharmacology in Medicine. 4th Edition. Edited by J.R. Di Palma. New York, McGraw-Hill, 1971.
18. Price, H.L., et al.: The uptake of thiopental by body tissue and its relation to the duration of narcosis. Clin. Pharmacol. Ther., 1:161, 1960.

## SUPPLEMENTARY REFERENCES

Albert A.: Relations between molecular structure and biological activity: stages in the evolution of current concepts. Annu. Rev. Pharmacol., 11:13, 1971.
Chasseaud, L.F., and Taylor, T.: Bioavailability of drugs from formulations after oral administration. Annu. Rev. Pharmacol., 14:35, 1974.
Ciaccio, E.I.: Intimate study of drug action. II: Fate of drugs in the body. In Drill's Pharmacology in Medicine. 4th Edition. Edited by J.R. Di Palma. New York, McGraw-Hill, 1971.
Condouris, G.A.: The natural laws concerning the use of drugs in man and animals. In Drill's Pharmacology in Medicine. 4th Edition. Edited by J.R. Di Palma. New York, McGraw-Hill, 1971.
Di Palma, J.R. (Ed.): Introduction; brief history. In Drill's Pharmacology in Medicine. 4th Edition. New York, McGraw-Hill, 1971.
Gero, A.: Intimate study of drug action. III: Mechanisms of molecular drug action. In Drill's Pharmacology in Medicine. 4th Edition. Edited by J.R. Di Palma. New York, McGraw-Hill, 1971.
Gillette, J.R., Davis, D.C., and Sasame, H.A.: Cytochrome P-450 and its role in drug metabolism. Annu. Rev. Pharmacol., 12:57, 1972.
Levine, R.R.: Pharmacology: Drug Actions and Reactions. 1st Edition. Boston, Little, Brown, 1973.
Rowland, M.: Drug administration and regimens. In Clinical Pharmacology: Basic Principles in Therapeutics. Edited by K.L. Melmon and H.F. Morrelli. New York, Macmillan, 1972.

# 3

## AUTONOMIC PHARMACOLOGY

Moment-to-moment existence in both health and disease depends upon the continuous integrity of a cycle of internal events that involves primarily the nervous systems. This cycle is illustrated in Figure 3.1 and consists of the following general phases: (1) the continuous sensing of both the external and internal environments. (2) the continuous flow of impulses to the central nervous system where the information received is integrated by specialized functional groups of neurons that are called vital centers. (3) before action is taken as to how the body might best be readjusted to compensate for the particular internal and external environmental changes, the facilitation or the inhibition by the higher centers of the brain of the huge variety of impulses or messages about to be dispatched. (4) passage of the flow of impulses along prescribed efferent nerve pathways out of the central nervous system by means of the somatic nervous system to the skeletal muscles; these somatic impulses initiate slight muscle tone adjustments or even command maximal contraction of skeletal muscle. (5) use of the two anatomical subdivisions of the autonomic nervous system (i.e., the sympathetic and the parasympathetic nervous systems) by the outward flow of efferent impulses on their way to smooth muscle cells, cardiac muscle cells, and gland cells. These outflowing autonomic impulses also can initiate slight muscle tone adjustments or secretory flow rates as well as command a maximal response. The skeletal muscles, the smooth and cardiac muscles, and the gland cells readjust to the body's best advantage for the moment and await the next change. Actually, what has been described is the simple reflex arc, a system which the body so well exemplifies.

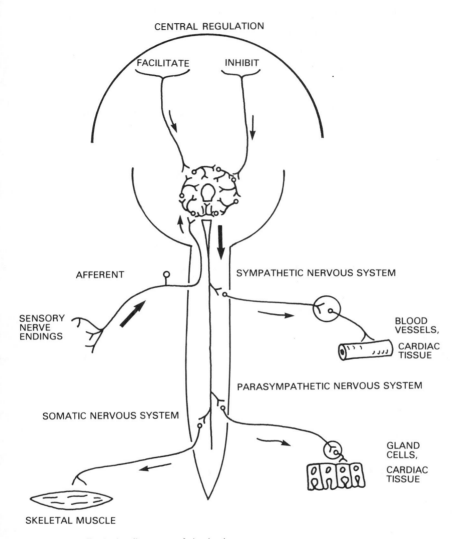

CENTRAL REGULATION

FACILITATE    INHIBIT

AFFERENT    SYMPATHETIC NERVOUS SYSTEM

SENSORY
NERVE
ENDINGS

BLOOD
VESSELS,

CARDIAC
TISSUE

PARASYMPATHETIC NERVOUS SYSTEM

SOMATIC NERVOUS SYSTEM

GLAND
CELLS,

CARDIAC
TISSUE

SKELETAL MUSCLE

**Figure 3.1**  Typical reflex arcs of the body.

A working knowledge of the autonomic nervous system is essential to the understanding of the effects of drugs that act upon the autonomic nerves and the innervated tissues. The autonomic drugs include agents administered by the dental hygienist and the dentist as well as drugs the patient is receiving through physician care. Certainly this is reason enough for acquiring a good grasp of the subject, but in addition many therapeutic agents that are not classified as autonomic drugs exert a variety of side effects through the autonomic nervous system. It is for this reason that autonomic pharmacology is in this introductory section on general principles that govern all drug action. Drugs that act at the different sites in the efferent, peripheral autonomic nervous system will be presented.

It is essential to pause and review certain anatomical and physiological landmarks or aspects before turning to the drug themselves.

## SELECTED ANATOMICAL FEATURES

As depicted diagrammatically in Figure 3.2, the autonomic nervous system consists of two subdivisions, the sympathetic and the parasympathetic. In each of these two subdivisions, between the

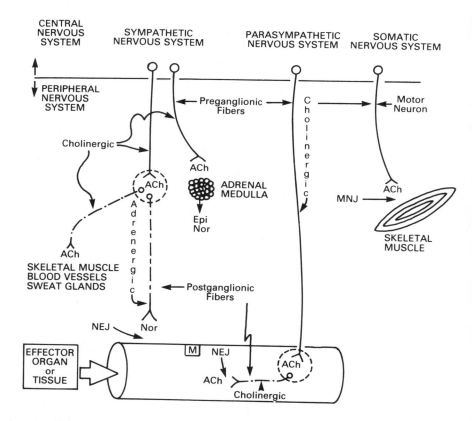

**Figure 3.2** Overview of the autonomic nervous system: M = noninnervated muscarinic cholinergic receptor; NEJ = neuroeffector junction; MNJ = myoneural junction. Cholinergic fibers release acetylcholine (ACh) at their endings, and adrenergic fibers release norepinephrine (Nor) at their endings.

point of exit from the central nervous system and the muscle or gland innervated, there are two neurons. The first neuron cell body is located in the central nervous system, and its axon runs to a ganglion where synaptic connection is made with the second neuron, which terminates at the effector or effector organ. The first neuron is the preganglionic nerve or fiber and the second, the postganglionic nerve or fiber.

In the parasympathetic division the preganglionic fibers leave the central nervous system at the cranial and sacral levels. At the cranial level the fibers exit with five of the cranial nerves; at the sacral level they run with the pelvic nerve. The parasympathetic ganglia are usually located close to or within the effector organ innervated.

In the sympathetic division the preganglionic fibers leave the central nervous system at the thoracic and upper lumbar levels of the spinal cord. They leave at the ventral root and proceed to synapse at only one of the several possible sympathetic ganglia. Some synapse with their postganglionic fibers in a paravertebral sympathetic ganglion; others bypass the paravertebral ganglia to synapse in a prevertebral sympathetic ganglion. Both types of sympathetic ganglia are located rather far away from the effector organs innervated.

Several additional anatomical features of the preganglionic and postganglionic fibers are of importance. In the parasympathetic division one preganglionic neuron usually synapses with only one or two postganglionic neurons, whereas in the sympathetic division it is not uncommon for one preganglionic fiber to synapse with up to twenty different postganglionic fibers. Parasympathetic preganglionic fibers are usually long relative to the length of the postganglionic fibers. In the sympathetic system the preganglionic and postganglionic fibers are both considered long. All preganglionic fibers in the autonomic system are myelinated, and all postganglionic fibers are nonmyelinated.

Knowing nature as a student of biology, one might suspect that there must be some exceptions in this nice, neat description. From an anatomical view there is one that must be understood, i.e., the autonomic innervation of the secretory cells of the adrenal medulla. These cells are directly innervated by only preganglionic sympathetic fibers. Anatomically, postganglionic sympathetic fibers do not exist. Pharmacologically, however, the medullary cells respond just as though they were postganglionic sympathetic fibers.

## SELECTED PHYSIOLOGICAL FEATURES

When parasympathetic fibers are stimulated, the resulting effects are discrete and localized. However, when sympathetic nerves are stimulated, the resulting effects may be either localized and discrete with only one effector responding or generalized or widespread. Thus, it may be said that the entire sympathetic system is capable of firing as a unit with effects seen in all parts of the body. During acute stress this is the case. The parasympathetic system fortunately does not fire as a unit.

A second important physiological feature of the autonomic nervous system is referred to as effector organ reciprocal innervation. It is well known that many effector organs are innervated by both sympathetic and parasympathetic fibers. In many of these dually innervated organs one division of the autonomic nervous system, when stimulated, causes an excitatory or motor response (contraction of muscle or secretion of gland cell) and the other division, when stimulated, causes an inhibitory response (relaxation of smooth muscle or inhibition of secretion). Through central control, when one division is increased in its activity, the other division shows decreased activity.

In the peripheral, efferent autonomic nervous system two major neurohumoral or chemical transmitters have been identified and accepted. These substances are biosynthesized, stored, and released by specific autonomic nerves. Cholinergic nerves release acetylcholine and adrenergic nerves release norepinephrine. Acetylcholine, as shown in Figure 3.2, is the chemical transmitter at the following sites: (1) the neuroeffector junction of the parasympathetic nervous system; (2) the synaptic junctions in ganglia of both sympathetic and parasympathetic nervous systems; (3) the neuroeffector junction between the preganglionic sympathetic nerve endings and the adrenal medullary secretory cells; (4) the neuroeffector junction between the postganglionic sympathetic nerve endings and the smooth muscle walls of the blood vessels in skeletal muscle as well as the postganglionic sympathetic nerve endings and the sweat glands. These two effectors are, therefore, innervated by sympathetic, cholinergic postganglionic fibers. Norepinephrine is the chemical transmitter at the neuroeffector junction of the sympathetic nervous system.

The next step in grasping an understanding of autonomic drugs is to acquire a working knowledge of the responses of selected, important effectors to autonomic nerve impulses. A general listing of such responses is found in Table 3.1. It is necessary to learn whether the sympathetic or parasympathetic innervation to each effector is excitatory or inhibitory. For example, stimulation of the sympathetic innervation to the sinoauricular node produces an increase in heart rate (excitatory response), whereas stimulation of the parasympathetic innervation to the same effector produces a slowing of the heart rate (inhibitory response). Another example would be the stimulation of the sympathetic innervation to the smooth muscle walls of the small intestine which produces a decrease in muscle tone (inhibitory response), whereas stimulation of the parasympathetic innervation to the same effector produces an increase in muscle tone (excitatory response). Finally, it is necessary to learn the class of autonomic agents to which the specific autonomic drug belongs. Atropine is categorized as a muscarinic, cholinergic blocker; phenylephrine is a directly acting, alpha-adrenergic stimulant. Therefore, with the information recommended, it is possible to develop quickly an adequate understanding of all autonomic drugs, including what their individual effects are upon effectors of the body through first dealing with learned generalities.

The adrenergic stimulants, in general, produce the effects listed in column B of Table 3.1 and the cholinergic stimulants, in general, produce the effects listed in column A. The adrenergic and cholinergic blockers may be expected to produce what appears to be a mild stimulation of the opposing innervation. Atropine, a muscarinic, cholinergic blocker, produces effects through dually innervated organs as if it were stimulating the adrenergic system; for example, the pupils dilate, the heart speeds, intestinal smooth muscle relaxes.

## CHOLINERGIC STIMULANTS

The body's own cholinergic stimulant is acetylcholine, and it will be considered here as the prototype. In the early 1920's, Otto Loewi performed his now classical experiment in which he used two isolated frog hearts as depicted in Figure 3.3. Electrodes were placed upon the vagus nerve to the first heart. The perfusate from the first heart was allowed to perfuse the second heart. The rate and force of myocardial contractions of each heart were recorded. Vagal stimulation to the first heart for 40 seconds produced asystole in the first heart immediately. Slowing of the second heart is observed in 15 seconds with arrest in 30 seconds. When stimulation ended, the first heart began to beat again in 20 seconds and the second heart in 45 seconds. The chemical substance that was liberated through vagal stimulation of the first heart and acted upon the second heart was identified as acetylcholine.

The biosynthesis of acetylcholine takes place in cholinergic nerves and includes the combination of choline to an activated acetyl group donated by coenzyme-A in presence of the enzyme, choline acetylase (or choline acetyltransferase). The acetylcholine thus formed is loosely bound to protein within vesicles in the

**Table 3.1. Effector Responses to Autonomic Impulses**

| Effector | Cholinergic Impulses Responses (Column A) | Adrenergic Impulses Receptor Type | Adrenergic Impulses Responses (Column B) |
|---|---|---|---|
| **Eye** | | | |
| Radial muscle iris | — | $\alpha$ | Contraction (mydriasis) |
| Sphincter muscle iris | Contraction (miosis) | | — |
| Ciliary muscle | Contraction for near vision | $\beta$ | Relaxation for far vision |
| **Heart** | | | |
| SA node | Decrease in heart rate | $\beta$ | Increase in heart rate |
| Atria | Decrease in contractility; increase in conduction velocity | $\beta$ | Increase in contractility and conduction velocity |
| AV node and conduction system | Decrease in conduction velocity; AV block | | Increase in conduction velocity |
| Ventricles | Decrease in contractility (?) | $\beta$ | Increase in contractility, conduction velocity, automaticity, rate of idiopathic pacemakers |

| Effector | | | |
|---|---|---|---|
| Blood vessels | | | |
| Coronary | Dilatation | $\alpha,\beta$ | Constriction; dilatation |
| Skin and mucosa | Dilatation | $\alpha$ | Constriction |
| Skeletal muscle | Dilatation | $\alpha,\beta$ | Constriction; dilatation |
| Salivary glands | Dilatation | $\alpha$ | Constriction |
| Lung | | | |
| Bronchial muscle | Contraction | $\beta$ | Relaxation |
| Bronchial glands | Stimulation | | Inhibition (?) |
| Intestine | | | |
| Motility and tone | Increase | $\alpha,\beta$ | Decrease |
| Sphincters | Relaxation | $\alpha$ | Contraction |
| Urinary bladder | | | |
| Detrusor | Contraction | $\beta$ | Relaxation |
| Trigone and sphincter | Relaxation | $\alpha$ | Contraction |
| Sex organs | Erection | | Ejaculation |
| Skin sweat glands | Generalized secretion | $\alpha$ | Slight, localized secretion |
| Salivary glands | Profuse, watery secretion | $\alpha$ | Thick, viscous secretion |

Source: Modified from Koelle, 1975.[1]
Note: The source should be examined for the many subtleties relating to the degree of control exerted by each type of impulse to each effector.

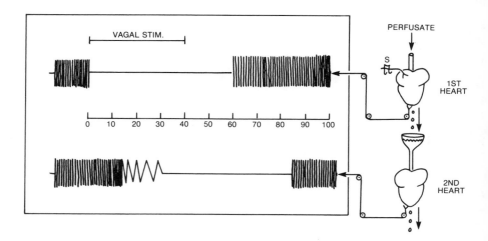

**Figure 3.3** Loewi's procedure for demonstrating the release of a vagus substance when vagus to frog heart was stimulated. The first heart is perfused and the nerve stimulated (S), whereupon the first heart is arrested. A chemical substance released by the first heart perfuses the second heart which causes a similar arrest in the second heart. (Adapted and redrawn from Koelle, 1975.[1])

cholinergic neurons. Following electrical or natural stimulation of the nerve, the arrival of the action potential at the nerve ending initiates the release of acetylcholine.

In man and many other species acetylcholine is stored in the body in the same cholinergic neurons. The majority of the neuronal acetylcholine is to be found in vesicles 300 to 600 angstroms in diameter which are located at the nerve ending. Moreover, the largest number of such vesicles is found close to or even part of the prejunctional membrane. A small amount of acetylcholine is also found in the axoplasm.

For the purposes of learning, it is important to recall where the cholinergic nerves that make, store, and release acetylcholine are distributed. They include both the preganglionic and post-ganglionic nerves of the parasympathetic system as well as the preganglionic nerves of the sympathetic system. In addition, there are anatomically sympathetic postganglionic fibers to sweat glands, skeletal muscle, and vascular smooth muscle that are cholinergic. Remember the motor neurons in the somatic nervous system are also cholinergic. In each case, when one of these cholinergic nerves is stimulated, acetylcholine is released as a transmitter, and it acts upon either postsynaptic membranes or postjunctional membranes to elicit an effect.

When the action potential arrives at the cholinergic nerve endings, the best evidence would indicate that calcium ions are taken up into the ending and there play a role in making the acetylcholine-containing vesicles adhere to the presynaptic membrane. During this latter process, it appears that a precise amount of acetylcholine (known as a quantum) is released to the outside of the nerve along with a return of the calcium ions.

The acetylcholine that is released under normal circumstances has an existence measured in microseconds. During that fleeting time, the molecule of acetylcholine interacts with its receptor and is inactivated through hydrolysis by the specific enzyme acetylcholinesterase. Consequently the choline is actively taken back into the nerve for further use in making acetylcholine, and the acetate enters the metabolic pool. Pharmacologically, it is the destruction of the transmitter by rapid hydrolysis that limits the duration of interaction between acetylcholine and its receptors.

A cholinergic receptor is that part of living tissue to which acetylcholine has affinity and to which acetylcholine transiently binds in order to exert its intrinsic activity that leads to the characteristic observable effects.

Early in autonomic pharmacology it was observed that injected acetylcholine produced at least two general types of actions. Small doses of acetylcholine caused effects which duplicated those produced by another chemical substance known as muscarine. Furthermore, it was noted that these effects of acetylcholine or muscarine rather faithfully duplicated the effects seen following the electrical stimulation of certain postganglionic parasympathetic innervations. This type of acetylcholine action, therefore, became known as the *muscarinic* action; the effects were called the muscarinic effects, and the receptors to which acetylcholine combined to produce the muscarinic effects came to be known as muscarinic receptors. These muscarinic receptors were then shown to be specifically blocked by the drug atropine. These muscarinic sites of acetylcholine action include (1) the neuroeffector junctions of the parasympathetic nervous system, and (2) the anatomically sympathetic but physiologically cholinergic postganglionic neuroeffector junctions found in the sweat glands and skeletal muscle blood vessels.

The second type of acetylcholine action requires higher doses (up to 100 times larger) than those necessary to produce the muscarinic effects. These nonmuscarinic effects appeared to duplicate many of the effects caused by yet another chemical substance known as nicotine. Nicotine's myriad effects had been exhaustively reported by the English physiologist, J.N. Langley, and were well known. This type of acetylcholine action became known as the *nicotinic* action; the effects were called the nicotinic effects. Many years later, these nicotinic receptors were further subdivided into two groups based upon anatomical location. These nicotinic sites of acetylcholine include (1) the ganglionic synapses of both the sympathetic and parasympathetic nervous systems, which includes the sympathetic preganglionic neuroeffector junction to secretory cells of the adrenal medulla, and (2) the myoneural junction.

## Cholinergic Receptor Activation

Postganglionic parasympathetic fibers innervate cardiac cells, smooth muscle cells, and secretory glands. When excited, each of these nerves releases acetylcholine which then acts upon muscarinic receptors on the effector to produce the characteristic effects. An examination of these characteristic effects (see Table 3.1) will indicate that in some instances acetylcholine's interaction with its muscarinic receptors leads to an inhibitory type of response, and in other instances acetylcholine's interaction with its muscarinic receptors leads to an excitatory type of response.

For example, the acetylcholine released from the ends of the stimulated right vagus interacts with the postjunctional membrane of the SA nodal fibers and produces a hyperpolarization of that membrane. The membrane becomes more negative on the inside in relation to the outside. It is known that in such membranes the acetylcholine causes the permeability of the membrane to increase selectively only to the smaller ions with radii up to about 5 angstroms. This selective increase would allow potassium ions to move out of the cell and chloride ions to move into the cells, but sodium ions would still be too large to pass. This makes the cell membrane more negative on the inside and, thus, hyperpolarized. Such a membrane would be more difficult to depolarize. Acetylcholine, in this instance, is raising the cell's threshold for excitability.

On the other hand, acetylcholine released from the ends of the stimulated vagus interacts with the postjunctional membrane on the smooth muscle cells of the duodenal wall and produces an increase in permeability to all ions, in particular sodium ions, and a depolarization of that membrane. Indeed, the membrane polarity first rises toward zero and then actually reverses polarity briefly before repolarization occurs. If the depolarization of the postjunctional membrane has been sufficient to reach the triggering threshold, an action potential is propagated and subsequent contraction of the smooth muscle fiber results.

Therefore, depending upon the state of the muscarinic receptor site, the acetylcholine will either produce hyperpolarization and an inhibitory response or depolarization and an excitatory response. Under normal conditions, the effectors will always manifest the same type of response to the interaction of acetylcholine with its muscarinic receptors.

The pharmacological effects of the prototype cholinergic stimulant, acetylcholine, may be observed upon various organ systems of the body. In general, the effects of parasympathetic innervation and acetylcholine are discrete and are essential to the adjustment of the body's background activities in order to accomplish better homeostatic position.

### Effects on Cardiovascular System

The right vagus (a parasympathetic nerve) innervates mainly the SA nodal tissue (the pacemaker cells), and the left vagus innervates mainly the AV nodal tissue. Both appear to innervate atrial muscle. There is limited and probably insignificant parasympathetic innervation of the ventricular muscle. When the vagi are stimulated and acetylcholine is released to act upon the muscarinic receptors in the heart, acetylcholine selectively increases the permeability of the SA pacemaker cells and the AV nodal tissue to potassium ions. The increased permeability leads to hyperpolarization and a decrease in the rate of discharge of the SA node and a decrease in the rate of conduction of impulses through the AV node. Sufficiently strong stimulation of the left vagus can actually produce heart block. The usual overt clinical response to increased vagal influence on the heart is bradycardia or slowing of the ventricular rate. Refer to Figure 3.4 to visualize the effects of acetylcholine upon the heart.

Acetylcholine's effects upon the atrial tissue include a decrease in the force of contraction, a decrease in the refractory period with an increase in conduction velocity, and an increase in atrial heart rate. Under experimental conditions vagal stimulation can produce atrial fibrillation, a rapid, ineffective rate of atrial rhythmic contractions. There is an overall decrease in myocardial activity as observed in a measurable decrease in oxygen consumption by the heart as a result of parasympathetic vagal stimulation.

Acetylcholine has definite vasodilating effects on most vascular beds. There are, however, a few vascular beds that have been proven to be innervated anatomically by postganglionic parasympathetic fibers. There is little doubt that muscarinic receptors exist on most vascular smooth muscle, even though these acetylcholine receptors are not innervated by the autonomic nervous system. Thus, acetylcholine causes vasodilation by acting on muscarinic

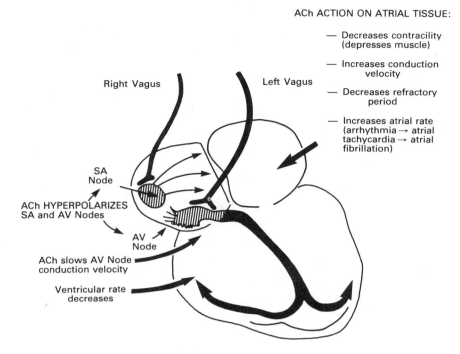

**Figure 3.4** Effects of acetylcholine (ACh) on mammalian heart: SA = sinoatrial; AV = atrioventricular.

receptors on vascular smooth muscle that are (1) not innervated by the autonomic nervous system as seen in the general vasculature; (2) innervated by postganglionic parasympathetic fibers as seen in the tongue and the penis; and (3) innervated by postganglionic sympathetic cholinergic fibers as seen in the skeletal muscle vasculature. The appropriate dose of acetylcholine administered intravenously may be expected to produce a fall in mean arterial blood pressure along with a brief period of bradycardia. It must be kept in mind that the normally functioning effective compensatory mechanisms would moderate these effects. These cardiovascular effects thus far described are blocked by atropine.

### Effects on the Eye

In the eye the parasympathetic postganglionic fibers, as depicted in Figure 3.5, innervate the sphincter muscle of the iris, as well as the ciliary muscle, which regulates the shape of the lens for accommodation. When these nerves are stimulated or acetylcholine is administered, the sphincter muscle contracts and the pupillary size becomes smaller. This is called miosis or acetylcholine's miotic effect. In addition, the ciliary muscle contracts, which in turn leads to relaxation of the suspensory ligaments of the lens, and the lens becomes more convex or adjusted for near vision.

Please note that acetylcholine and drugs that mimic its muscarinic effects have a secondary effect upon the eye that is important to understand. When the sphincter muscle of the iris contracts, the canals of Schlemm becomes less obstructed mechanically which allows for better drainage of the intraocular fluid from the anterior chamber. In the common disorder known as glaucoma, it is desirable, indeed essential, to keep the canals as patent as possible.

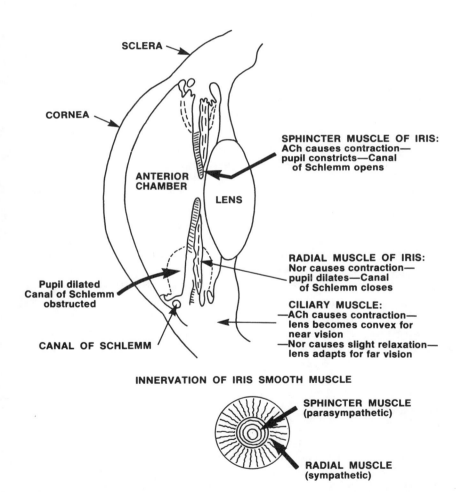

**Figure 3.5** Effects of acetylcholine (ACh) on the eye: Nor = norepinephrine.

### Other Effects

Many gland cells in the digestive system and respiratory system are innervated by postganglionic parasympathetic fibers. When these fibers are stimulated or acetylcholine is administered, the gland cells secrete. This is of importance in dentistry in that an adequate salivary flow is essential for oral health. Most sweat glands are innervated by postganglionic sympathetic cholinergic fibers; therefore, the sweat glands are also stimulated to secrete by acetylcholine. These muscarinic secretory effects of acetylcholine are blocked by atropine.

Parasympathetic innervation to the gastric and upper small intestine smooth muscle leads to contraction of the walls and relaxation of the sphincters. In general, the results are an increase in tone, motility, and secretion.

Stimulation of the postganglionic parasympathetic fibers to the urinary bladder produces contraction of the detrusor muscle and simultaneous relaxation of the trigone and sphincter, resulting in evacuation of the bladder.

The effects of acetylcholine thus far described are those exerted through its muscarinic sites of actions which are blocked by atropine. There are two other effects of acetylcholine which are nonmuscarinic and not blocked by atropine and which result from the action of acetylcholine upon its nicotinic sites of action. First, acetylcholine stimulates the release of epinephrine and norepinephrine from the secretory cells of the adrenal medulla, as well as stimulates the cholinergic receptors at the myoneural junction in skeletal muscle. Both of these receptor types are classified as nicotinic, but the former is specifically blocked by the competitive acetylcholine antagonist, hexamethonium, whereas the latter is specifically blocked by another competitive acetylcholine antagonist, d-tubocurarine.

Three groups of drugs increase the actions of the cholinergic neurotransmitter, acetylcholine, or imitate its actions. (1) The choline esters include acetylcholine and several synthetic substitutes and act directly upon the cholinergic receptors. (2) The cholinomimetic agents include drugs such as pilocarpine which are not choline esters but act directly upon the cholinergic receptors. (3) The cholinesterase inhibitors or anticholinesterase agents potentiate the effects of acetylcholine, both that which is released endogenously and that which is administered.

CHOLINE ESTERS. The effects of acetylcholine have been described and are shown in profile with three other choline esters in Table 3.2. Acetylcholine is only rarely used in human therapeutics

### Table 3.2. Comparison of Cholinergic Stimulants

| Examples | Susceptibility to Cholinesterase | | Pharmacological Actions | | | | | |
|---|---|---|---|---|---|---|---|---|
| | | | Muscarinic | | | | | Nicotinic |
| | Acetyl- | Pseudo- | Cardiovascular (Heart and Blood Vessels) | Gastrointestinal Smooth Muscle | Urinary Bladder | Eye (topical) | Antagonism by Atropine | |
| **Choline Esters:** | | | | | | | | |
| Acetylcholine (Miochol) | +++ | ++ | ++ | ++ | ++ | + | +++ | ++ |
| Methacholine (Mecholyl) | + | — | +++ | ++ | ++ | + | +++ | + |
| Carbachol (Carcholin) | — | — | + | +++ | +++ | ++ | + | +++ |
| Bethanechol (Urecholine) | — | — | ± | +++ | +++ | ++ | +++ | — |
| **Cholinomimetics:** | | | | | | | | |
| Pilocarpine | — | — | (—) Prominent action on the salivary & sweat glands | ++ | ++ | ++ | +++ | + |

Source: (in part) Modified from Koelle, 1975.[1]
Note: — = no action; +++ = strong action.

and then only locally in the eye for its miotic effect. The reason for this is undoubtedly the drug's diffuseness of actions when administered intravenously and its rapid hydrolysis and inactivation by plasma cholinesterase. A number of synthetic choline esters have been investigated, but only a few are actually on the market today. Perhaps the three most often used are methacholine, carbachol and bethanechol.

Methacholine (Mecholyl) is far less affected by the cholinesterases than is acetylcholine and thus methacholine has more practical duration of action in man. Very little difference is observable between acetylcholine's effects and methacholine's effects with the exception that methacholine produces little if any detectable nicotinic effects. Methacholine at one time was used to treat selected cases of paroxysmal auricular tachycardia, but the drug is difficult to control in its effects. It is still available today for use in the local treatment of vasospastic conditions of the limbs by the iontophoretic route or as an ointment. It is not used in the treatment of glaucoma, salivary disorders, or lower intestinal dysfunctions.

Carbachol (Miostat) is not inactivated by either acetylcholinesterase or plasma cholinesterase and possesses a prolonged duration of action. In contrast to methacholine, carbachol produces the most pronounced nicotinic action and is the least affected by atropine. Carbachol's usefulness in therapeutics is reserved today for only local treatment of glaucoma. When instilled in the eye, the miotic effect is long lasting.

Bethanechol (Urecholine) is the most often systemically used choline ester. It is similar to methacholine in its pharmacological profile and possesses not only fewer nicotinic properties but also less muscarinic cardiovascular activity. Therefore, the drug is used orally as well as subcutaneously to treat postoperative smooth muscle sluggishness such as seen in terms of abdominal distention, urinary retention, or gastric retention.

CHOLINOMIMETICS. The cholinomimetics are naturally occurring alkaloids that are not choline esters and hence are not acted upon by cholinesterase. Only two such agents are mentioned; pilocarpine is obtained from the South American shrub, *Pilocarpus jaborandi*, and muscarine is found in a number of mushrooms such as *Amanita muscaria*.

Muscarine is not used in therapeutics today and is of historical interest only. Its effects are purely those of a muscarinic stimulant.

Pilocarpine is commercially available and still widely used by local instillation in the eye for treatment of glaucoma. Pilocarpine is predominantly a muscarinic stimulant with what appears to be a greater selectivity for sweat glands and salivary cells. It would be helpful in dentistry to have available a specific salivary secretagogue to use in cases of xerostomia which results as a common side effect of many drugs. Unfortunately, systemic pilocarpine is not sufficiently selective for this use, and the problem must be dealt with on a local basis.

ANTICHOLINESTERASE AGENTS. Whereas the choline esters and cholinomimetics act through a direct stimulation of the cholinergic receptors, the anticholinesterase drugs exert their effects indirectly. By inhibiting cholinesterase, which limits the action of acetylcholine, the endogenously released transmitter is allowed to accumulate and to produce its usual effects for a more prolonged time period. Recalling where the cholinergic nerves are in the body and what they innervate will give the best indication of what may be expected in terms of effects when an anticholinesterase is administered.

The anticholinesterase agents have a fascinating history which involved man's search for more terrorizing ways to hurt his fellowman. The highly toxic substances known as the nerve gases developed for the purpose of chemical warfare are anticholinesterase poisons. There are several valid therapeutic uses for the anticholinesterase agents, and the discussion to follow serves as a basis for these more appropriate uses.

In general terms, there are two major classes of anticholinesterase agents, the reversible group and the irreversible group. The reversible anticholinesterase agents included only the betel nut alkaloid, physostigmine (also known as eserine) for over a century. Physostigmine is a lipid-soluble, tertiary amine and carbamic acid ester which easily crosses the blood-brain barrier to produce some of its most pronounced effects on central nervous system cholinesterase. Neostigmine (Prostigmin) is a purely synthetic prototype of a large group of reversible anticholinesterase drugs available today. Neostigmine is similar in its mechanism of action to physostigmine; however, neostigmine is a quaternary ammonium compound, charged at physiological pH, and does not cross the blood-brain barrier. Therefore, neostigmine's effects are restricted to reversibly inhibiting peripherally located cholinesterase. Both physostigmine and neostigmine combine with the enzyme acetylcholinesterase and are themselves hydrolyzed in a manner similar to that of acetylcholine, but the rate of hydrolysis for these reversible inhibitors is very, very slow relative to that of acetylcholine's hydrolysis.

There is adequate evidence to indicate that there are two active sites on the enzyme, acetylcholinesterase. One is the negatively charged anionic site, and the other is called the esteratic site. As depicted in Figure 3.6, acetylcholine binds to the active site by an electrostatic link with its positively charged nitrogen atom and through hydrogen bonds between the agent's methyl groups and the enzyme protein surface. This binding orients the ester portion of the acetylcholine to the esteratic site where covalent bonding occurs. The next step in this process is termed cleavage wherein the ester link is broken and choline is released from the enzyme which is now acetylated. In the presence of water the active enzyme is once again rapidly generated with a release of acetate.

The reversible anticholinesterase agent, neostigmine, binds essentially in a similar manner to that of acetylcholine. Cleavage takes place quickly, but the final hydrolysis of the remaining carbamylated enzyme takes place decidedly more slowly in comparison to the hydrolysis of acetate, and the active enzyme is regenerated. Hence neostigmine is classed as a reversible inhibitor.

The irreversible anticholinesterase agents are organophosphorus compounds and, no one would deny, some of the most lethal chemicals made by man. The prototype of this class is diisopropyl

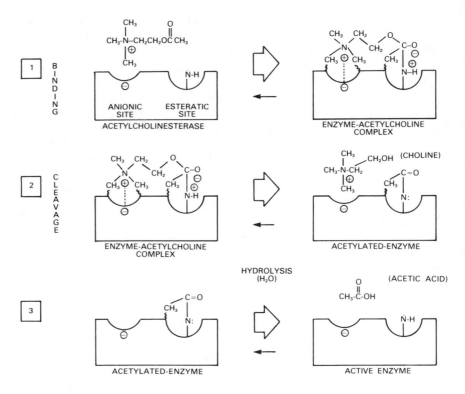

**Figure 3.6** Hydrolysis of acetylcholine. (Adapted and redrawn from Koelle, 1975.[2])

phosphorofluoridate (isoflurophate, DFP, Floropryl). Essentially what these agents do is to phosphorylate the enzyme to produce a stable compound. As shown in Figure 3.7, DFP binds only to the esteratic site in an irreversible manner so that the enzyme is lost to the body. The DFP duration of action depends then on how long it will take the body to biosynthesize new acetylcholinesterase.

It does not take too much imagination to foresee that anticholinesterase agents can have potentially profound and widespread effects throughout the body. These drugs combine with both the specific acetylcholinesterase and the much less specific circulating plasma or pseudocholinesterase and inhibit their actions. However, the effects of the drugs are thought to be due to only the inhibition of specific acetylcholinesterase. As yet, little is understood concerning a physiological function for plasma cholinesterase.

Both the reversible and irreversible agents produce qualitatively similar effects and can be considered as a group. They differ from one another greatly in their quantitative aspect. If each drug is administered over a wide dosage range intravenously, each can be shown to cause the same gamut of effects. The effect of some disappears with time; that of others persists. The innervated cholinergic receptor sites, both muscarinic and nicotinic, are so ubiquitous throughout the body it is difficult to predict beforehand which of the possible effects will predominate. Indeed, which effects predominate depends on a number of factors. Remember, these effects can all be understood in the light of the drug's allowing an excess, endogenously released amount of acetylcholine to act upon its receptors. The actual effects depend upon the dose, the absorption, and the distribution to the various areas where the cholinergic receptors are located.

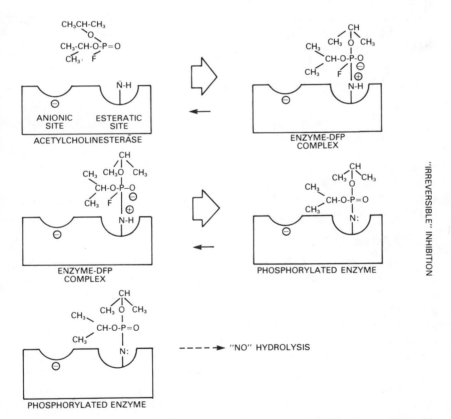

**Figure 3.7** Combination of isofluorophate (DFP) with acetylcholinesterase. In reality, hydrolysis does occur, but so slowly it is of little significance. (Adapted and redrawn from Koelle, 1975.[2])

Owing to their lipid solubility and ability to gain access to the central nervous system both physostigmine and DFP have their therapeutic usefulness practically limited to local instillation in the eye for glaucoma. However, in the last several years physostigmine has found a new application in being used parenterally in the reversal of unusual, bizarre, hallucinatory effects which can occur following administration of diazepam.

The charged, quaternary ammonium, reversible anticholines-terase agents which neostigmine exemplifies have a number of therapeutic and diagnostic uses. Although neostigmine does lead to peripheral muscarinic effects, its major effects are seen at the myoneural junction. In order to restrict its actions to the myoneural site, atropine is administered before the neostigmine in order to block the muscarinic receptors. Neostigmine actually has a dual effect at the myoneural junction. It reversibly inhibits acetyl-cholinesterase located at the site and thereby allows released acetylcholine to accumulate. Neostigmine also directly stimulates these nicotinic cholinergic receptors.

## ANTICHOLINERGIC AGENTS

Cholinergic blocking agents are usually classified into three groups. There are the antimuscarinic agents which inhibit acetyl-choline's effects at the muscarinic site of action. Secondly, there are the ganglionic blocking agents which inhibit acetylcholine's nicotinic effects at autonomic ganglia. Lastly, there are the skeletal muscle relaxants which inhibit acetylcholine's nicotinic effects at the myoneural junction. Only the first two types of anticholinergic agents will be discussed.

### Atropine

Cholinergic blocking agents that specifically antagonize the actions of acetylcholine and other drugs at the muscarinic choliner-gic receptor are useful agents in therapeutics. The classical drug or prototype of the antimuscarinic agents is the naturally occurring alkaloid, atropine, from the plant known as *Atropa belladonna*.

Various products of the deadly nightshade plant have been in use for many centuries. Today, through extensive structure activity relationship (SAR) studies, there exists an enormous number of fully synthetic substitutes for atropine. In general terms, the substi-tutes serve little advantage over the older alkaloids and differ from the older atropine essentially only in a quantitative sense. There-fore, atropine will be presented as the representative of the entire group.

Atropine's mechanism of action may be explained as a competitive antagonist. Both acetylcholine (the agonist) and atropine (the antagonist) possess high affinity for the muscarinic cholinergic receptor. Whereas acetylcholine also possesses high intrinsic activity leading to the appropriate effector response, atropine possesses little if any intrinsic activity. When atropine is administered, it attaches to the muscarinic receptors and prevents acetylcholine from reaching these receptors. A sufficient amount of acetylcholine can be administered or allowed to accumulate endogenously (through the use of anticholinesterase agents) which can override the atropine blockade.

Atropine does not inhibit acetylcholine's biosynthesis or release from cholinergic nerves, nor does it interfere with its inactivation by acetylcholinesterase. Atropine simply attaches itself to the muscarinic receptors and prevents acetylcholine's access to these receptors.

Although atropine can be shown to have, under special experimental conditions, a blocking effect at much higher doses at the nicotinic cholinergic sites, this is clinically insignificant in terms of atropine's use in dentistry.

In learning the effects of atropine-like drugs on the various organ systems of man, at least several factors emerge as paramount in importance. The muscarinic receptor sites in the body do not have uniform sensitivity to atropine. Some are more easily blocked than others. Therefore, atropine's clinical effects can best be summarized in terms of dose administered.

Secondly, to understand atropine's actions the dynamic nature of the postganglionic, cholinergic innervations to the organs of the body must be appreciated. Remember, atropine blocks only the effects of another substance, in this case acetylcholine released from these specific cholinergic fibers or other administered muscarinic stimulants. If acetylcholine is not being released, then there is nothing for atropine to block. An example is in order. Owing to training mainly, young adults who are especially active in sports have at rest a relatively high vagal tone. Acetylcholine is continuously being released and slowing the heart rate. In young children and adults over 50 years of age, there is little vagal tone to the heart at rest. Therefore, it may be expected that atropine's effect on the heart rate will be most obvious in the young adult whose heart rate routinely increases in the presence of atropine.

A third rule of thumb to keep in mind when learning atropine's effects is that most of the organ systems are dually innervated by the autonomic nervous system. Moreover, these innervations are most often in opposition, and when one side of the dual innervation is blocked the other side predominates. Therefore, in many instances the effects of atropine would appear as a mild stimulation of the adrenergic innervations.

A general description of the effects of atropine in man follows. These effects are categorized in terms of five oral dose ranges.

ORAL DOSAGE OF 0.2 TO 0.4 MG. One of the first effects of atropine that can be observed clinically is its inhibitory action upon salivary flow. Because the salivary secretory system is sensitive to atropine, these glandular smooth muscle cells are under continuous cholinergic impulse bombardment to secrete. This inhibitory effect is also manifested by the bronchial secretions and also by the eccrine sweat secretions. It is in this lowest dosage range that the drug is specifically used to treat what is called nocturnal sweats as well as to premedicate surgical patients in order to reduce airway secretions. It is at this dosage level that dentists utilize the antisialagogue activity of atropine or drugs like atropine in order to reduce the salivary flow so that a dry field may be present for the taking of impressions.

ORAL DOSAGE OF 0.5 TO 1.0 MG. The effects of atropine upon the cardiovascular system and, in particular, effects upon the heart begin to emerge at this dosage range. Keep in mind that there are few vascular beds receiving cholinergic impulses when the patient is at rest! At this dosage level there are often seen first a slight slowing of the heart rate which is thought to be due to a central effect and then the beginning of cardioacceleration from the antagonism of the effects of the vagal innervation.

The drug is used to increase the heart rate, especially during surgical procedures when the presenting bradycardia is thought to be due to a hyperactive carotid sinus reflex. In addition, the blocking effects of atropine upon the sphincter muscle of the iris begin to appear when the pupillary diameter increases.

ORAL DOSAGE OF 1.0 MG. At this level the effects of atropine on the eye are manifest. Dilation of the pupil (mydriasis) is observed along with the paralysis of accommodation (cycloplegia). These effects are useful in refraction procedures for corrective lenses. Keep in mind that atropine also causes an increase in intraocular fluid pressure owing to its ability to obstruct mechanically the canals of Schlemm.

In addition, at this dosage level atropine's central therapeutic usefulness is seen in its ability to reduce the tremors and rigidity of the Parkinson syndrome.

ORAL DOSAGE OF 1.0 TO 2.0 MG. Dryness of the mouth and upper respiratory tract is certain at these doses. Moreover, palpitations, mydriasis, and cycloplegia are apparent. The antimuscarinic effects of atropine next become obvious upon the cholinergic innervations to the smooth muscle walls of the gastrointestinal tract as well as the urinary system. The atropine-insensitive, gastric secretory system now begins to show the inhibitory effects of the drug. At these higher doses patients take the drug to ameliorate the environment of their ulcer lesions or it is prescribed to reduce ureteral spasms (spasmolytic or antispasmodic effect) which may accompany urinary tract infections.

ORAL DOSAGE OF 5.0 TO 10.0 MG. The definite toxic symptoms of atropine poisoning may be seen at this level. They include central nervous system stimulation in terms of hallucinations, delirium, and hyperpyrexia followed by central nervous system depression with coma and death of the victim in respiratory failure.

Atropine overdosage may be best remembered by the mnemonic: dry as a bone (decreased secretions); hot as a hare (increased body temperature); red as a beet (face flushing); mad as a hatter (central stimulation); and blind as a bat (mydriasis; cycloplegia).

## Other Antimuscarcinic Agents

There are an enormous number of drugs in the category of atropine-like agents. They may be subdivided into two groups: the other few belladonna alkaloids and the large number of fully synthetic atropine substitutes. For the purposes of general dentistry and dental hygiene only several commercially available products will be mentioned.

Scopolamine is a closely related, naturally occurring alkaloid which differs mainly quantitatively from atropine in its effects. At clinical dosage levels, scopolamine has a more obvious depressant effect upon the central nervous system. This property makes this antimuscarinic agent more preferred at times when premedication for surgical procedures in the adult is indicated, since the double benefit of central depression along with reduced airway and salivary secretions may be desirable. Scopolamine's central effects also include the production of considerable amnesia which may also be a desired action. In generaly dentistry, scopolamine is utilized in intravenous sedation procedures in combination with other drugs.

Of the many fully synthetic atropine substitutes only one, methantheline (Banthine), will be mentioned because this drug is widely used in an antisialagogue in prosthodontics and orthodontics. Methantheline in oral dosage effectively reduces salivary flow for a brief and more reasonable duration than does atropine. However, methantheline does possess mild ganglionic blocking activity (antinicotinic effect), and postural hypotension as a side effect must be considered.

## Contraindications for Antimuscarinic Agents

Atropine and atropine-like drugs should be used only with considered caution, if at all, in the dental patient who in addition to his dental problems is diagnosed as having glaucoma. Atropine's mydriatic effect has the tendency to stuff the iridic tissue into the narrow angle and thereby reduce mechanically the outward flow of intraocular fluid through the canals of Schlemm.

Furthermore, the dental patient with cardiovascular disease should be given atropine-like drugs only after consultation with the patient's physician in that the antimuscarinic action can unmask sympathetic dominance which may be an intolerable stress upon an already compromised circulatory system.

Drugs with antimuscarinic activity must not be used in elderly men who are experiencing prostatic hypertrophy, since atropine's effects upon the urinary system are in the same direction, namely, the production of further urinary retention.

Lastly, children may respond to atropine with more central excitatory effects including hyperpyrexia than observed in the adult. Caution, therefore, must be used in considering the use of atropine in the prepuberty age group.

## ADRENERGIC STIMULANTS

The sympathetic nervous system serves a dual role in the homeostasis of bodily processes. In the usual case, the sympathetic nervous system is the efferent arm of nervous pathways monitoring and readjusting many organ systems minute by minute. An example of this function is the maintenance of cerebral blood flow by sympathetically-mediated constriction of the blood vessels in the legs when the body's position is changed from supine to erect.

The ability of the sympathetic nervous system to function as a unit as a component of the stress response is of particular importance in dentistry, since many patients approach a pending dental office appointment with some degree of anxiety. In addition, there is obvious stress imposed by the dental or dental hygiene procedure itself. This response of the sympathetic nervous system, as well as the administration of drugs that modify or mimic it (sympathomimetic agents), is involved in a great many of the clinical situations in which the practitioner must modify usual procedures, including use of certain drugs.

The sympathetic component of the stress response can be summarized as being directed toward the mobilization and use of energy stores. Glucose and free fatty acids are released into the general systemic circulation. Respiration is stimulated and the bronchioles dilate. Heart rate and force of contraction are increased. Vasoconstriction occurs in visceral areas, while blood vessels in the skeletal muscle are dilated, shunting blood away from visceral areas into the skeletal muscles. At the same time gastrointestinal function in inhibited.

### Chemical Transmitters of the Sympathetic (Adrenergic) Nervous System

The chemical substances, epinephrine and norepinephrine, which mediate the efferent effects and the response to stress belong to the chemical class known as catecholamines. The two compounds are identical in chemical structure except that epinephrine has a methyl group attached to the amino nitrogen. Because of this close structural similarity, it is not surprising that epinephrine and norepinephrine have many pharmacological actions in common, even though the relatively small structural difference due to the methyl group results in several interesting pharmacological differences that will be discussed.

These two substances are distributed chiefly in the adrenergic nerve terminal (norepinephrine) and the chromaffin cells of the adrenal medulla (primarily epinephrine). As shown in Figure 3.8 both are synthesized from the amino acid, tyrosine, by a common series of chemical reactions catalyzed by certain enzymes. It should be noted that the intermediate, dopamine, has a physiological role of its own, apparently acting as a chemical transmitter in certain central neuronal pathways.

The rate limiting step in the synthesis of both epinephrine and norepinephrine is the hydroxylation of tyrosine which is catalyzed by the enzyme, tyrosine hydroxylase; inhibition of this enzyme leads to rapid depletion of catecholamine stores. Another important characteristic of the enzymes involved in the synthesis of epinephrine and norepinephrine is their relative lack of specificity. Molecules, structurally similar to the intermediates of epinephrine and norepinephrine synthesis, may enter the synthetic pathway shown in Figure 3.8 and act as substrates for the respective enzymes. The resulting formation of structural analogs of the components of catecholamine synthesis can significantly alter adrenergic function.

Metabolic inactivation of both epinephrine and norepinephrine occurs by the action of one, or both, of two enzymes, catechol-0-methyl transferase (COMT) and monoamine oxidase (MAO). In general, COMT, which is located primarily in the liver and kidneys, is more important in metabolizing catecholamines present in the blood. These include exogenously administered catecholamines, as well as epinephrine released from the adrenal

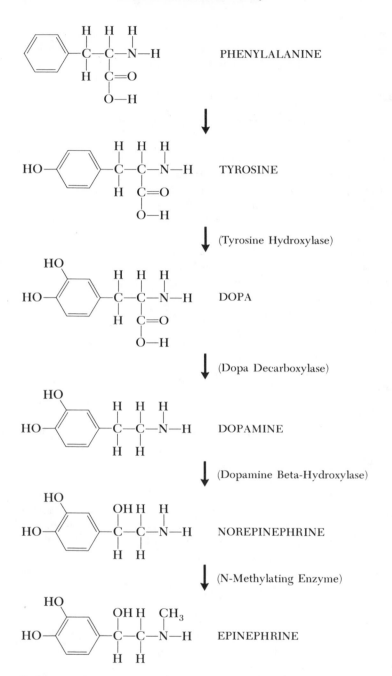

**Figure 3.8**   Synthesis of norepinephrine and epinephrine. (Redrawn from Kolle, 1975.[1])

medulla and a portion of the norepinephrine released from adrenergic nerve terminals. On the other hand, MAO, which is located in the mitochrondria of the adrenergic nerve terminal, is generally more important in the metabolic disposition of monoamines that make their way by various mechanisms into the adrenergic nerve. MAO also plays an important role in metabolizing monoamines within the central nervous system.

### Function of the Adrenergic Nerve Terminal

A thorough understanding of the physiology of the adrenergic nerve terminal is imperative if one is to understand the pharmacological effects of the stimulants and inhibitors of adrenergic function. Figure 3.9 is a diagrammatic representation of the adrenergic nerve terminal. Norepinephrine exists within the terminal in three pools or compartments. Two of these pools are found within the electron dense synaptic vesicles (granules) from which norepinephrine is released by the nerve action potential. The greatest portion of this norepinephrine is tightly bound to adenosine triphosphate (ATP) in a ratio of ATP:norepinephrine of 1:4. This norepinephrine pool has been given the name of reserve pool. A second pool, the intragranular mobile pool, is composed of unbound norepinephrine which is in equilibrium with the norepinephrine of the reserve pool. The norepinephrine that is released by the nerve action potential appears to come primarily from the intragranular mobile pool. Coupling of release of norepinephrine to the nerve action potential occurs through a calcium-requiring process that remains to be elucidated in detail. As norepinephrine is released from the intragranular mobile pool, it is replaced by norepinephrine from the reserve pool. A third pool of norepinephrine is found within the cytoplasm of the adrenergic nerve terminal and is the source of norepinephrine which is released (or displaced) by certain drugs such as tyramine. This norepinephrine pool has been named the cytoplasmic mobile pool.

Termination of the effects of norepinephrine released by adrenergic nerve activity occurs by a different type of mechanism from that terminating cholinergic nerve activity. In contrast to metabolic breakdown of released acetylcholine by acetylcholinesterase, MAO and COMT normally play only a minor role in terminating sympathetic nerve activity. Rather, the adrenergic nerve has a unique uptake process that pumps released norepinephrine back into the adrenergic nerve terminal. This process has the characteristics of a carrier-mediated active transport process and is efficient enough to pump (recapture) a large portion of the

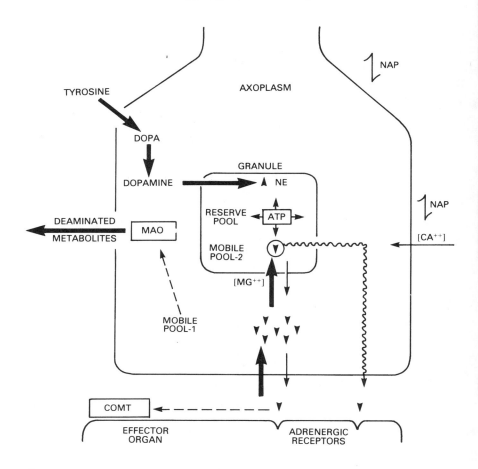

**Figure 3.9** Adrenergic nerve terminal: NAP = nerve action potential; MAO = mono-amine oxidase; COMT = catechol-O-methyltransferase; NE = norepinephrine; ATP = adenosine triphosphate; ▼ = norepinephrine. For explanation, see text. (Redrawn from Koelle, 1975.[1])

norepinephrine released by the nerve impulse back into the cyto-plasm of the adrenergic nerve terminal, terminating adrenergic activity. This uptake mechanism also influences the concentration of norepinephrine in equilibrium with its receptors and, thus, the magnitude of effect produced at any given moment. It should be noted that other substances structurally similar to norepinephrine may also bind to this carrier-mediated process, thus competing with norepinephrine for its carrier and inhibiting its uptake.

The norepinephrine which is pumped back into the nerve terminal enters the cytoplasmic mobile pool. A portion of this recaptured norepinephrine may be broken down by MAO, which serves to regulate the concentration of monoamines within the cytoplasm, but the preponderance of cytoplasmic norepinephrine is pumped back into the granule by an even more efficient active uptake process. This norepinephrine resupplies the intragranular mobile and reserve pools, allowing the adrenergic nerve to maintain its ability to fire tonically as long as these uptake processes are functioning. The ability of the adrenergic nerve to fire tonically for long periods is aided by continual synthesis of new norepinephrine, although this is a much slower process and cannot support long-term nerve activity alone.

It should be understood that the description of adrenergic nerve activity is oversimplified and much has been deleted in an attempt to aid basic understanding of adrenergic nerve function. Actual adrenergic nerve activity is, of course, much more complicated and less clear-cut.

### Adrenergic Receptors

As in the case of the parasympathetic nervous system, two distinct receptors are responsible for mediating the effects of adrenergic agents. These receptors were identified by studying the pharmacological effects of a related series of adrenergic agonists in various biological systems. The characteristics of the effects and associated relative potencies of the agonists formed two distinct profiles. In one case, adrenergic agonists studied usually produced excitation or stimulation of the tissue with epinephrine being the most potent and isoproterenol the least potent (Figure 3.10); in the other case, the agonists usually produced inhibition or relaxation of the tissue with isoproterenol being the most potent and norepinephrine the least potent (see Figure 3.11). Ahlquist concluded that the former type of effect was mediated by a distinct type of receptor, which he called the *alpha* adrenergic receptor, and that the latter type of effect was mediated by a second, also distinct, receptor, which he called the *beta* adrenergic receptor. Subsequent similar studies utilizing selective beta receptor antagonists have shown that there are at least two distinct types of beta adrenergic receptors—the beta$_1$ receptors in the heart and the beta$_2$ receptors in the peripheral vasculature.

Based upon the above information the following general rule may be made for the nonmetabolic adrenergic effects: drugs that act via alpha adrenergic receptors stimulate, whereas drugs that act via beta adrenergic receptors inhibit or relax living tissue. Like most general rules, this one too has several important exceptions, including these: (1) the beta adrenergic receptors of the heart stimulate,

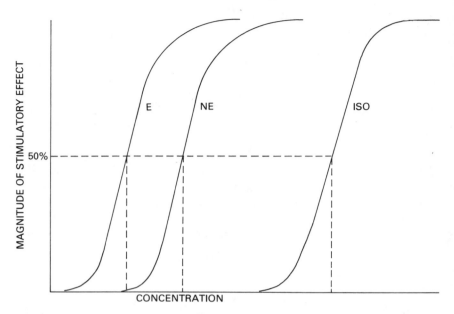

**Figure 3.10** Potency characteristics of alpha adrenergic effects: E = epinephrine; NE = norepinephrine; ISO = isoproterenol.

e.g., increase both the rate and force of contraction of heart muscle; and (2) the alpha adrenergic receptors of the smooth muscle of the intestine inhibit, e.g., decrease intestinal smooth muscle tone.

## Effects of Adrenergic Agonists

By learning the exceptions and applying the general rule for nonmetabolic adrenergic effects in other cases, it is possible to predict many of the nonmetabolic pharmacological effects an adrenergic agent will produce when it is given to a patient. To make such a prediction requires that the predictor (1) knows the relative distribution of alpha and beta adrenergic receptors in the important tissues and organ systems (Table 3.1); and (2) knows the type of adrenergic activity the given agent possesses, i.e., is it a pure alpha adrenergic agent, a pure beta adrenergic agent, or does it have both types of activity? With respect to the latter, isoproterenol is the prototype for drugs possessing only beta adrenergic activity at usual doses, and phenylephrine is the prototype for drugs possessing only alpha adrenergic activity at usual doses. Norepinephrine might qualify for this latter role, except that it is quite potent in interacting with the beta adrenergic receptors of the heart. Finally, epinephrine is the classic agent possessing both significant alpha and beta adrenergic activity.

HEART. Epinephrine has profound effects on the heart. Basically, these effects are on (1) the myocardial cells (positive inotropic effect), (2) the pacemaker cells of the sinoatrial (SA) node (positive chronotropic effect), and (3) the cells of the ventricular conduction system (arrhythmogenic effect). Through the beta receptors of the myocardial cells, epinephrine increases the force with which these muscle cells contract, resulting in an increase in the amount of blood pumped out by the heart with each beat. This usually results in an increase in the cardiac output, although other effects of epinephrine, such as increased arterial pressure and decreased cardiac filling owing to an accelerated heart rate, oppose the increase in stroke volume. The increase in the force of contraction results in an increase in work done by the heart and an increase in oxygen consumption. These latter two factors do not increase equally, however, and the amount of work done for a given amount of oxygen consumed (the efficiency) is decreased. The decrease in cardiac efficiency usually results in a relative hypoxia.

Through the beta receptors of the pacemaker cells of the SA node, epinephrine greatly increases the heart rate by increasing the rate of intrinsic depolarization (increases automaticity). In addition, epinephrine increases conduction of impulses through the atrioventricular (AV) node and, in cases of depressed conduction, improves conduction through the Purkinje system of the ventricle.

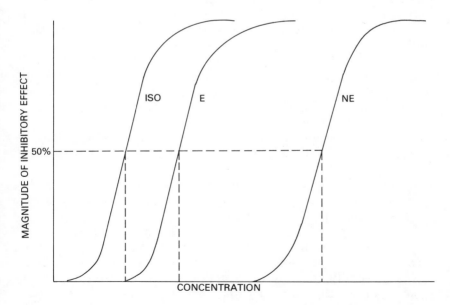

**Figure 3.11** Potency characteristics of beta adrenergic effects: E = epinephrine; NE = norepinephrine; ISO = isoproterenol.

The effects of epinephrine on the electrical properties of the conduction system of the ventricle are such that latent pacemaker cells are actuated, and high doses may cause ventricular extrasystoles and other arrhythmias, including ventricular fibrillation.

PERIPHERAL VASCULAR SYSTEMS. In most of the vascular beds of the body, alpha adrenergic receptors appear to predominate; the notable exception is the vasculature of the skeletal muscles which possess significant populations of both types of adrenergic receptors. Thus, application of the general rule would predict that alpha adrenergic agents will produce vasoconstriction in most vascular beds, while beta adrenergic agents will produce vasodilation in skeletal muscle blood vessels but will have little effect in most other vascular beds. Agents, like epinephrine, that have both alpha and beta adrenergic activity can produce vasoconstriction, vasodilation, or both depending on the vascular bed and the dose. These effects are most important in, although not limited to, the smooth muscle of the smaller arterioles and precapillary sphincters.

In the skeletal muscle vascular bed the influence of dose on the effects produced by an adrenergic agent with mixed alpha and beta activity is demonstrated by the effects of epinephrine. The beta adrenergic receptors appear to be more sensitive (have a greater affinity) to epinephrine than the alpha adrenergic receptors. Epinephrine in small doses increases blood flow (indicating vasodilation) in the human calf and forearm, but large doses reduce it (indicating vasoconstriction). This can be interpreted to indicate that more beta than alpha receptors are activated at the lower doses. With even larger doses epinephrine causes an initial vasoconstriction which is followed by vasodilation as the tissue level of epinephrine falls. Norepinephrine in similar doses causes a somewhat similar biphasic response except that the dilation is less pronounced. Isoproterenol, as expected, produces a marked vasodilation of the blood vessels of the skeletal muscle.

In cutaneous and mucous membrane vascular beds, epinephrine causes constriction of the blood vessels. In mucous membranes the initial vasoconstriction and resulting decongestion are usually followed by vasodilation and rebound congestion, caused in part by reactive hyperemia. Norepinephrine is also quite potent in producing vasoconstriction in these vascular beds.

In the splanchnic vascular beds, both epinephrine and norepinephrine cause vasoconstriction in the renal, hepatic, mesenteric, and uterine tissues when given in moderately high doses. Generally, isoproterenol produces no demonstrable vasodilation in these vascular beds, although there is one report of a local renal dilator response to isoproterenol after intraarterial injection.

Also, in normal humans, continuous intravenous infusion of low doses of epinephrine (0.1 $\mu$g/kg/min) decrease splanchnic resistance and increase hepatic blood flow.

In salivary glands stimulation of the respective sympathetic nerves innervating these vascular beds results in vasoconstriction. It is generally agreed that this vasoconstriction is mediated by alpha adrenergic receptors. The presence of beta adrenergic receptors in the blood vessels supplying the submaxillary gland has also been suggested by several studies; the physiological significance of these receptors, if any, remains to be defined.

In several vascular beds, any direct effects of epinephrine are exceeded by its other effects or by autoregulatory controls. For example, cerebral blood flow is closely related to systemic blood pressure; consequently, infusion of epinephrine in doses that raise the systemic blood pressure also increase cerebral blood flow, even though epinephrine has little direct effect on the cerebral blood vessels. Similarly, although epinephrine can be shown to constrict pulmonary vessels under the proper circumstances, epinephrine, after systemic intravenous infusion of moderately high doses, increases pulmonary pressure primarily through its effects on the heart and the systemic great veins. Epinephrine-induced constriction of the large veins (an alpha effect) increases the return of blood to the left atrium. This, combined with an epinephrine-induced increase in the heart's cardiac output, shunts a greater amount of blood into the pulmonary circulation, increasing the pulmonary pressure and passively dilating the small pulmonary blood vessels. The direct effect of epinephrine on the coronary arteries can be either constriction or dilation, but constriction usually predominates in man. Here too, however, any direct effect is obscured by a powerful local vasodilation caused by metabolites produced as a result of the relative hypoxia that accompanies the increased force of myocardial contraction caused by epinephrine.

CARDIOVASCULAR SYSTEM AS A WHOLE. The pharmacological effects of epinephrine, as the prototype adrenergic stimulant having both alpha and beta activity, have been discussed with respect to individual elements of the cardiovascular system. The reader must be cognizant of the complicating factors that operate to modulate the effects of adrenergic agents on the cardiovascular system as a whole. Epinephrine's net effect on total peripheral resistance will be the algebraic sum of its beta-mediated vasodilation and its alpha-mediated vasoconstriction, with the former predominating at lower doses. Agents with primarily alpha activity (such as norepinephrine) will produce only vasoconstriction and will tend to cause a greater increase in overall peripheral resistance than epinephrine at comparable moderate doses. Since diastolic blood pressure is closely related to peripheral resistance, it follows that norepinephrine typically causes a greater rise in diastolic blood pressure than comparable moderate doses of epinephrine. The greater rise in diastolic pressure is usually accompanied by a greater rise in the mean blood pressure which, in turn, influences the changes in heart rate caused by these two agents. It should be remembered that it is the mean blood pressure that is monitored by baroreceptors of the aortic and carotid arches. As a result, the elevation of systolic, diastolic, and mean blood pressure caused by intravenous infusion of norepinephrine is accompanied by reflex (vagal) slowing of the heart rate, even though norepinephrine has some direct beta-mediated positive chronotropic effect on the heart. On the other hand, intravenous infusion of epinephrine, although significantly increasing systolic pressure, causes a smaller rise in, and may even decrease, diastolic pressure. Similarly, there is less change in the mean blood pressure and less vagal slowing of the heart. The latter, in combination with the strong direct positive chronotropic effect of epinephrine, results in a significant elevation of heart rate. Of course, the effects of a primarily beta adrenergic stimulant (such as isoproterenol) differ still further from those of norepinephrine. Intravenous infusion of isoproterenol causes a significant drop in peripheral resistance and diastolic blood pressure, as well as a drop in the mean blood pressure. The decrease in mean blood pressure decreases the degree of vagal tone on the heart which, in combination with the strong direct positive chronotropic effects of isoproterenol, results in a significant increase in heart rate.

From the preceding discussion, it should be apparent that the effects of epinephrine on the cardiovascular system as a whole are diverse and much dependent on the dose and method of administration. It should be emphasized, however, that epinephrine is the most potent pressor agent known. Consequently, even relatively small doses of epinephrine, when administered intravenously at a rapid rate, can cause elevation of heart rate and blood pressure. The pressor effect may contribute to the cardiac arrhythmias that often occur after such intravenous administration of epinephrine.

It is especially important that this principle is understood by the dentist and dental hygienist, since they repeatedly inject epinephrine as part of their local anesthesia procedure. After subcutaneous or intramucosal administration, epinephrine is absorbed slowly because of the local vasoconstriction produced and, consequently, usually has no significant effect on the cardiovascular system. On the other hand, if an intramucosal dose of epinephrine is inadvertently injected into a vein, the rapid distribution of this relatively large intravenous dose may cause significant stress on the cardiovascular system, especially if it is already compromised by disease.

RESPIRATORY SYSTEM. Epinephrine causes a brief, centrally mediated stimulation of respiration which is sometimes preceded by a brief period of apnea. Epinephrine's most significant effects on the respiratory system, however, are the results of its effects on the smooth muscle of the bronchi and the blood vessels of the bronchial mucosa. Epinephrine and other beta adrenergic agonists are powerful bronchodilators, especially when the bronchial smooth muscle is already contracted (as in asthma or anaphylaxis). Through its alpha receptor-mediated construction of the vessels within the bronchial mucosa, epinephrine also increases vital capacity by decreasing mucosal congestion. The effects of adrenergic agonists on bronchial secretions are negligible, any decrease in secretion being due primarily to decreases in blood flow to the secretory glands.

GASTROINTESTINAL SYSTEM. The effects of adrenergic agents on gastrointestinal smooth muscle, in general, result in inhibition of function. The smooth muscle of the wall of the stomach and small intestine is relaxed, decreasing both tone and motility. This relaxation of gastrointestinal smooth muscle appears to be mediated both by alpha and beta receptors, the alpha receptors in this case being an exception to the general rule for alpha receptor effects. Usually, although the effect is somewhat dependent on preexisting tone, the smooth muscles of the various gastrointestinal sphincters are contracted by epinephrine. The effects of adrenergic agents on gastrointestinal glands are insignificant.

EYE. The effects of acetylcholine on the eye have been described in detail; epinephrine acts in opposition to acetylcholine. Epinephrine causes contraction (alpha receptors) of the radial muscle of the iris, resulting in mydriasis or dilation of the pupil. Conversely, it relaxes (beta receptors) the ciliary muscle, increasing the tension exerted on the lens by the suspensory ligaments and thus decreasing the angle of curvature of the lens.

URINARY BLADDER. Epinephrine and other adrenergic agonists produce urinary retention. The mechanism of this effect is a beta-mediated relaxation of the smooth muscle of the walls of the fundus of the bladder accompanied by an alpha-mediated constriction of the smooth muscle of the trigone and sphincter.

CENTRAL NERVOUS SYSTEM. Epinephrine usually has no effect on the central nervous system when given in therapeutic concentrations, although in some people it may cause restlessness, apprehension, tremor, and headache. The powerful CNS stimulatory effects of noncatechol adrenergic agonists will be discussed in more detail later.

UTERUS. The effects of epinephrine on the smooth muscle of the uterus are complex and will not be discussed in detail. Both alpha and beta receptors are present in the myometrium, the relative proportions varying with species as well as other factors. Both nonpregnant and pregnant human uterus are contracted by epinephrine in vitro. In vivo, the response to epinephrine varies with the dose and state of gestation. In the late stages of pregnancy, epinephrine usually decreases uterine tone and contractions, especially at lower doses.

SALIVARY GLANDS. Adrenergic agonists can stimulate an increase in salivary flow, but the characteristics of this stimulation differ significantly from that induced by cholinergic agonists. Adrenergic agonists are much less effective in increasing the flow rate, and the salivia is a thick, mucous type of secretion. The characteristics of the pharmacodynamics involved suggest that the increased salivation caused by adrenergic agonists and sympathetic nerve stimulation is mediated by alpha adrenergic receptors. (Epinephrine is most potent, isoproterenol the least potent in stimulating salivary flow; the response can be antagonized by alpha adrenergic receptor blocking agents.)

The role played by the sympathetic nervous system in modulating normal salivary flow, if any, remains to be determined. The effect of sympathetic nerve stimulation on individual salivary glands varies with the particular animal species. In man, the submaxillary gland is considered to be most significantly influenced by sympathetic nerve stimuli; the human parotid gland apparently does not respond.

In addtion to the alpha adrenergic receptor-mediated stimulation of salivary flow, beta adrenergic receptors have been suggested to mediate an increase in salivary secretion of the rat submaxillary gland, as well as an increase in salivary flow and protein content both from the human submaxillary and parotid glands. The significance of this beta-mediated increase in salivation is not known; at least part of this phenomenon may be an indirect result of increased blood flow to the glands.

METABOLIC EFFECTS. Through activation of a membrane-bound enzyme, adenyl cyclase (a beta effect), epinephrine and other catecholamines have important effects on several aspects of intermediary metabolism. Carbohydrate metabolism is affected by several different mechanisms, both direct and indirect. Epinephrine changes the activity of a number of enzymes involved in glycogen synthesis and storage, the net result being an increase in mobilization of glycogen stores into utilizable glucose (in the liver) and lactate (in skeletal muscle). By actions on other metabolic pathways, synthesis of new glucose from amino acids and lactate is stimulated. These actions are supported by an alpha receptor-mediated inhibition on insulin secretion by the pancreas, since insulin acts to antagonize many of the effects of catecholamines on carbohydrate metabolism. Epinephrine also activates an enzyme that increases the breakdown of triglycerides in adipose tissue, thus releasing free fatty acids and glycerol into the blood where they can act as additional energy sources.

## Sympathomimetic Agents

Drugs may mimic sympathetic activity by acting either directly via the adrenergic receptors or indirectly by actions at the level of the adrenergic nerve terminal; some drugs act both directly and indirectly. The effects of agents that act directly via adrenergic receptors have been described in detail.

The mechanisms of action of indirectly acting agents were alluded to in the section on the function of the adrenergic nerve terminal. Indirectly acting sympathomimetics act either by blocking re-uptake of norepinephrine into the adrenergic nerve terminal or by displacing norepinephrine from the cytoplasmic mobile pool within the nerve terminal. Indirectly acting sympathomimetics, although producing effects in many ways similar to directly acting sympathomimetics, also differ in some respects: (1) Since true indirectly acting agents produce their effects via norepinephrine, as a group they (like norepinephrine) produce primarily alpha responses except for some beta effects on the heart. (2) Unlike directly acting agents that require only the presence of adrenergic receptors, indirectly acting agents require the presence of sympathetic innervation in order to produce their effects. (3) In addition, unlike directly acting agents that repeatedly cause the same magnitude of response with repeated administration of the same dose at short intervals, indirect agents that act by releasing norepinephrine from the adrenergic nerve cause a decreasing magnitude of response with repeated administration of the same dose at short intervals. This phenomenon is called tachyphylaxis. (4) The indirectly acting agents are effective when given orally, whereas many of the directly acting agents generally are not effective when given orally. The same structural difference that imparts indirect action to these agents prevents their metabolism by COMT, increasing their oral effectiveness. (5) Finally, after parenteral administration, indirectly acting agents have a shorter onset and longer duration of action than the directly acting catecholamines. The longer duration of action is also a result of a lower susceptibility to catabolism by COMT.

Cocaine, a local anesthetic and central nervous system stimulant, is the prototype of indirectly acting sympathomimetic agents that block the active uptake of norepinephrine and other catecholamines into the adrenergic nerve terminal. As described before, this blocking increases the amount of agonist in equilibrium with its receptor, increasing or potentiating its effects. Blockade of reuptake of released norepinephrine by cocaine has been suggested as the mechanism of action of various effects of cocaine, including vasoconstriction (an effect unusual for local anesthetics) and even its central nervous system stimulating effects. Other drugs possess this action, and in many cases it explains their side effects but does not account for their major therapeutic effect. The tricyclic antidepressants also block adrenergic reuptake, an effect that explains their potentially serious potentiation of adrenergic agents (hypertensive crisis, arrhythmias). Whether this effect is also responsible for their antidepressant effects is not certain, although many agents that increase the concentration of adrenergic neurotransmitters at central nervous system synapses have stimulatory effects. The tricyclic antidepressants are discussed in greater detail in Chapter 15.

Amphetamine, a noncatecholamine sympathomimetic, is the prototype for indirectly acting drugs that cause a relatively rapid release or displacement of norepinephrine from the cytoplasmic mobile pool of the adrenergic nerve terminal. Peripherally amphetamine causes a sustained pressor effect, increasing both systolic and diastolic blood pressure. Heart rate and force of contraction are increased, although compensatory reflexes may subsequently slow the heart rate. If the dose is large enough, arrhythmias may occur. Urinary retention and difficulty in micturition as a result of contraction of the urinary bladder sphincter may occur in individuals taking amphetamine.

Amphetamine and its congeners are most widely used and abused for their effects on the central nervous system. Indeed, these agents are the most powerful central nervous system stimulants among the sympathomimetic agents. The more important central effects of amphetamines include (1) stimulation of the medullary respiratory center, (2) reversal of drug-induced central nervous system depression (analeptic effect), (3) a decrease in appetite (anorectic effect), and (4) a decrease in fatigue. The latter, along with the psychic effects of amphetamine, is intimately linked to the high abuse liability of the amphetamine derivatives. The psychic effects of the amphetamines vary with the dose as well as the mental and emotional state of the individual. Generally there is increased wakefulness and alertness; mood elevation, sometimes even euphoria; and restlessness. The ability of amphetamine to improve physical performance and delay fatigue has led to the widespread use of these agents by those who wish to maintain performance of simple mental tasks, although users of the agents do not decrease the frequency of mistakes. Studies have also shown that amphetamines delay the onset of fatigue while maintaining adequate task performance. The amphetamines have the remarkable ability to restore performance of tasks requiring prolonged concentration which has been reduced by fatigue and lack of sleep. It should be noted, however, that the artificial prolongation of performance is followed by fatigue, prolonged sleep (especially REM, rapid eye movement, sleep), and often, periods of depression.

The types of activity and major clinical uses of selected sympathomimetic agents are summarized in Table 3.3. It should be noted that ephedrine and metaraminol not only have significant direct actions via the beta adrenergic receptors but also cause release of norepinephrine from adrenergic nerve terminals. The effects of ephedrine on the cardiovascular system are qualitatively similar to those of epinephrine, but ephedrine is much less potent and its effects last up to ten times as long as those of epinephrine. The same is true for the relaxation of bronchial smooth muscle by ephedrine. Ephedrine has effects on the central nervous system that are similar to, but much less dramatic than, those of amphetamine. It is effective orally.

Levonordefrin is used as a vasoconstrictor in several local anesthetic preparations, and claims have been made that it causes less cardiac stimulation than epinephrine. Although levonordefrin is less potent than epinephrine, both in its alpha and beta effects, studies in animals have shown that levonordefrin does stimulate the heart at adequate doses. Its effects have also been shown to be potentiated by cocaine. Carefully controlled trials in man comparing the effects of levonordefrin and epinephrine on blood pressure and the heart at equieffective local vasoconstrictor doses remain to be performed.

### Theraputic Uses of Sympathomimetic Agents

The sympathomimetic agents have a wide range of clinical applications; only those considered to be of primary importance for the dentist and dental hygienist will be discussed.

LOCAL VASOCONSTRICTION. Topical application of epinephrine is effective in controlling minor bleeding from arterioles and capillaries. It should be noted that such topical application of

**Table 3.3.    Clinical Uses of Important Sympathomimetic Drugs**

| Type | Drug Name | Clinical Uses | | |
|------|-----------|-------------|---|---|
| | | $\alpha$-Receptor | $\beta$-Receptor | CNS |
| Directly acting | Epinephrine | A,P,V | B,C | |
| | Norepinephrine | P | | |
| | Isoproterenol | | B,C | |
| | Nordefrin | V | | |
| | Phenylephrine | N,P | | |
| | Methoxamine | N,P | | |
| | Isoxsuprine | | Vd | |
| Indirectly acting | Tyramine* | | | |
| | Amphetamine | | | CNS |
| | Methamphetamine | | | CNS |
| Mixed acting | Ephedrine | N,P | B,C | |
| | Metaraminol | P | | |

Source: Modified from Innes and Nickerson, 1975.[3]
(*) Tyramine is the prototype, but it is not used clinically.

*ALPHA ($\alpha$) ACTIVITY*
A    = allergic reactions
N    = nasal decongestant
P    = pressor
V    = local vasoconstrictor

*BETA ($\beta$) ACTIVITY*
B    = bronchodilator
C    = cardiac stimulant
Vd  = vasodilator

CNS = central nervous system stimulant

epinephrine to an injured or denuded area of the oral mucosa may result in significant systemic absorption and, as a result, stimulation of the cardiovascular system. The amount of absorption, of course, depends upon the concentration administered and the area to which it is administered.

Topical application of epinephrine to highly vascular tissue, such as the gingiva and the nasal and pharyngeal mucosa, causes vasoconstriction, blanching, and a decrease in blood content of the tissues. As a result tissue volume decreases. This effect has led to the advocation of topical application of relatively high concentrations of epinephrine to the gingival tissue to produce retraction (see Chapter 11). Again it should be noted, however, that such application can lead to significant systemic absorption of epinephrine. The use of topical sympathomimetic agents to produce nasal decongestion is widespread. Disadvantages include short duration of action, irritation, and rebound after congestion. To avoid these disadvantages, oral administration of longer acting noncatecholamines can be used but is usually not as effective as topical application.

The most important use of the adrenergic vasoconstrictors in dentistry is their inclusion in local anesthetic preparations for the purpose of retarding absorption and increasing the duration of local anesthesia. By tradition, epinephrine (1:200,000 to 1:50,000) is the most widely used adrenergic vasoconstrictor for this purpose. In these concentrations epinephrine causes effective local vasoconstriction but has the potential disadvantage of placing the heart under increased stress through its beta adrenergic effects. Other adrenergic vasoconstrictors included in combination with local anesthetics and their respective concentration include norepinephrine (1:30,000), levonordefrin (1:20,000), phenylephrine (1:2,500).

CARDIAC AND PRESSOR EFFECTS. Adrenergic agents are useful in treating hypotensive episodes, including shock. In almost all such instances administration of a sympathomimetic agent is limited only to a temporary emergency measure. Norepinephrine and other sympathomimetic pressor agents have been used to treat shock from various etiologies in an attempt to improve circulation to vital organs by raising the blood pressure. The effectiveness of this treatment has been questioned on the basis that increased vasoconstriction will decrease blood flow (which is probably already diminished by high sympathetic tone) to vital organs. An exception to this argument is cardiogenic shock in which the decreased blood pressure is a direct result of inadequate cardiac output. In most cases an effective vasopressor agent can raise the blood pressure in myocardial shock, increasing coronary flow to still viable areas of the myocardium. Although some experts advocate the use of vasopressor agents that also stimulate the heart directly through beta adrenergic action, it should be noted that in any hypotensive episode, resulting myocardial hypoxia may predispose the heart to the arrhythmogenic properties of beta adrenergic agents.

VASODILATION. The use of orally effective, long-acting beta adrenergic agents has been advocated for the improvement of blood flow in areas in which flow has been reduced by disease. The effectiveness of such agents in causing further dilation of blood vessels which are likely to be maximally dilated by local factors has been questioned.

BRONCHODILATION. The catecholamines, epinephrine and isoproterenol, are the most effective agents in the treatment of acute bronchospasm. Isoproterenol is usually given by inhalation, epinephrine by inhalation or subcutaneous administration. In disease associated with chronic bronchospasm, such as asthma, longer acting beta adrenergic agents, such as ephedrine, are often effective in preventing bronchospastic attacks but have little effect in reversing the attack once it has begun.

ANAPHYLAXIS. Epinephrine, injected subcutaneously, is the drug of choice for the emergency treatment of acute hypersensitivity reactions to drugs and other antigens. It acts to maintain patency of the airways by physiologically antagonizing the bronchospasm of anaphylaxis (direct beta receptor-mediated bronchodilation) and by decreasing the edema of the glossopharyngeal areas (alpha receptor-mediated local vasoconstriction). Epinephrine supports the blood pressure through its beta receptor-mediated stimulation of the heart and its alpha receptor-mediated vasopressor effects.

CENTRAL NERVOUS SYSTEM EFFECTS. Ephedrine and the amphetamine derivatives are the sympathomimetic agents used most often for their effects on the central nervous system. The effects of amphetamine on fatigue have been discussed. Amphetamines have been used to counteract drug-induced central nervous system depressions and are effective in lessening depression in moderate cases. Their effectiveness in large overdosage of central nervous system depressants is questionable. Amphetamines are widely used for their anorectic effect. Although these agents effectively depress the appetite of many patients, they cannot be relied upon alone to produce weight loss. In addition, their potentially serious adverse effects and abuse liability require that their use in weight loss be kept to a minimum and carefully monitored.

## Sympatholytic Agents

Drugs that block sympathetic nerve activity can be divided into two groups: (1) agents interfering with the chemical mediation of the nerve impulse—adrenergic neuron blocking agents, and (2) agents blocking adrenergic receptors—adrenergic receptor blocking agents or, simply, adrenergic blocking agents.

Drugs interfere with adrenergic postganglionic nerve activity through several different mechanisms. Two of the clinically more important such agents are guanethidine and reserpine. Both agents cause a depletion of transmitter from peripheral adrenergic neuronal terminals—guanethidine displaces norepinephrine from its storage sites, and reserpine blocks norepinephrine uptake into the storage granule. Prolonged administration of both agents causes a depletion of catecholamine from peripheral tissue. In addition, reserpine causes a significant reduction of catecholamine content in the brain and the adrenal medulla. Guanethidine differs further from reserpine in preventing release of norepinephrine by the nerve action potential before significant depletion of norepinephrine has occurred.

Both guanethidine and reserpine prevent the response to postganglionic adrenergic nerve stimulation and the administration of indirectly acting sympathomimetic agents. They do not prevent the response to directly acting adrenergic agonists and may even potentiate the response to many of these agents (especially norepinephrine and epinephrine). Although reserpine was used in the past as an antipsychotic agent, both guanethidine and reserpine find their most important present clinical use in treatment of essential hypertension (see Chapter 14).

The clinically useful adrenergic receptor blocking agents act as competitive pharmacological antagonists at the receptor level. The alpha adrenergic receptor antagonists include phenoxybenzamine and phentolamine. The blockade caused by phenoxybenzamine differs from that of phentolamine in that the former apparently involves more than an easily reversible binding of the parent compound to the alpha receptor. Phenoxybenzamine consequently has a longer onset and duration of action. Nevertheless, both drugs cause a decrease in the number of alpha receptors available for interaction with the agonist at any given moment.

The prototype of the beta adrenergic receptor antagonists is propranolol. This agent effectively blocks the beta receptors in most bodily tissues at comparable doses. Other, more selective, beta adrenergic blocking agents have recently been introduced. For example, practolol blocks the beta receptors in the heart in concentrations that have little effect on the beta receptors of the peripheral vasculature.

The alpha adrenergic receptor blocking agents block the response to postganglionic adrenergic nerve stimulation and the response to administration of indirectly acting adrenergic agonists (the heart is an exception to this statement since such responses are mediated through beta receptors; in the heart beta receptor antagonists are required to prevent the response to postganglionic adrenergic nerve stimulation as well as to administration of indirectly acting sympathomimetics). Both alpha and beta blocking agents prevent the response to administration of directly acting alpha and beta agonists, respectively. In general the dose required to prevent the response to administration of these directly acting agonists is lower than that required to prevent the response to the appropriate postganglionic adrenergic nerve stimulation. The adrenergic receptor blocking agents find their greatest clinical use in the treatment of various cardiovascular diseases (see Chapter 14).

## GANGLIONIC AGENTS

As the last topic for consideration in autonomic pharmacology, a few highlights of the ganglionic stimulating and blocking agents will be presented. This topic is included not because these particular autonomic drugs will ever be prescribed by the dentist or dental hygienist in the treatment or prevention of oral disease or.that the practitioner is called upon to alter drastically his own treatment plan for the few patients who would actually be taking a ganglionic blocking agent. There are two good reasons however. No discussion of autonomic pharmacology could ever be considered complete at the minimum level without at least an attempt to put the ganglionic agents into the entire picture. Furthermore, there will be numerous times when a particular drug used regularly by the dental practitioner has as one of its side effects the ability to inhibit ganglionic transmission or drugs being taken by the dental patient will have as one of their side effects a ganglionic blocking activity. Whoever treats such a patient must understand the relative importance of this fact.

The only other major site of action for drugs in the peripheral, efferent autonomic nervous system is the ganglion, and, of course, this site of action exists in both the parasympathetic and sympathetic subdivisions. Drugs that stimulate the postganglionic nerves at the ganglionic level and those that block transmission through the autonomic ganglia produce distinctive, predictable effects in man.

The easiest way to understand what the effects of the ganglionic agents might be requires the learning of four useful principles or rules. Keep in mind that these rules have the tendency to greatly oversimplify a sophisticated, complex physiological process (ganglionic transmission) in order to establish an initial grasp concerning what effects drugs that alter the process might produce. For the purposes of this discussion then these principles apply: (1) All ganglionic stimulating agents and all ganglionic blocking agents will be considered to act equally upon both parasympathetic and sympathetic ganglia. (2) Once a ganglionic stimulant has stimulated the ganglia, and if the dose administered was sufficient, there will inevitably follow a period of some degree of ganglionic blockade. (3) In general terms, the effects caused by a ganglionic stimulating agent in man closely mimic the effects that would follow the simultaneous electrical stimulation of all the excitatory autonomic innervations to all the organ systems, regardless of whether the excitatory innervation is anatomically sympathetic or parasympathetic or whether it is physiologically adrenergic or cholinergic. (4) In general terms, the effects caused by a ganglionic blocking agent in man closely mimic the effects that would follow

the simultaneous cutting of all the predominating autonomic innervations to all the organ systems, regardless of whether the predominating innervation is anatomically sympathetic or parasympathetic or whether it is physiologically adrenergic or cholinergic.

In terms of the singly innervated effectors (those with only
parasympathetic or only sympathetic innervation) it might be
expected to find some effectors whose single autonomic innervation, when stimulated, leads to an inhibitory response (see Figure
3.12). These are few! In man none perhaps is of great significance.
On the other hand and still in terms of singly innervated effectors,
there are to be found in man a number which when stimulated lead
to an excitatory response. The following are cited as representative
examples: the sphincter muscle of the iris is innervated only by the
parasympathetic system, and muscle contracting (excitatory) response results from stimulation; the radial muscle of the iris is
innervated only by the sympathetic system, and muscle contraction
results from stimulation; and the adrenal medullary secretory cells
are innervated only by the sympathetic system, and a secretory,
excitatory response results from stimulation.

In terms of dually innervated effectors—those innervated by both
subdivisions of the autonomic nervous system—it may be predicted
(as opposed to expected), based upon experimental evidence, that
ganglionic stimulation will result in excitation preferentially over
inhibition. Therefore, every smooth muscle contracting response,
every excitatory type of cardiac response, and every increase in
glandular secretory rate listed in Table 3.1 will be produced by the
ganglionic stimulating agent.

A closer look at rule (4) allows the effects of ganglionic blocking
agents to be predicted in man. Except for several unusual effectors,
it could be just as accurately learned that the general effects of
ganglionic blocking agents closely mimic the effects that would
follow the simultaneous cutting of all the excitatory autonomic
innervations (rather than the predominating autonomic innervations), because most predominating innervations of dually innervated effectors in man at rest are excitatory. However, the following
representative exceptions are noted: (1) Young adults manifest high
vagal tone to the SA node which allows an inhibitory type of
response (slowing of the heart rate) to predominate at rest. (2) The
smooth muscle sphincters of the upper gastrointestinal tract have a
lower tone at rest owing to predominant parasympathetic innervation that produces this inhibitory type of response (relaxation of
intestinal, sphincter smooth muscle). Keeping in mind these exceptions, it can be said that every smooth muscle relaxing response,
every inhibitory type of cardiac response, and every decrease in

## 1. SINGLY INNERVATED EFFECTORS

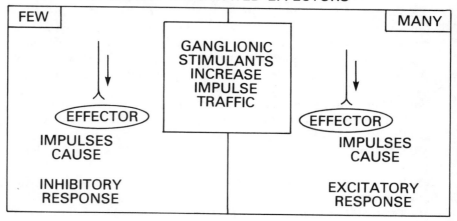

## 2. DUALLY INNERVATED EFFECTORS

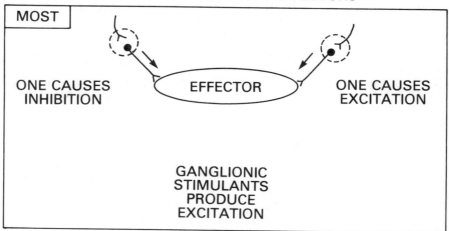

**Figure 3.12** Action of ganglionic stimulants on singly and dually innervated effectors.

glandular secretory rate listed in Table 3.1 will be produced by the effective dose of a ganglionic blocking agent.

### Ganglionic Stimulating Agents

For the purposes of this discussion little needs to be added regarding drugs that specifically stimulate autonomic ganglia. They have, as a drug group, no single therapeutic use. The body's own ganglionic stimulant is acetylcholine which is released from the ends of all preganglionic fibers into the ganglionic synapse. After diffusing across the 100 to 150 angstroms of the synaptic cleft, the acetylcholine combines with its nicotinic receptors located on the postsynaptic membrane of the postganglionic fiber. The result of this transient combination is the brief depolarization of the post-synaptic membrane with a subsequent discharge of the post-ganglionic fiber. It is believed that acetylcholine only depolarizes its nicotinic receptors at the ganglionic level and does not act through hyperpolarization as sometimes observed at the muscarinic receptors at the neuroeffector junctions.

It is only of historical interest that the prototype ganglionic stimulant, nicotine—the alkaloid of the tobacco plant—was one of the first known chemical substances to be shown to act specifically upon the autonomic nervous system. The early work of Traube in 1862 and the classic investigations of the English physiologist, J.N. Langley, at the end of the last century established nicotine as an autonomic drug. Like acetylcholine, nicotine and the few other known ganglionic stimulants produce a transient depolarization of the postsynaptic membrane's nicotinic receptors that causes the postganglionic fibers to fire. If the dose is properly selected, ganglionic stimulation is all that results, and the manifested clinical signs are the expressions of all the excitatory innervations to the body's effectors. The generally unpleasant experience that results may be easily confirmed by anyone who recalls smoking of tobacco for the first time.

### Ganglionic Blocking Agents

The ganglionic blocking agents were once held in high esteem as widely used drugs in the treatment of arterial hypertension; how-ever, because of their lack of specificity for inhibition of transmission through sympathetic ganglia and thus their myriad undesirable side effects that result from parasympathetic ganglionic blockade, the ganglionic blocking agents have now been reserved for selected and infrequent use.

There are two types of ganglionic blocking agents, based upon their induced clinical effects, but both types eventually share the same mechanism of action. The first type of ganglionic blocking agent is exemplified by nicotine (and all other ganglionic stimu-lants) and it is referred to as depolarizing blockers. These drugs first stimulate the nicotinic receptors by depolarization and, when the dose is sufficiently large and depolarization is persistent, allow the normal transmission through the ganglia to be interrupted. Before the drug's complete effects disappear, however, the ganglionic blockade converts from the prolonged depolarizing type to a second type of blockade, namely, ganglionic transmission blockade by competitive, nondepolarization of the nicotinic receptors. This general type of ganglionic blocking agent really has no therapeutic use, since stimulation precedes blockade of the ganglia.

The second type of ganglionic blocking agent is exemplified by the prototype, hexamethonium, and these agents are known as nondepolarizing, nonstimulating, competitive blockers of acetylcholine's nicotinic receptors at the autonomic ganglia. The actual ganglionic blocking agents still in use today are of this type. Hexamethonium produces clinical effects in complete accordance with rule (4). The lack of selectivity leads to the undesirable side effects of postural hypotension, dry mouth, paralytic ileus, impotence, and a host of lesser problems.

Two drugs of the hexamethonium type are used, albeit infrequently, in the following manner: trimethaphan (Arfonad) is used parenterally to reduce the degree of predictable hemorrhage in a variety of surgical procedures; mecamylamine (Inversine) is used orally in the final stages of chronic arterial hypertension, usually in combination with other antihypertensive agents; and, lastly, mecamylamine has some therapeutic efficacy in selected cases of acute pulmonary edema.

## REFERENCES

1. Koelle, G.B.: Neurohumoral transmission and the autonomic nervous system. *In* The Pharmacological Basis of Therapeutics, 5th Edition. Edited by L.S. Goodman and A. Gilman. New York, Macmillan, 1975.
2. Koelle, G.B.: Anticholinesterase agents. *In* The Pharmacological Basis of Therapeutics, 5th Edition. Edited by L.S. Goodman and A. Gilman. New York, Macmillan, 1975.
3. Innes, I.R., and Nickerson, M.: Norepinephrine, epinephrine, and the sympathomimetic amines. *In* The Pharmacological Basis of Therapeutics, 5th Edition. Edited by L.S. Goodman and A. Gilman. New York, Macmillan, 1975.

## SUPPLEMENTARY REFERENCES

Aviado, D.M.: Sympathomimetic Drugs. Springfield, Ill., Charles C Thomas, 1970.
Carrier, O. Jr.: Pharmacology of the Autonomic Nervous System. Chicago, Year Book Medical Publishers, 1972.
Levy, B., and Ahlquist, R.P.: Adrenergic drugs. *In* Drill's Pharmacology in Medicine. 4th Edition. Edited by J.R. Di Palma. New York, McGraw-Hill, 1971.
Maxwell, R.A.: Adrenergic blocking drugs, adrenergic neuron blocking drugs, and drugs altering biochemical mechanisms in adrenergic neurons. *In* Drill's Pharmacology in Medicine. 4th Edition. Edited by J.R. Di Palma. New York, McGraw-Hill, 1971.
Nickerson, M., and Collier, B.: Drugs inhibiting adrenergic nerves and structures innervated by them. *In* The Pharmacological Basis of Therapeutics. 5th Edition. Edited by L.S. Goodman and A. Gilman. New York, Macmillan, 1975.

Root, W.S., and Hofmann, F.G. (eds.): Physiological Pharmacology, Vol. 3, The Nervous System—Part C: Autonomic nervous system drugs. New York, Academic Press, 1967.

Root, W.S., and Hofmann, F.G. (eds.): Physiological Pharmacology, Vol. 4, The Nervous System—Part D: Autonomic nervous system drugs. New York, Academic Press, 1967.

Waser, P.G. (ed.): Chloinergic Mechanisms. New York, Raven Press, 1975.

PART **//**

# DRUGS USED BY THE DENTAL HYGIENIST

# 4

## LOCAL ANESTHETICS

No other single group of drugs is more widely administered in dentistry than the local anesthetics. The methods of administration require specialized training and such skills, for the orofacial region, are not usually shared by the physician. Although local anesthetics have been applied topically for some time, it is only in recent times that many states have authorized the dental hygienist to inject local anesthetics. This authority is a milestone in the developing dental hygiene profession, and the added responsibility involves a thorough understanding of the essential pharmacology of these drugs.

### HISTORICAL BACKGROUND

For centuries the natives of the Peruvian and Bolivian Andes have chewed the leaves of the shrub, *Erythroxylon coca*. They still do today. Especially the laborers, who must farm their alta plano land 12,000 to 14,000 feet above sea level, clear new fields of heavy rocks, or carry their harvested crops over the high mountain passes, may be found consuming a large quantity of the shrub's leaves. It is estimated that approximately 20 million pounds of the leaves are chewed by approximately 2 million natives which means 10 pounds of leaves per year per person. If they are asked why they chew the leaves, they will say it is just a habit, it makes them feel better, their loads seem lighter, the air is easier to breathe, or its keeps away the aches and pains and allows them to withstand the cold winds that continuously blow at that level.

Intrigued with these effects, a Swiss chemist brought some of the leaves from Peru to the famous German chemist, Albert Niemann. In 1860, Niemann succeeded in isolating the alkaloid, cocaine, from the leaves and noted that when one tasted the powder, the taste sense was lost as well as the sense of pain. Such was the first description given to the world's first local anesthetic as a single chemical entity.

Twenty years later one of Niemann's former students carried the studies further and noted that when cocaine was infiltrated subcutaneously the skin became insensitive to all stimuli applied to it. Von Anrep, however, was more interested in the drug's effects than in its therapeutic usefulness, although he was the first to suggest the possibility.

Four years after Von Anrep's paper was published, two well-known Viennese physicians reported their experiences with cocaine. Sigmund Freud was concerned mainly with its systemic effects upon the central nervous system, and Carl Koller was more intrigued with its local anesthetic effects in the eye. Koller stated in 1884 that a few drops of 2% cocaine solution in the conjunctival sac completely anesthetized locally for over an hour. The eye surgeons almost instantly began using the new drug.

In the same year in the United States, R.J. Hall first reported cocaine's usefulness as a local anesthetic in dentistry. The dental profession, however, did not ever widely accept cocaine and no doubt had not forgotten the fate of the two dentists (Wells and Morton) who first demonstrated the clinical effectiveness of nitrous oxide and diethyl ether in the 1840's. In this instance, dental conservatism paid off for the patient's sake, because the severe toxicity of injected cocaine with its high dependence liability soon had claimed many victims.

Wrought by many failures but pursuing a deliberate plan for many years, Einhorn finally reported in 1909 that he had synthesized in 1904 the diethylaminoethyl ester of para-aminobenzoic acid, which he named procaine.[1] He described its nondependence-producing, local anesthetic properties.

But dentistry was not going to fall for the old story again, so for another almost 40 years painful dentistry prevailed. It was only shortly after the second world war that procaine really began to be used widely and routinely in dentistry. About 25 years later it was estimated that dentists alone in the United States were administering almost one million local anesthetic injections each day. For an excellent review of the development of local anesthetics, the article by Liljestrand is recommended.[2]

## GENERAL CHARACTERISTICS

A local anesthetic is a drug which, when administered locally close to a nerve in both an effective and a nontoxic concentration, causes a reversible blockade of impulse transmission within the nerve in that local region.

Local anesthetics possess a number of general features. They will produce the described effect regardless of whether the drug is infiltrated into an area under the skin, painted on mucous membranes, injected into the fluid compartment surrounding the spinal cord, or placed near any nerve. Furthermore, the properly selected local anesthetic in an effective concentration will block impulse conduction in any kind of nerve, be it motor, sensory, or autonomic. The drug temporarily blocks nerve conduction in both nonmyelinated and myelinated fibers. It is often well to remember that the local anesthetics that are so widely used by injection in dentistry are general depressants of all cellular membrane activity, including that of cardiac, smooth, and skeletal muscles.

In terms of dentistry it is of interest that these drugs are most often used not to treat an oral disease or any disease, but these agents are administered to prevent pain-producing treatment procedures from being interpreted as painful by the patient. The patient is made more comfortable during the procedure, less anxious, or fearful and, it is hoped, more willing to return for treatment and preventive instructions. In addition, under the influence of these drugs the patient is less likely to exhibit the typical physical responses to pain, such as jerking the head or closing the mouth, and thus the patient will not injure himself or the practitioner during a procedure.

Local anesthetics as used in dental hygiene are administered usually in such a way that the drug's site of administration and the drug's site of action coincide. An important goal in the dental use of the local anesthetics is to avoid the rapid absorption of the drug into the systemic circulation. This, of course, is in contrast to most instances of drug use in which much time and effort are expended to get the drug into the systemic circulation. Indeed, the proper administration of these drugs requires considerable clinical skill.

## THE SITE AND MECHANISM OF LOCAL ANESTHETIC ACTION

It seems only reasonable that if the practitioner must administer the local anesthetic as near its site of action as possible, then what is understood to be the site of action is important. Irrefutable evidence shows, and all would agree, that the site of action for the local anesthetic must be the nerve itself. These drugs exert their local anesthetic action by binding reversibly to certain parts of the neuronal conducting membrane. Recent research would indicate that these certain parts include the sodium rapid transit channels that pierce the membranes.

It now becomes essential to picture a section of an axon with its conducting membrane surrounding the axoplasm. Figure 4.1 de-

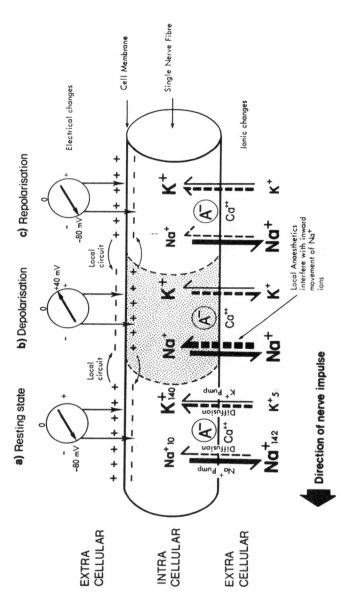

**Figure 4.1** Diagram of single nerve fiber to illustrate electrical (upper surface) and ionic (lower surface) changes that occur during conduction of nerve impulse (central shaded area) passing in the direction from right to left, i.e., (c) to (a). (a) Resting state: extracellular concentration of sodium ions (Na⁺) greatly exceeds intracellular concentration, although the opposite is true for potassium ions (K⁺). (Indicated by relative size of symbols; actual amounts in mEq/liter are also shown). Active transport of ions is indicated by continuous arrows (→) and diffusion by broken arrows (---→). The presence of intracellular indiffusible and negatively charged protein anions (A⁻) and extracellular calcium ions (Ca⁺⁺) which are essential components are also shown. (b) Depolarization: reversal of membrane polarity caused by transient inward rush of Na⁺ is followed by outward movement of K⁺. (c) Repolarization: sodium pump extrudes excess of intracellular Na⁺, and this is followed rapidly by inward movement of K⁺. The presence of local electrical circuits at junctions between normal and depolarized segments of nerve are indicated by semicircular arrows. Local anesthetics are believed to block nerve conduction by interfering with inward movement of Na⁺ which is essential for normal transmission. (This diagram is an oversimplification of a complicated process: for further details see text.) (Reprinted by permission from Walton, J.G., and Thompson, J.W.: Pharmacology for the Dental

picts, in terms of the ionic theory of nerve conduction, what happens to a segment of axon when an impulse passes. It will be noted that at rest the ions are distributed on each side of the conducting membrane so that the higher concentration of sodium ions is found on the outside and the higher concentration of potassium ions is found on the inside. Calcium ions are loosely bound to the outer surface. The outside is positively charged in relationship to the inside of the membrane which is negatively charged.

In even more diagrammatic form, Figure 4.2 shows the proposed structure of a segment of the membrane with its lipid and protein arrangements, as well as water-filled pores or channels that functionally are believed to exist, even though the microanatomical evidence is only now being accumulated. The size or caliber of these water-filled pores when the membrane is at rest is known. Hydrated sodium ions whose diameter is 6.8 angstrom units cannot pass through the membrane, but hydrated potassium ions whose

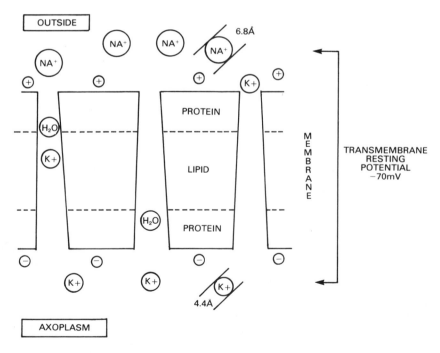

**Figure 4.2** Structure of segment of resting conducting membrane showing protein-lipid arrangement of layers and water-filled pores through the membrane. Approximate diameters of hydrated ions are indicated in angstrom units. See text for further details.

diameter is 4.4 angstrom units can pass along with water and chloride ions. Calcium ions are too large to pass. It would appear that when the membrane is at rest calcium ions may play a significant role in keeping the sodium ions on the outside. It is suggested that calcium ions bind loosely to the negatively charged phosphate groups of two phospholipid molecules within the sodium rapid transit channels.

When the impulse comes along the conducting membrane, the local circuit in some as yet unclear way causes a momentary reconfiguration of the membrane's outer surface. More specifically, the arrival of the action potential causes calcium ions to be released from their usual binding site; when this occurs, the pore entrance becomes sufficiently large for sodium cations to rush down both their concentration as well as electrostatic gradients into the axoplasm. The membrane is quickly depolarized, oppositely polarized (negative outside to positive inside), and then the segment repolarizes in the opposite direction with the help of the energy-consuming sodium pump mechanism.

It is believed by many that the local anesthetic molecule substitutes for calcium ions by mass action. The receptor sites have a greater affinity for the local anesthetic ion than for calcium ions. With the local anesthetic molecules substituted for calcium ions the arrival of the impulse is unable to remove the local anesthetic cation from the rapid transit channels, with the result that sodium ions do not enter the axoplasm, nor does there follow any other reaction which normally results from sodium's inward movement. It is an experimental fact that calcium cations and local anesthetic cations compete with one another. When the local anesthetic is in place, an increase in the external calcium ion concentration promptly reverses the local anesthetic action. Moreover, if the usual calcium ion concentration surrounding a nerve is reduced, far less local anesthetic is required to block conduction.

Although a sufficiently high concentration of the local anesthetic is next to the conducting membrane, the arrival of impulses at that segment of nerve does not result in a sudden influx of sodium cations, and hence the nerve fails to generate an action potential. As the concentration of local anesthetic dissipates, the calcium ions replace the drug and function is restored. Three characteristic features of the drug's action are (1) the drug blocks local conduction by preventing the generation of a local action potential; (2) the drug obstructs the inward flow of sodium cations through the conducting membrane; and (3) the drug produces a nondepolarizing (or stabilizing) block of impulse transmission, which means that the membrane remains polarized, essentially unchanged in the presence of the drug. The resting membrane potential is unaffected because the resting ionic permeability is unaltered. The drugs do not affect neuronal metabolism significantly in clinically used concentrations.[4]

## CLASSIFICATION OF LOCAL ANESTHETICS

It is essential for the dental hygienist to have some understanding of the classification of local anesthetics. The reason is not academic but urgently practical. Evidence, both basic and applied, confirms the fact that a patient may show hypersensitivity (or allergic) reactions to a local anesthetic. It is known, moreover, that such a patient will manifest a cross-sensitivity to other local anesthetics of the same chemical series but usually not show cross-sensitivity to those local anesthetics in another chemical series. It is necessaary, therefore, to realize that there are two major chemical groups of injectable local anesthetics. One group is called the esters, and the other group the amides. The classification shown in Table 4.1 is one of many and is based upon nitrogen content, water solubility, and chemical linkage.

The nonnitrogenous group includes a number of aromatic alcohols that are not used in dentistry as injectable agents. They are used topically, if at all. Each is extremely irritating to living tissue and produces a rapid denaturation of cellular protein which is the basis for their local anesthetic action. In addition to chlorobutanol such agents as phenol, cresol, benzyl alcohol, menthol, and eugenol are included.

### Table 4.1. Classification of Local Anesthetics
### Council on Dental Therapeutics Accepted Preparations

| Nonnitrogenous | Nitrogenous | | | |
| | Water Insoluble | Water Soluble | | |
| | | Ester | Amide | Ketone |
| (Aromatic Alcohols) | (Esters) | (Acid Salts) | (Acid Salts) | (Acid Salts) |
| Chlorobutanol* (Dentalone) | Benzocaine* (Americaine) | Procaine (Novocain) | Lidocaine (Xylocaine) | Dyclonine* (Dyclone) |
| | | Tetracaine (Pontocaine) | Mepivacaine (Carbocaine) | |
| | | Propoxycaine (Ravocaine) | Prilocaine (Citanest) | |
| | | Butacaine* (Butyn) | | |

*These drugs are only used topically owing to high toxicity when injected.

The nitrogenous group is divided into water-insoluble and water-soluble agents. The nitrogenous, water-insoluble group consists (practically) of only one agent, benzocaine, which is one of the most widely marketed local anesthetics for topical administration only. The local anesthetic to be found in most over-the-counter preparations is benzocaine.

The nitrogenous, water-soluble group includes the local anesthetics most commonly injected in dental hygiene. There are two exceptions, butacaine and dyclonine, both of which are used for surface local anesthesia only because of their greater toxicity upon injection. Thus, the injectable local anesthetics in dentistry may be conveniently subdivided into the esters and the amides. Figure 4.3 depicts the general structural formula for local anesthetic activity, which includes the aromatic end that confers lipid solubility characteristics to the compound, another end involving an amino group that confers water solubility characteristics to the compound, and a link between these two ends that gives the chemical identification to the two groups.

When the patient has a history of hypersensitivity to an ester type of local anesthetic, the patient may be expected to be hypersensitive also to all other ester types of local anesthetics. The procedure to follow for such a patient is to elect to use one of the amide types of local anesthetics.

## FACTORS INFLUENCING EFFECTIVE CONCENTRATION AT SITE OF ACTION

The local anesthetics are weak organic bases, poorly soluble in water, and unstable in an aqueous medium. If a local anesthetic such as procaine is treated with hydrochloric acid, the highly water-soluble, stable acid salt is formed as depicted in Figure 4.4. When procaine hydrochloride is dissolved in water, the drug exists in two forms because of dissociation: the noncharged, nonionized form and the charged, cation form. How much of the local anesthetic exists in each form depends on the local anesthetic's $pK_a$ (or negative log of the drug's dissociation constant) and the pH of the aqueous solution. If the local anesthetic's $pK_a$ is known, the familiar Henderson-Hasselbalch expression may be used to determine the relative concentration of the two forms at any specific pH.

In order for the local anesthetic to diffuse efficiently through the aqueous extracellular tissue spaces from the tip of the needle to the nerve's conducting membrane, it is helpful to have as much of the local anesthetic as possible in its water-soluble, cation form. When the drug reaches the lipoid nerve sheath (or any lipoid membrane which needs to be crossed), it is essential to have as much of the

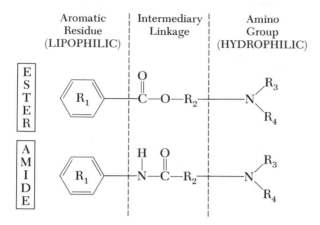

**Figure 4.3** Common structural formula for local anesthetic activity. $R_1$ to $R_4$ = moieties that may be varied slightly and still maintain a compound with local anesthetic activity.

local anesthetic as possible in its noncharged, nonionized lipid-soluble form so that it will diffuse down the concentration gradient across the sheath into the periaxonal space. Then, once the local anesthetic is inside the sheath, and in accordance with one theory, it is necessary to have as much of the local anesthetic as possible in its cationic form because it is this charged form that directly interacts with the local anesthetic receptor to produce the desired effect. Changes in tissue-buffering capacity (pH of aqueous solution in which drug is dissolved) alter the relative amounts of the local anesthetic in its two forms and hence alter the drug's penetrability to its site of action. As the pH becomes more acidic, the equilibrium moves toward the charged cation form; or as the pH becomes more alkaline, the equilibrium shifts toward the non-charged, nonionized form sometimes called the free base. It is necessary to grasp this point in order to understand why a local anesthetic solution injected into an inflamed tissue is more than likely not to produce an adequate level of local anesthesia. Figure 4.5 illustrates the normal situation on the left in which the extracellular tissue space (outside the nerve sheath) has a pH of 7.3 and the periaxonal tissue space (inside the nerve sheath) has a pH of 7.0. In these usual circumstances, a 2 ml cartridge of 2% lidocaine hydrochloride (containing 40 mg of the drug) would hypothetically distribute itself across the nerve sheath as cation and base in the amounts shown. On the right of this same figure, there is depicted the contrasting situation in which the tissue is inflamed so that the local extracellular tissue space has a buffering capacity at pH

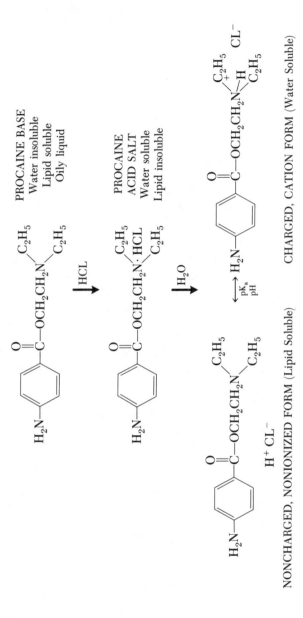

**Figure 4.4** Solubility of procaine forms and dissociation into noncharged and charged (nonionized and ionized, respectively) forms in aqueous solution: $pK_a$ = negative log of dissociation constant.

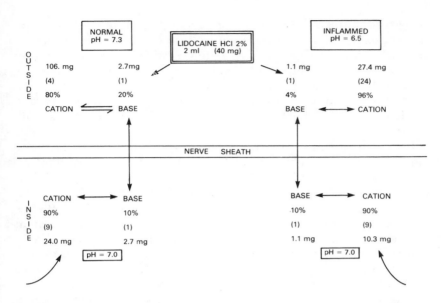

**Figure 4.5** Infiltration of local anesthetic for normal (on left) and for the inflamed (on right) tissue showing distribution of drug concentrations in both base and cation forms on both sides of nerve sheath. Note larger amount of cation form on inside of nerve sheath under normal tissue pH; see text for further details.

6.5. The same amount of the drug injected into the more acidic tissue would cause the drug to distribute across the nerve sheath in the amounts shown. Compare the relative amounts of the drug in each form on each side of the nerve sheath.[5]

The local anesthetic's action is terminated by its diffusion from the area down its concentration gradient. If the anesthetized nerve is in a highly vascular tissue, the drug will rapidly leave the site by entering the blood stream.

## SYSTEMIC EFFECTS OR SIDE EFFECTS

Regardless of the means of administration for a local anesthetic, the definite possibility exists for the occurrence of what may be called systemic or side effects. These systemic effects produced by the local anesthetic result when an effective concentration of the drug is reached at some site in the body other than the desired local site of action. From the dental hygienist's point of view, any and all systemic effects are side effects and unwanted. It is to be understood, of course, that once the drug has been administered into the tissues, all of it must sooner or later enter the systemic circulation, be passed through the liver, and eventually be eliminated from the body, usually by way of the kidneys into the urine. In the usual, carefully placed injection of the drug, systemic effects are rarely observed. Furthermore, under these usual circumstances the circulating blood concentration of the local anesthetic rises slowly to a low level, certainly below an effective concentration at any one particular site for the local anesthetic to exert an overt systemic effect.

It is well to know the other systems which the local anesthetic most commonly might alter so that the appropriate patient responses may be predicted. These systems involve primarily the central nervous system and the cardiovascular system.

CENTRAL NERVOUS SYSTEM SIDE EFFECTS. Local anesthetics have a definite action upon the complex, functional neuronal mechanisms that make up the central nervous system. When slowly injected intravenously in man, the local anesthetics can produce a wide range of effects that vary from mild euphoria (a false state of well being) to generalized seizures, coma, and death.

It is of some considerable interest that local anesthetics when given intravenously may produce anticonvulsant effects in man. Lidocaine has been shown to protect or to inhibit convulsions when given at a dose of 2.5 mg per kilogram of body weight at the rate of 45 mg per minute.[6] This experimental fact should give the dental hygienist some questions to ponder.

As the blood level of the local anesthetic is rising, the patient may show the following signs of central nervous system involvement, but not necessarily in the order listed: dizziness, throbbing sensation in the head, ringing of the ears, blurring of vision, numbness and tingling in the extremities, warm and flushed skin, and a dreamy state or perhaps hysteria.

These signs are a warning of the increasing concentration of the drug in the blood and herald, possibly, generalized seizures of the grand mal type. In nonconvulsant levels, it has been observed recently that the components of man's limbic system are the first area of the brain to manifest excitable responses. Is it not interesting that the amygdala followed by the hippocampus receives a large part of the brain's blood flow, and that local anesthetics may cross the blood-brain barrier more easily in the amygdala than elsewhere? When given in these subconvulsant doses, there appear drug-induced, localized abnormal discharges which are first confined to the amygdala and hippocampus and are difficult to distinguish from epileptogenic focal discharges of a patient with temporal lobe epilepsy. Indeed, the patient's behavioral and electrical manifestations closely resemble those of the psychomotor epileptic. When the drug is administered to the epileptic patient, he experiences his usual seizure with typical apprehension, various unusual sensations, changes in consciousness level, confusion, fixed glaze, and other signs.

It is well known that the partial seizures of focal epilepsies can easily spread along normal neuronal paths to the rostral portion of the brain stem reticular formation and there trigger the bilaterally synchronous pattern of generalized seizure of the grand mal variety. The neural path between the amygdala in the limbic system and the brain stem reticular formation is now clearly identified; thus, it is not surprising that when the local neuronal discharges become of sufficiently high voltage and frequency they spread to produce a generalized seizure.

The question is how does the local anesthetic in increasing concentration in the limbic system produce this focus of increasing hyperexcitability in the amygdala? Because of the preferential depression of inhibitory functions by local anesthetics elsewhere in the nervous system rather than early depression of facilitory functions, it is believed that the local anesthetic depresses certain limbic areas that normally send inhibitory impulses continuously to the facilitory areas of the amygdala. With these inhibitory areas eliminated, amygdala hyperexcitability results, producing at first what closely resembles human psychomotor seizure and perhaps, with sufficient inhibitory suppression, a spread of the discharge to the rostral brain stem reticular formation resulting in an overt seizure. If the increasing drug concentration is changed in its rate or degree of development, it is possible that all functional areas, both inhibitory and facilitory, are depressed. Depression would result in the clinical picture of sedation or even coma.

CARDIOVASCULAR SYSTEM SIDE EFFECTS. Local anesthetics also produce recognizable effects upon the cardiovascular system. This is no surprise when a local anesthetic's mechanism of action is recalled: the drug should interefere with the activity of any tissue in which impulse transmission is involved. The heart with its intricate impulse conduction system is a prime target for a drug such as the local anesthetic. General myocardial depression may be expected and, indeed, sudden cardiac arrest and death have followed the infiltration of a local anesthetic. The cardiac depressant effect produced by local anesthetics is predictable and apparently dose dependent. This is the basis for one of the medical uses of lidocaine, a popular local anesthetic used by the dental hygienist. No doubt all local anesthetics have some effect upon vascular smooth muscle. Once again this response would be a natural consequence of the drug's mechanism of action. The expected response is smooth muscle relaxation both via a direct effect upon the contraction mechanism of the muscle cell and via an indirect effect upon the contraction mechanism of the muscle cell and via an indirect effect upon the nervous system which is bringing impulse messages for contraction. The first local anesthetic, cocaine, confused this issue, since cocaine not only is an excellent local anesthetic but also a strong vasoconstrictor. Still today cocaine is the only local anesthetic with obvious arteriolar constricting properties. Other local anesthetics, as used by the dental hygienist, produce some degree of arteriolar vasodilation. At the systemic level, this adds up to the possibility of cardiovascular collapse if the blood levels of the drug rise too high or too quickly. At the local tissue level, the vasodilating effect will shorten the duration of effective local anesthesia and increase the risk of too rapid systemic absorption.

OTHER SIDE EFFECTS. Much has also been reported regarding the depressant effect of local anesthetics upon transmission at the myoneural junction. However, unless an enormous amount of drug is injected intravenously and rapidly, little myoneural depression can be observed in man.

## TOXICITY AND FATE

It must be realized that local anesthetics are certainly not innocent, innocuous substances that can be injected into living tissue or arbitrarily sprayed or painted over mucous membranes without concern for the possibility that the practitioner may accidently place the drug directly into the systemic circulation or may inject the drug a sufficient number of times in a short time interval so as to have a large amount absorbed. For selected dental procedures these compounds have no equal for their benefits exerted locally upon a nerve, but they also produce systemic effects that can be not only serious, but even fatal. The large majority of systemic or side effects can be reduced to a minimum by a combination of healthy respect for the drug, adequate patient history, proper administrative techniques, and good oxygenation of the patient. In accordance with general principles of pharmacology, the systemic side effects of the local anesthetics are closely related to the drug's blood level, i.e., the higher the blood level and the longer it remains elevated, the greater the chance of actual toxic effects.

Toxicity to local anesthetics is also known to occur when just a minute amount of the drug comes in contact with the hypersensitive or allergic patient. The allergic reaction to local anesthetics, including everything from contact dermatitis to anaphylactic shock, is relatively rare and almost, but certainly not exclusively, limited to the ester type of local anesthetic. There are definitely patients the dental hygienist will treat who are allergic to the amide type of local anesthetic (e.g., lidocaine, mepivacaine, and prilocaine) and who respond predictably and normally to the ester type local anesthetic (e.g., procaine, propoxycaine, and tetracaine). The reverse is equally true. Furthermore, there are even those few people who are actually allergic to both the ester and the amide types of agents. They are indeed unfortunate!

Local anesthetics themselves are practically free of cytotoxicity when used in the usual commercial concentrations, but be warned against allowing these drugs to come into contact with certain metal ions, especially copper, or local irritation may result. If the local anesthetic solution is in any way cloudy or discolored or contains crystals or particulate matter, it should be discarded and never considered for use in the patient.

Local anesthetics are changed by the body and thereby have their activity terminated by one or two general pathways. The esters are usually rapidly hydrolyzed in the blood by the plasma esterases (probably plasma pseudocholinesterase). The prompt cleavage of the esters when the circulation is reached serves as an inherent safety device against the too rapid accumulation of active ester. Nonetheless, it is possible to overwhelm the process, with the result being a variety of the discussed systemic side effects.

The pathway of metabolism for the amide type of local anesthetic is more complex and less understood. Because the amides rely upon the hepatic enzymes for their biotransformation, patients with a history of severe liver disease should not receive one of the amides without careful consideration and consultation with the patient's physician.

## PREPARATIONS

Characteristics, properties, and effects produced by all local anesthetics that should be of interest to the dental hygienist have been considered in general terms. It is now necessary to examine some essentials regarding the individual drugs that are in fact used by the dental hygienist as local anesthetics.

With practically every class of drugs there are too many individual drugs about which something specific could be stated. For the purposes of this text, there will be no succumbing to such an indulgence. The actual number of individual local anesthetic names will be severely limited, and only those found in accepted preparations of the Council on Dental Therapeutics will be described in any further detail. More than adequate information regarding all individual local anesthetics available may be found in the American Society of Hospital Pharmacists' Formulary.[7] At this point the local anesthetic preparations will be divided into two groups, the injectable agents and the topical or surface agents.

INJECTABLE LOCAL ANESTHETICS. The local anesthetic drugs that are injected by the dental hygienist have a number of characteristics in common as products. Each local anesthetic is in the form of its hydrochloride salt dissolved in an aqueous solution. The clear, sterile solution is usually 1.8 ml in volume and is housed in a cartridge (dental disposable unit) ready for insertion into the appropriate syringe.

The commercial local anesthetic solution contains other substances. There would not seem to be uniformity regarding these substances, but the following are not uncommon:

1. sodium chloride (to make solution isotonic)
2. sodium hydroxide (to adjust pH to between 6 and 7)
3. methylparaben (to act as preservative, 0.1%)
4. sodium metabisulfite (to act as antioxidant when vasoconstrictor is also present; 0.05%)
5. adrenergic agonist (to act as local vasoconstrictor)

These additives must not be overlooked, since some patients are hypersensitive to methylparaben in particular. Furthermore, should the patient have the solution injected accidentally into the systemic circulation, it will be necessary for the dental hygienist to distinguish between the systemic effects produced by the local anesthetic and those produced by the other ingredients, especially the highly active adrenergic agonist that may be included as vasoconstrictor.

The infiltrated local anesthetics begin to manifest their desired effect almost at once and, when precisely placed, produce their peak effect in 5 to 7 minutes. Their duration of effective action varies, depending upon the specific local anesthetic preparation, from less than 1 hour to longer than 2 hours. To be more exact than this is not possible at the present time.

The Council on Dental Therapeutics has accepted only six individual local anesthetics for injectable purposes.[8] These are found in thirteen preparations, as shown in Table 4.2, which are made by a variety of manufacturers. There is little doubt that the three amide products (lidocaine, mepivacaine, and prilocaine) with and without vasoconstrictors are the most popular in dental hygiene. The amides would appear to have a lower incidence in hypersensitivity reactions, greater stability in solution (longer shelf life), higher frequency of successful local anesthesia, and a realistic duration of action for dental hygiene procedures. In fact, the only

justification for using one of the ester types of injectable preparations today is for the dental hygiene patient who has a history of
allergic reactions to the amide type of local anesthetic or who
cannot tolerate one of the amides for some other specific reason.
However, when an ester type is needed, it is needed and no amide
will suffice. Of the three ester types accepted by the Council on
Dental Therapeutics, perhaps the most popular is the product
known as Ravocaine and Novocain with Neo-Cobefrin. Local anesthesia induced by procaine alone simply does not have sufficient
duration for most dental procedures.

SURFACE LOCAL ANESTHETICS. Some special features characteristic of the local anesthetics used for surface or topical administration deserve attention. The question may be asked by the dental
hygienist whether one could not dismantle a cartridge containing
any one of the injectable local anesthetics and use that solution
directly or by means of a cotton-tipped applicator to achieve surface
local anesthesia of the oral mucous membrane. It will be noted by
examining Table 4.1 that several local anesthetics listed are not
injectable agents.

There are three differences between the surface and injectable
local anesthetic agents to be discussed. Generally speaking, it
requires a higher concentration of the same local anesthetic for
topical anesthesia than it does for infiltration to obtain a quantitatively similar drug effect. It may be recalled that when a local
anesthetic solution is injected there is heavy reliance upon the
injected tissue's buffer capacity to bring the pH of the injected
solution as close to neutrality as possible. This is absolutely
essential in order to establish (according to the Henderson-
Hasselbalch expression) a larger amount of local anesthetic base or
noncharged form, which is highly lipid soluble. This is the form
necessary to cross the lipoid membranes, including the nerve
sheath, in order to reach the site of action. Unfortunately the
mucous membrane surface has a poor buffering capacity, certainly
nothing like that of the extracellular tissue space. When the rather
acidic, injectable local anesthetic solution comes into contact with
the surface cells, it essentially establishes a mucous membrane
surface pH the same as that of the local anesthetic solution. Under
these conditions very little lipid-soluble drug is available to cross
the cell membrane and head for the sensory nerve ending lying
nearby. Thus, the same local anesthetic solution with its acidic pH
can be infiltrated and lead to adequate local anesthesia but may
show no effect when it is applied topically.

According to general principles, however, all is not lost; there are
several possibilities. In the past, practitioners have alkalinized

## Table 4.2. Local Anesthetics for Injection Council on Dental Therapeutics Accepted Preparations

| | Commercial Names* | Anesthetic Concentration (%) | Other Active Components | | Chemical Class | Approximate Duration of Action | Maximal Safe Dosage (mg) |
| | | | Name | Concentration | | | |
|---|---|---|---|---|---|---|---|
| Procaine HCl | Novocain | 2 | — | — | Ester | < 1 hour | 1,000 |
| | | 2 | Epinephrine | 1:50,000 | | | |
| | | 4 | Phenylephrine | 1:2,500 | | | |
| Lidocaine HCl | Lidocaine Xylocaine Doricaine Lidocaton Octocaine Prolido | 2 | — | — | Amide | 1–2 hours | 500 |
| | | 2 | Epinephrine | 1:50,000 | | > 2 hours | |
| | | 2 | Epinephrine | 1:100,000 | | | |
| Mepivacaine HCl | Carbocaine Isocaine Mepivacaine | 3 | — | — | Amide | < 1 hour | 500 |
| | | 2 | Neo-cobefrin | 1:20,000 | | > 2 hours | |
| Prilocaine HCl | Citanest | 4 | — | — | Amide | 1–2 hours | 600 |
| | Citanest Forte | 4 | Epinephrine | 1:200,000 | | > 2 hours | |
| Tetracaine HCl | Pontocaine Tetracaine | 0.15 | Novocain Neo-cobefrin | 2% 1:20,000 | Ester | > 2 hours | 100 |
| Propoxycaine HCl | Ravocaine | 0.4 | Novocain Neo-cobefrin | 2% 1:20,000 | Ester | 1–3 hours | 200 |
| | | 0.4 | Novocain Levophed | 2% 1:30,000 | | | |

*Available in cartridges (dental disposable units) of 1.8 ml.

their topical anesthetic solutions so that tissue buffer capacity could be ignored. Both experimentally and clinically this practice has been of little usefulness because these particular local anesthetics become more and more unstable as alkalinity increases (most of the drugs will actually precipitate out of aqueous solution). The other possibility is to increase the amount of the drug applied and by the laws of mass action a greater amount of the drug will be available to cross the membranes to the site of action. Therefore, the preparations for topical administration are usually in a higher concentration than those used for injection, if the drug is injected at all.

There is a second major difference between the topical and infiltration routes for the use of a local anesthetic in dental hygiene. It has been clearly shown and confirmed that more systemic reactions occur to local anesthetics applied topically to mucous membranes than occur to infiltrated solutions of the drugs.[9] These systemic responses are all unwanted from the dental hygienists' point of view and are an expression of the drug's effects when it acts upon the other tissues of the body when an effective drug concentration is achieved at the distant sites. By actually measuring the blood level of local anesthetic following application to mucous membrane, it was found that topical anesthetic solutions give blood levels within minutes greater than those following slow intravenous infusion and comparable to those following rapid intravenous injection; there is certainly more rapid rise to peak and a higher peak than what results from proper infiltration.[10]

The third difference presented by the topical local anesthetics is still an enigma. For reasons yet to be adequately explained, the addition of epinephrinelike vasoconstrictors or any other type of vasoconstrictor thus far tested to the topical local anesthetic solution has only insignificant influence upon the onset of action or duration of action of a local anesthetic. Nor does the vasoconstrictor delay the systemic absorption of the local anesthetic.

Table 4.3 lists the pertinent information regarding the six individual topical local anesthetics accepted by the Council on Dental Therapeutics at this time.[8] As noted, these drugs appear in a large number of commercial products for the specific use of producing topical or surface local anesthesia.

## VASOCONSTRICTOR USED WITH DENTAL LOCAL ANESTHETICS

The duration of action of the local anesthetic is dependent primarily upon how long the active form of the molecule can remain at an effective concentration in equilibrium with the receptors on the conducting membrane. As has been discussed, the drug

## Table 4.3. Local Anesthetics for Topical Use
### Council on Dental Therapeutics Accepted Preparations

| | Commercial Names (Manufacturer) | Anesthetic Concentration (%) | Selected Other Components | | Chemical Class | Maximal Safe Dosage (mg) |
| | | | Name | Concentration (%) | | |
|---|---|---|---|---|---|---|
| Benzocaine | Benzocaine Ointment with Oil of Cloves (Novocol) (Oradent) | 20 | clove oil, lanolin, petrolatum | 2.0 | Ester | + |
| | Benzodent (Vick) | 20 | eugenol, 8-hydroxyquinoline, petrolatum, sodium CMC* | 0.4 0.1 | | |
| | Cora-Caine Analgesic Adhesive (Coralite) | 14 | aluminum hydroxide, zinc oxide, petrolatum, gum karaya, flavor, color | 2.0 0.5 | | |
| | Getz Surgical Dressing (Teledyne) | 6 | chlorobutanol, guaicol, oil of wintergreen, lanolin, beeswax, petrolatum | 5.0 1.0 | | |
| | Gingicaine (Hassler) | 22 | flavor, polyethylene glycol (solution) | — | | |
| | Hurricane Gel (Beutlich) Hurricane Solution (Beutlich) | 22 | flavor, polyethylene glycol | — | | |
| | Lorvicaine Dental Ointment (Lorvic) | 20 | eugenol, 8-hydroxyquinoline, petrolatum, lanolin, acacia | 0.45 0.1 | | |

124

| | Product (Manufacturer) | % | Other Ingredients | % | Type | |
|---|---|---|---|---|---|---|
| Benzocaine | Orabase Emollient with Benzocaine (Hoyt) | 20 | paste of gelatin, pectin, sodium CMC* in polyethylene and mineral oil gel base | — | Ester | + |
| | Paracain (Proco-Sol) | 10 | flavors, color, propylene glycol | — | | |
| | Topical Anesthetic (Oradent) | 16 | chlorobutanol, DSSS†, peppermint & clove oil, polyoxyethylene sorbitan monolaurate, glycol | 5.0, 1.0, 0.155, 23.4 | | |
| Tetracaine HCl | Cetylite Liquid Topical Anesthetic (Cetylite) Cetylite Spray Topical Anesthetic (Cetylite) | 2 | benzocaine, butylaminobenzoate, benzalkonium chloride, cetyldimethylethyl-ammonium bromide, water-soluble base (spray-metered nozzle) | 14.0, 2.0, 0.5, 0.005 | Ester | 80 |
| | Topical Anesthetic Aerosol Spray (Graham) | 2 | benzocaine, chlorobutanol, benzalkonium chloride, glycol base, propellants (metered nozzle) | 12.0, 2.0, 0.5, 65.0 | | |
| | Novol-Benzocaine-Tetracaine Solution (Novocol) | 1 | benzocaine, essential oils, water soluble base | 20.0, 0.3 | | |
| | Topicale Liquid (Premier) Topicale Ointment (Premier) | 2 | benzocaine, benzalkonium chloride, flavor, glycol base | 18.0, 0.1 | | |

## Table 4.3. Continued

| | Commercial Names (Manufacturer) | Anesthetic Concentration (%) | Selected Other Components | | Chemical Class | Maximal Safe Dosage (mg) |
|---|---|---|---|---|---|---|
| | | | Name | Concentration (%) | | |
| | Topicale Spray (Premier) | 2 | benzocaine, benzalkonium chloride flavor, dipropylene glycol base, propellants (metered nozzle) | 17.0 0.5 65.0 | | |
| Butacaine | Dental Ointment Butyn 4% and Metaphen 1:1,500 (Abbott) | 4 (as base) | nitromersol, eugenol, menthol, petrolatum, anhydrous lanolin, white beeswax | 0.067 0.1 0.5 | Ester | ++ |
| Lidocaine | Lidocaine Liquid 5% Flavored (Graham) Xylocaine Liquid 5% Flavored (Astra) | 5 | propylene glycol, glycerin, flavor | — | Amide | 200 |
| | Lidocaine Ointment 5% Flavored (Graham) Xylocaine Ointment 5% Flavored (Astra) | 5 | polyethylene glycol 1500 and 4500, propylene glycol, flavor | — | | |
| | 10% Xylocaine Dental Spray (Astra) | 10 | ethyl alcohol, polyethylene glycol 400, cetylpyridium chloride propellants (metered dose valve) | 7.13 20.79 0.01 60.6 | | |

| | | | | | Ketone | 300† |
|---|---|---|---|---|---|---|
| | Xylocaine Viscous (Astra) | 2 (as HCl) | sodium CMC*, methylparaben, propylparaben, flavor, and water | 2.5<br>0.07<br>0.03 | | |
| Dyclonine HCl | Dyclone Solution 0.5% (Dow) | 0.5 | chlorobutanol | 0.3 | | |
| Chlorobutanol | Dentalone (Parke, Davis) | 38.5 | clove oil, methyl salicylate, cinnamon oil, cinnamic aldehyde | 63.4<br>2.5<br>5.0<br>5.0 | Aliphatic | ++ |
| | Sedative Dressing (Crutcher) | 4.0 | benzocaine, Peruvian balsam, eugenol | 4.0<br>46.0<br>46.0 | | |

*CMC: carboxymethylcellulose; †DSSS: dioctylsodiumsulfosuccinate; ‡This figure is probably too low and is based upon one report; (+) = This figure does not seem to be available but must be relatively larger than for other topical agents; (++) = This figure is not available.

127

has already made a journey from the tip of the needle in the tissue to the receptors in accordance with the physicochemical principles of passive diffusion. Since there is nothing holding the local anesthetic molecules at the receptor sites, the drug continues to diffuse passively in all directions (from areas of its higher concentration to those of its lower concentration). How fast the drug will diffuse from the desired site determines duration of effective action.

The local anesthetic is more rapidly removed from highly vascular tissue because the blood passing through the area contains (practically) no local anesthetic. Therefore, the drug quickly diffuses into the circulation.

Slowing or reducing the blood flow through the site of administration (and, in this case, the site of action) would logically inhibit the diffusion of the drug and prolong the local anesthesia. It is now well known, of course, that the application of cold (resulting in vasoconstriction) prolongs local anesthetic action and application of warmth (resulting in vasodilation) shortens effective anesthesia.

Over 70 years ago, cocaine was widely used not only topically but also by infiltration. Upon injection cocaine produced a prompt blanching of the tissue, and its vasoconstrictor properties have been well confirmed. Unfortunately, the majority of the synthetic local anesthetics do not possess vasoconstrictor activity but actually cause local vasodilation to varying degrees. The drug then will shorten its own local anesthetic duration by increasing the blood flow at the injection site. Shortly after procaine's introduction during the first decade of this century, many attempts were made to improve the drug's brief duration of action, since it possessed so much potential as a safe drug in comparison to cocaine. One procedure, which Heinreich Braun called his "chemical tourniquet," was to add a small amount of epinephrine to the local anesthetic solution.[2] The actions of this adrenergic agonist greatly prolong the duration of effective local anesthesia.

The rationale for the addition of vasoconstrictors to local anesthetics has changed little since Braun's day, namely, to constrict the arterioles in the area of the injection in order to reduce the blood flow through the area. By so doing (it is believed) the local anesthetic would have a longer time to reach its effective concentration and its site of action and thus lead to a more intense and longer local anesthesia. In yet other words, by reducing the local blood flow, the rate of absorption of the local anesthetic would be suppressed. Secondarily, this reduced rate of absorption would reduce the chance of the blood concentration of the drug reaching a level that would produce unwanted systemic effects.

## Table 4.4. Local Vasoconstrictors for Local Anesthetics Council on Dental Therapeutics Accepted Preparations

| | Commercial Name | Concentration Used in Local Anesthetic Solutions | Recommended Maximum Amount* | Percentage† Alpha/Beta Stimulant Activity |
|---|---|---|---|---|
| Epinephrine, U.S.P. | Adrenalin Epinephrine | 1:200,000–1:50,000 | 0.2 mg | 50/50 |
| Levarterenol Levarterenol bitartrate, U.S.P. | Levophed | 1:30,000 | 0.34 mg | 90/10 |
| Levonordefrin, N.F. | Neo-Cobefrin | 1:20,000 | 1.0 mg | 75/75 |
| Phenylephrine HCl, U.S.P. | Neo-Synephrine HCl Phenylephrine HCl | 1:2,500 | 4.0 mg | 99/1 |

*These amounts are recommended for the healthy dental outpatient only; the doses must be much less (or none at all) for patients with cardiovascular problems.
†These percentage ratios are approximate only.

Over the years as newer local anesthetics have been introduced the manufacturer has made his drug available in combination with at least one concentration of a vasoconstrictor. Since epinephrine was the traditional vasoconstrictor, few other vasoconstrictors have been examined. Until a little over 10 years ago, only adrenergic agonists were tested.

In the United States today the dental local anesthetic solutions that the dental hygienist will be administering include only the adrenergic type of vasoconstrictor as shown in Table 4.4. It should be pointed out that of the hundreds of epinephrine analogs few have been studied to determine which is not only the most effective but also the safest to use with the local anesthetic. Only four adrenergic vasoconstrictors are available in the commercial products, namely epinephrine, levarterenol (Levophed), levonordefrin (Neo-Cobefrin) and phenylephrine (Neo-Synephrine). Even these four adrenergic vasoconstrictors, approved by the Council on Dental Therapeutics,[8] have undergone scanty fundamental study regarding their comparative value for the task, and certainly well-controlled clinical investigations on the comparative effectiveness and safety of these four are nonexistent.

The question could be raised, if it is only local vasoconstriction that is desired, why are four different drugs necessary? Anyone of these four adrenergic agonists should be able to accomplish the desired amount of vasoconstriction when injected in equiconstrictor amounts in the local anesthetic solution. If the pharmacologist were to select the adrenergic agonist best suited to accomplish the one objective of local vasoconstriction, the drug of choice would be the purest alpha adrenergic receptor stimulant of direct action. That drug (of the four accepted by the Council on Dental Therapeutics) would be phenylephrine. Epinephrine, which is by far the most commonly included vasoconstrictor, possesses both alpha and beta adrenergic receptor stimulating properties. The danger arises when the local anesthetic solution along with the epinephrine is accidentally deposited in the vascular system. The patient's systemic response will involve as serious a problem (or more so) from the epinephrine acting upon the heart as from the unwanted local anesthetic effects. Phenylephrine does not stimulate the beta adrenergic receptors in the heart.

## REFERENCES

1. Einhorn, A., and Uhlfelder, E.: Ueber den p-Amino-benzoesaure-diathylamino-und Piperiodoathylester. Justus Liebigs Ann. Chem., 371:131, 1909.
2. Liljestrand, G.: The historical devleopment of local anesthesia. In International Encyclopedia of Pharmacology and Therapeutics. Section 8, Local Anesthetics, Vol. 1. Edited by P. Lechat. Oxford, Pergamon Press, 1971.

3. Walton, J.G. and Thompson, J.W.: Pharmacology for the Dental Practitioner. London, British Dental Association, 1970.
4. deJong, R.H.: Physiology and Pharmacology of Local Anesthesia. Springfield, Ill., Charles C Thomas, 1970.
5. Ritchie, J.M.: The mechanism of action of local anesthetic agents. *In* International Encyclopedia of Pharmacology and Therapeutics. Section 8, Local Anesthetics, Vol. 1. Edited by P. Lechat. Oxford, Pergamon Press, 1971.
6. Bohm, E., Flodmark, S., and Petersen, I.: Effect of lidocaine (Xylocaine) on seizure and interseizure electroencephalograms in epileptics. Arch. Neurol. Psychiat., *81*:550, 1959.
7. Reilly, M.J. (ed.): American Hospital Formulary Service. Washington, D.C., American Society of Hospital Pharmacists, 1976.
8. Accepted Dental Therapeutics. 36th Edition. Chicago, American Dental Association, 1975.
9. Adriani, J., and Zepernick, R.: Clinical effectiveness of drugs used for topical anesthesia. J.A.M.A., *188*:711, 1964.
10. Adriani, J., and Campbell, D.: Fatalities following topical application of local anesthetics to mucous membranes. J.A.M.A., *162*,:1527, 1956.

## SUPPLEMENTARY REFERENCES

Bennett, C.R.: Monheim's Local Anesthesia and Pain Control in Dental Practice. 5th Edition. St. Louis, Mosby, 1974.
Covino, B.G., and Vassallo, H.G.: Local Anesthetics. New York, Grune & Stratton, 1976.
Dal Santo, G. (ed.): Biotransformation of Local Anesthetics, Adjuvants and Adjunct Agents. Boston, Little Brown, 1975.
Ritchie, J.M., and Cohen, P.J.: Cocaine, procaine and other synthetic local anesthetics. *In* The Pharmacological Basis of Therapeutics. 5th Edition. Edited by L.S. Goodman and A. Gilman. New York, Macmillan, 1975.
Ritchie, J.M., and Greengard, P.: On the mode of action of local anesthetics. Annu. Rev. Pharmacol. *6*:405, 1966.

# 5

## LOCAL ANTIINFECTIVES

An important responsibility for all health practitioners, including the dental hygienist, is to prevent the spread of infectious disease. Any practitioner who treats patients must have a clear understanding of infectious microorganisms and how to reduce the number of microbes in the office environment. Toward this end the dental hygienist must apply a knowledge of the methods for sterilizing as well as for partially reducing the number of microorganisms in the area. Chemical substances known as local antiinfective agents (antiseptics and disinfectants) are used so casually and routinely in many situations today it may be difficult to accept that they are drugs. Be aware; the local antiinfective agents are drugs! The dental hygienist must learn what the limits of expectation should be for these agents.

### CLASSIFICATION AND TERMINOLOGY

The large general class of drugs known as the antimicrobial agents may be divided into two large subgroups, depending upon the primary route of administration for the drug and, to a lesser extent, the drug's relative, selective toxicity (see Figure 5.1). Local antiinfective agents are administered only topically, and their action is relatively less selective (more nonspecific) than that observed for the systemic antiinfectives. The systemic antiinfectives or chemotherapeutic agents will be considered in Chapter 10.

Local antiinfective agents are antimicrobials which, when applied topically in the proper manner, either destroy or inhibit the growth of pathogens. Because of their systemic toxicity these agents are never administered internally. In addition to their widespread use on living tissue, some local antiinfective agents are used to

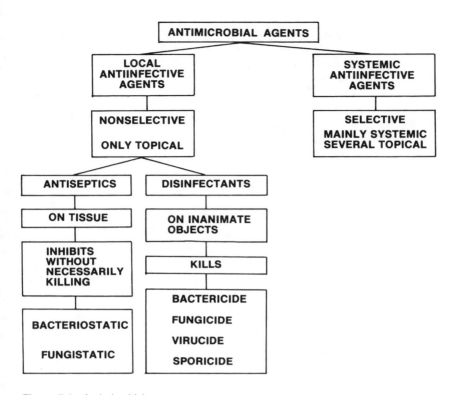

**Figure 5.1** Antimicrobial agents.

destroy or inhibit the growth of pathogens on inanimate objects such as surgical instruments or certain materials that come into contact with the patient. Traditionally the local antiinfectives are divided into two subgroups, the antiseptics and the disinfectants.

An antiseptic is a local antiinfective agent that stops or inhibits the growth of microorganisms without necessarily killing them. An antiseptic is the type of local antiinfective that is used on living cells.

A disinfectant is a local antiinfective agent that kills pathogenic microorganisms. It is the type of local antiinfective that is used on inanimate objects.

Bacteriostatic and fungistatic agents are examples of antiseptics. Bactericides, fungicides, virucides, and sporicides are examples of disinfectants.

The local antiinfectives are a fascinating conglomeration of drugs. Unfortunately, since the advent of chemotherapy pharmacologists appear to have lost all interest in research in the field.

Even bacteriologists must believe their further development is a morbid subject. For a class of drugs all take for granted, perhaps one should keep in mind the fact that of all the drugs taken by human beings, the local antiinfectives still stand first when it comes to frequency of use, not only in all practitioners' offices but also in hospitals, as well as in the home. Speaking of the home, more Americans are buying local antiinfectives over the counter every year. For mouthwashes and gargles alone (only two of the types of commercial products that contain local antiinfectives) the public spent approximately $241 million in 1971, $245 million in 1972, and $253 million in 1973.[1]

## USEFULNESS OF LOCAL ANTIINFECTIVES

Although often never given a thought, the only rational use for a local antiinfective agent in dental hygiene is to prevent infection. If this basic purpose for the drug group is kept well in mind, it is possible to define briefly how the local antiinfectives are used by the profession.

Many dental hygienists use a disinfectant to reduce the number of microorganisms adhering to nonpenetrating instruments. These are instruments which when placed in the patient's mouth do not break through the tissue surface or do not come in contact with the patient's blood. All instruments that do penetrate tissue or contact the patient's blood must be sterilized before reuse. There is no justification today to resort to disinfecting agents for any instrument that can and should be sterilized or that can be purchased in a sterile condition, used, and then discarded. No known local antiinfective solution is a "cold sterilizing solution." No such thing yet exists! To sterilize an instrument it must be exposed to one of the well-known sterilization processes. At best a carefully selected disinfectant solution can, if used exactly according to directions on the labeling, reduce the number of microorganisms on the instrument, but none can remove all forms of life from the instrument. These are facts to be accepted, and once this stage of understanding is reached, the rational use of local antiinfectives may begin.

Some instruments cannot be sterilized (at least as yet) without at the same time making them less functional or indeed nonfunctional. These instruments must then be treated with a disinfectant with the full understanding that the micoorganisms will probably be reduced in number but certainly never eliminated altogether.

Dental hygienists may apply a soothing antiseptic solution to the gingival sulcus after oral prophylaxis or after scaling. Once again the only purpose for so doing is to reduce transiently the number of microorganisms in the oral cavity and thus to prevent infection.

Keep in mind that the Council on Dental Therapeutics states that there is inadequate evidence to show there is any specific benefit from such a nonselective change in the oral microbiota.[2] Perhaps the use of warm water would mechanically remove an equivalent number of microorganisms.

Many dentists may be observed using an antiseptic solution in their treatment of minor soft tissue lesions in the oral cavity. This practice might prevent systemic infection, but the chances are slim. The antiseptics will not be killing a large number of microorganisms or even inhibiting the growth of others if the drug is allowed to be diluted, remains in contact too short a time, or is itself inactivated on the spot. Furthermore, the organisms reached (and hence affected) by the antiseptic will be only those on the surface that is swabbed. Few of these drugs can be expected to penetrate tissue at the lesion site or elsewhere when it is just not possible for them to do so, as their mechanism of action will confirm. Once again let it be clearly understood, there is nothing improper about using an antiseptic in this manner to try to prevent or curtail the local infection so long as the practitioner fully realizes that at best the agent is only reducing the number of surface micoorganisms.

Although to a lesser extent today, endodontists will be observed using an antiseptic (or disinfectant) to reduce the number of pathogens from within the hard tooth structure, the root canal.

## COMMON CHARACTERISTIC

The volume of pharmacology on the older local antiinfectives is almost overwhelming, and after a careful study of the specific properties of these agents there is a common characteristic that can be identified. Almost without exception local antiinfective agents have a great affinity for protein. They interact with protein regardless of whether it is microbial protein or man's tissue protein, and a great variety of agents have been demonstrated to act by one or more of the following general mechanisms: (1) it binds to microbial enzyme protein, leading to vital enzyme inhibition; (2) it binds to microbial membrane protein, leading to an alteration of the permeability characteristics; or (3) it binds rapidly to all protein, leading to protein coagulation and thus cellular death. Regardless of the mechanism, these drugs possess a very broad spectrum of antimicrobial action and are considered to be nonselective.

## FACTORS INFLUENCING EFFECTIVENESS

A number of factors influence the action and the effectiveness of the local antiinfective agents, and it is essential for the dental hygienist to understand these constraints if the drugs are to be used for anything other than ritualistic ceremonies.

CONCENTRATION. The concentration of the drug surrounding the microorganisms is critical, and a slight change in the concentration will alter effectiveness greatly. For example, it is not uncommon for a bactericidal concentration of a disinfectant to become so low that at best it exerts only bacteriostatic effects. Therefore, in the use of these agents clinically, the labeling instructions for preparation and use must be followed precisely and with the most accurate of measuring instruments available.

EXPOSURE TIME. The desired effect of these agents is greatly dependent upon how long the effective concentration surrounds the microorganisms to be destroyed. These drugs do not act unless they are in direct contact with the microorganisms. If the drug acts by inhibition of microbial enzymes or alteration of membrane permeability a little more time will usually be required for the drug's full effect than if the agent acts by coagulating protein. Under clinical situations in the oral cavity such antiseptic solutions are constantly being diluted and also (like any drug) passively diffusing away in all directions from the site of administration.

MICROBIAL PROTEIN CONCENTRATION. If the amount of drug and the exposure time are held constant, the desired effect is produced in relationship to how many microorganisms are actually present. Each of the local antiinfectives is far more effective in destroying or inhibiting a small number of pathogens in contrast to a large number.

PROTEIN DEBRIS CONCENTRATION. The antimicrobial effect is also strongly influenced by the amount of organic material or protein debris (pus, cell fragments) in the area of application. Keep in mind that these drugs nonspecifically bind to all protein.

In marked contrast to most systemically administered antiinfective agents, for example, the antibiotics, local antiinfective agents are nonspecifically lethal to all cells. In only a few instances does the effective concentration of one of the locally applied agents exert little or no effect upon the host's cells. In their applied concentrations these drugs can seriously inhibit the activity of leukocytes. This is a sobering thought while the patient is being deluged by mouthwashes, gargles, throat sprays, and other antiseptic applications by well-meaning health practitioners.

## ANTISEPTICS AND DISINFECTANTS

Tables 5.1 and 5.2 summarize the activity of selected antiseptic and disinfectant preparations utilized in dental hygiene.

### Table 5.1. Relative Antimicrobial
### Effectiveness of Local Antiinfectives

| Class Name | Prototypes | Relative Effectiveness | | | |
|---|---|---|---|---|---|
| | | Vegetative Bacteria | Bacterial Spores | Fungi | Viruses |
| Alcohols | Ethyl alcohol | G | N | F | N |
| Iodine preparations | 2% Iodine solution or 2% Iodine tincture (50% alcohol) | VG | P | G | G |
| | Povidone-Iodine solution (an iodophor) | G | P | P | G |
| Mercury preparations | Nitromersol solution (Metaphen) | P | N | P | P |
| Quaternary ammonium compounds | Benzalkonium chloride (Zephiran) | VG | N | G | N |
| Oxidizing agents | Hydrogen peroxide solution | G | P | P | G |
| Aldehydes | Glutaraldehyde (Cidex) | VG | VG | G | G |
| Phenolic compounds | Hexachlorophene (pHisoHex) | F* | N | G | N |

Note: N = no effect; P = poor effect; F = fair effect; G = good effect; VG = very good.
*The agent is effective only against gram-positive bacteria in concentrations used.

ALCOHOLS. There are only two aliphatic alcohols of interest, ethyl alcohol and isopropyl alcohol, both of which are commercially available in 70% by weight concentrations. Their major usefulness is for skin antisepsis. Neither can remove more than about 75% of the microorganisms from the skin even following 5 minutes' exposure. The alcohols are mainly effective (bactericidal) against bacterial vegetative forms, have no effectiveness against spore forms, and have an unpredictable effect upon viruses. Against vegetative forms of fungi, the alcohols show fair activity, but there are other much more efficient antifungal agents. Since the alcohols have no effect on spores, alcohol cannot be used to disinfect surgical instruments. Spores may easily contaminate the solution, the instrument, and subsequently the patient.

The local application of alcohol to lesions of the oral soft tissues is not recommended, since the drug produces intense stinging, tissue irritation, and a coagulum of precipitated protein under

**Table 5.2. Antiseptics and Disinfectants**

| Class Name | Prototypes | Antiseptics[a] | | | | Disinfectants[a] (Instruments) | | Probable Mechanism of Action |
| | | Mucous Membranes | | Skin | | | | |
| | | E. Conc (%) | E. Time (min) | E. Conc (%) | E. Time (min) | E. Conc (%) | E. Time (min) | |
| --- | --- | --- | --- | --- | --- | --- | --- | --- |
| Alcohols | Ethyl alcohol | 70 | 0.5 | 70 | 2–5 | * | * | Denatures microbial protein |
| Iodine preparations | 2% Iodine solution or 2% Iodine tincture (50% alcohol) | 2 (soln) | 0.5 | 2 (tinc) | 2 | * | * | Iodinates vital microbial enzyme protein |
| | Povidone-Iodine solution (an iodophor) | 1 | 0.5 | 1 | 2 | * | * | |
| Mercury preparations | Nitromersol solution (Metaphen) | 0.2 | 0.5 | 0.5 | 5 | * | * | Inhibits sulfhydryl enzymes (bacteriostatic only!) |
| Quaternary ammonium compounds | Benzalkonium chloride (Zephiran) | 0.13 | b | 0.13 | 7 | 0.13 | 180 | Alters permeability characteristics of microbe |
| Oxidizing agents | Hydrogen peroxide solution | 3 | c | * | * | * | * | Oxidizes vital microbial chemicals |
| Aldehydes | Glutaraldehyde (Cidex) | * | * | * | * | 2 | 10[d] | Interacts with amino groups on proteins |
| Phenolic compounds | Hexachlorophene (pHiso-Hex) | * | * | 1–3 | 7 | * | * | Alters permeability characteristics of certain microbes |

a = E. CONC is effective concentration of drug to produce effects identified; b = The exposure time for benzalkonium to produce its maximum effect upon mucous membranes is not available; c = The exposure time for hydrogen peroxide to produce its maximum effect upon mucous membranes is not known; d = In order for glutaraldehyde to kill some bacterial spores an exposure time of 10 or more hours may be required; * = Agent not used routinely for this category.

which microorganisms can grow. Such a practice is acceptable in England.[3] The alcohols are believed to act by denaturing microbial protein, a process for which water must be present. It has been known for sometime that 70% alcohol is more toxic to phagocytic cells (leukocytes) than to a variety of bacteria. On the positive side, the alcohols (specifically, ethanol and isopropanol) possess a low level of allergenicity.

IODINE PREPARATIONS. Antiseptics that contain iodine or that slowly release iodine may be the most effective available today. Iodine has some activity against all microorganisms, but as is true for all local antiinfectives the bacterial spores are fairly resistant. Iodine is not used as a disinfectant for instruments, whereas iodine in an aqueous 2% solution may be applied to mucous membranes for a period of 30 seconds with a large reduction in pathogens. Glycerin with 2% iodine may be even more appropriate for irritated oral mucous membranes. The mechanism of action is proposed to be the iodination of microbial enzyme protein. The iodophors are complexes of iodine with surface-active agents that may have some weak antibacterial activity of their own. The iodophors do not stain, nor have they been shown to sting or irritate oral soft tissue. Some individuals are hypersensitive to iodine, and, of course, no iodine-containing drug or iodine-releasing drug should be administered to such an individual.

MERCURY PREPARATIONS. Contrary to three quarters of a century's advertising superlatives about the antiseptic adequacy of the organic mercurial compounds, these drugs are at their best not very effective and are only bacteriostatic in action. Their activity is due to the slow release of ionic mercury which combines with sulfhydryl groups of enzymes in both the microorganisms and in the patients. Unfortunately the combination of mercury and the sulfhydryl group is not stable, and the active enzymes may be regenerated by a number of naturally occuring substances readily found in the body. Therefore it is possible for the organic mercurial antiseptic to inhibit the growth of bacteria on the mucous membrane; then the patient swallows or absorbs in some other way the inhibited bacteria which are reactivated (capable of causing disease) after entrance to the body is achieved. Furthermore, mercurial antiseptics also cause inhibition of leukocytes which is undesirable. They are not the safest of the antiseptics available and certainly not the most effective. There are patients for whom mercury is allergenic, and these persons should not be exposed to the mecurial antiseptics.

QUATERNARY AMMONIUM COMPOUNDS. The quaternary ammonium compounds are also cationic surface-active agents. They each possess a high molecular weight lipophilic cation. They should not be confused with the anionic surface-active agents, which include the common soaps. The quaternary ammonium compounds are effective bactericidal agents for vegetative forms of many microorganisms. However, that is all that can be said for the group. Perhaps they are best suited for sanitizing agents or as disinfecting agents for office furniture and other materials in the office with which the patient may come in contact. The quaternary ammonium compounds have no effect upon bacterial spores or upon viruses such as the one that produces hepatitis. No doubt many cases of viral hepatitis could be directly traced to instruments that have been stored in what misleadingly is called the "cold sterilizing" solution of a quaternary ammonium compound. The mechanism of action is thought to be more than just the ability to be attracted to protein and the alteration of the permeability characteristics of the microbe. Although the compounds seem to affect both gram-positive and gram-negative microorganisms, the drugs do have some reported deleterious effects upon human tissue.

OXIDIZING AGENTS. Hydrogen peroxide is an example of an oxidizing agent that possesses brief antiseptic activity in contact with living tissue. It interacts almost instantly with the ubiquitous tissue enzyme, catalase, which converts the drug to water and gaseous oxygen. It is actually the release of gaseous oxygen which mechanically loosens and moves tissue debris that gives hydrogen peroxide its uniqueness. Because its action is so transient, the drug is practically useless as a skin antiseptic and should not be used for the disinfection of instruments. Hydrogen peroxide is rapidly destroyed in the presence of any organic matter. It is an ingredient in popular over-the-counter mouthwashes, and the dental hygiene patient must be warned against the continuous use of such mouthwashes, since hypertrophied filiform papillae will result. The condition produced is aptly named black hairy tongue. When the drug is stopped, the condition disappears. Hydrogen peroxide has other uses in dentistry.

ALDEHYDES. A mixture of the oldest disinfectants and the newest disinfectants may be found in this group. The newest, glutaraldehyde (Cidex), would appear to have good potential as a disinfectant for instruments (e.g., the handpiece) that cannot be sterilized by physical means. Since it produces irritation of the skin and mucous membranes, it must never be used on these tissues. Indeed, any item stored (no longer than 24 hours) in glutaraldehyde must be rinsed with sterile water or alcohol before contact with living tissue. Although most bacteria, fungi, and viruses are killed by an appropriately prepared solution (activated by means of adding the buffer that comes with the commercial product) with an exposure time of 10 minutes, bacterial spores will require an exposure time of 12 hours or longer. It must be remembered that as yet there is no specific evidence to indicate that the drug will kill the causative agent of viral hepatitis. Formaldehyde is too irritating to be allowed to contact living soft tissue; however, it does find other uses in dentistry.

PHENOLIC COMPOUNDS. Only one such drug, hexachlorophene, will be considered, owing to its widespread use for many years. Hexachlorophene is most commonly combined with anionic surface-active agents (soaps) for skin antisepsis. In contrast to the cationic surface-active agents with which the anionic compounds are absolutely incompatible, hexachlorophene is effective only against gram-positive bacteria and has no effect upon gram-negative microorganisms. This fact, along with the evidence that hexaclorophene has no sporicidal or virucidal properties, should certainly severely limit the usefulness of this weak antiseptic in dental hygiene. With prolonged hand washing with hexachlorophene (2 to 3%) the number of gram-positive microorganisms can be shown to be cumulatively reduced. The drug should not be relied upon to be as effective as the standard preoperative hand-scrubbing techniques learned in the student's early training in dental hygiene.

## REFERENCES

1. Goldberg, J.H. (ed.): 1976 Marketing Guide. Oradell, N.J., Medical Economics, 1976.
2. Accepted Dental Therapeutics. 36th Edition. Chicago, American Dental Association, 1975.
3. Kay, L.W.: Drugs in Dentistry. 2nd Edition. Bristol, John Wright & Sons, 1972.

## SUPPLEMENTAL REFERENCES

Burnett, G.W., Scherp, H.W. and Schuster, G.S.: Oral Microbiology and Infectious Disease. 4th Edition. Baltimore, Williams and Wilkins, 1976.
Darlington, R.C.: Topical oral antiseptics, mouthwashes and throat remedies. *In* Handbook of Non-Prescription Drugs. 1973 Edition. Edited by G.B. Griffenhagen and L.L. Hawkins. Washington, D.C., American Pharmaceutical Association, 1973.

# 6

## FLUORIDES

Scopp succinctly defines the complex disease of dental caries or tooth decay as "a bacterial infection that develops when the mineral components of enamel dissolve in acids formed by bacterial accumulation on the tooth surfaces."[1] Almost needless to say, tooth decay is of paramount concern to every dental hygienist. Although at the present time the dental hygienist may not be allowed to treat dental caries, the dental hygienist is an important member of the health team involved in the prevention of carious lesions. Through patient education, effective oral hygiene techniques, and the use of anticariogenic fluorides, the dental hygienist strives daily to reduce the incidence of this most prevalent condition.

The role of inorganic fluorides in the prevention of tooth decay is widely known and accepted as an incontestable fact by a large majority of scientists, practicing dentists, dental hygienists, and the informed public. In this chapter only the pharmacological aspects of inorganic fluoride are considered. Immediately, some may argue that fluoride is not a drug; it is an essential nutrient, an essential mineral such as calcium or phosphate or iron. No stand will be taken for or against such an argument because it adds nothing to our understanding of fluorides and may inhibit some from the proper use of the substance. Fluoride and drugs in general do have characteristics in common and therefore the subject of fluorides is included.

Fluoride ions are chemical substances that produce effects upon living tissues. These effects are predictable in relationship to the amount of fluoride in contact with the living tissue, and these effects may be divided into, generally speaking, beneficial and nonbeneficial. Furthermore, in man fluoride can be shown clinically to act as a bona fide therapeutic agent because it alters the course of an existing disease (osteoporosis). In addition, fluoride can be shown experimentally and clinically to act as an effective preventive agent in man because it significantly reduces the incidence of a commonly occurring disease, dental caries.

The interest of everyone in fluoride is growing exponentially in recent years. A number of excellent specifically applicable reviews are now available in language we all can understand.[2-6]

## MECHANISM OF ACTION

Although there is no doubt regarding the anticariogenic effectiveness of fluoride when administered systemically during the formation and mineralization of the teeth or when administered topically after the teeth have erupted, just exactly how fluoride produces this beneficial effect is unknown.

Of the many known effects of fluoride ion at least two would appear to result directly in the prevention of tooth decay as we understand the process at this time. Fluoride ion exerts an action upon the hydroxyapatite crystal of enamel and causes through its physical presence a decrease in the solubility of enamel in acids, stabilization of the crystalline structure by providing additional and stronger hydrogen bonds, and a promotion of the remineralization or hardening of the enamel surface.

The second action that fluoride ion exerts is upon the bacteria of dental plaque. There is a growing body of evidence to show that the concentration of fluoride ion in the immediate vicinity of the dental plaque organisms can be sufficiently high to inhibit vital microbial enzyme systems and thereby alter the usual pattern of growth and acid production which leads to tooth decay.[7] Although the high concentration of fluoride in surface enamel and in plaque may be unavailable, since it is in a bound form, it is now known that when attacked by acid (from the bacterial fermentation process) the fluoride may be released in ionic form and kill the bacteria. In terms of topical fluoride application there is no question but that the fluoride ion concentration applied is bactericidal. The correct use of fluoride-containing prophylactic pastes has been shown to reduce the actual number of *Streptococcus mutans*, the most virulent caries-producing oral streptococcus. Once again exactly how fluoride ion leads to this change in plaque flora is not fully understood. Many other viable proposed mechanisms are offered to explain fluoride's anticariogenic effectiveness, and the true mechanism may most likely involve a combination of many.

## PHARMACOKINETICS OF FLUORIDE ION

ABSORPTION. Fluoride is a ubiquitous substance and finds its way into the systemic circulation of man by a variety of routes. The major site of absorption is the gastrointestinal tract, with more being absorbed from the large surface of the upper small intestine than from the stomach. Studies have shown that following the ingestion of soluble fluoride over 80% is usually absorbed within 90 minutes. No energy appears to be required as fluoride passively diffuses down its concentration gradient from the lumen of the intestine to the lumen of the blood vessels.

In areas where there is less than 0.1 ppm fluoride in the drinking water adults absorb approximately 1.0 mg per day. Moreover, in areas where there is an optimum of fluoride in the drinking water (0.8 to 1.2 ppm F) adults absorb approximately 2.5 mg per day, but there is a wide variation from individual to individual in each of the areas.

The second most common route of absorption for fluoride is from the air via the lungs. In days past, workers in steel and aluminum plants which used fluoride in their processes absorbed large amounts of fluoride from the heavy laden air. In some instances so much fluoride was absorbed via the lungs that toxic effects of fluoride were manifested. Today through proper safety devices fluoride no longer is a serious hazard for these workers.

DISTRIBUTION. After the fluoride ion reaches the systemic circulation, it is destined to be deposited in bone or be excreted in the urine. According to Newbrun the blood contains approximately 0.1 ppm fluoride ion with 85% of this bound.[2] This leaves only 0.02 to 0.05 ppm fluoride as ionic form to distribute throughout the body. The saliva contains only 0.01 to 0.02 ppm fluoride ion. It is estimated that the total adult body may contain 2.6 grams of fluoride with 95% in the skeleton. Thus, fluoride deserves its label of "bone seeker." When the individual is remodeling bones and developing tooth structures, more of the ingested fluoride will be deposited in hard tissue. During middle age most of the ingested fluoride is excreted.

EXCRETION. Fluoride ion is excreted from the body by way of the urine, feces, and sweat, the routes being given in the order of importance. The urinary level of fluoride ion is a faithful indicator of the amount of fluoride ion ingested. There is a direct relationship between the amount of fluoride in the drinking water and the amount found in the urine. Except during hot weather the amount of fluoride ion lost through sweating is minimal. Fluoride not absorbed from the gastrointestinal tract is lost in the feces. As the individual grows older, the proportionate amount of fluoride deposited in the skeleton becomes less and the proportionate amount excreted in the urine becomes more.

## TOXICITY

Fluoride ion is no different from any other chemical entity or drug; it has both beneficial and nonbeneficial effects which it can produce upon living tissue. Let it be understood from the outset that the beneficial effects of fluoride in man far outweigh the various and rarely occurring toxic effects. The best known beneficial effects of fluoride are as an anticariogenic agent in the prevention of dental decay and as an antiosteoporotic agent. All of the other effects that have been reported to result from the action of fluoride ion may be considered as unwanted, undesirable, or, in many cases, toxic side effects.

ACUTE TOXICITY. Acute toxicity refers to the nonbeneficial effects produced by a single overwhelming overdose of fluoride. The lowest reported lethal oral dose of sodium fluoride in man is 75 mg per kg of body weight, and the lowest reported toxic oral dose of sodium fluoride in man is 4 mg per kg of body weight.[8] The relationship of fluoride dose or concentration to toxic effect is shown in Table 6.1 as adapted from the work of H.C. Hodge.[2] Without treatment the victim may be expected to live 2 to 4 hours and show almost immediately the following obvious symptoms: nausea, vomiting, diarrhea, intense lower intestinal cramping, profuse salivation, thirst, and sweating. Before death the patient will show cardiovascular collapse and coma; death usually is the result of respiratory failure. Thus far there are few studies relating the human toxic effect to blood levels of fluoride. It is reported that inorganic serum fluoride concentrations of $175\,\mu M$ to $750\,\mu M$ have been shown in fatal cases of fluoride intoxication.[4] It is possible to reduce the toxic blood levels of fluoride by extracorporeal hemodialysis.

### Table 6.1.  Toxic Responses to Fluoride

| Concentration or Dose of Fluoride | Time | Toxic Effect |
|---|---|---|
| 2 ppm or more | during tooth formation | dental fluorosis |
| 8 ppm | years | 10% osteosclerosis |
| 20–80 mg/day or more | years | crippling fluorosis |
| 50 ppm | years | thyroid changes |
| 100 ppm | months | growth retardation |
| More than 125 ppm | months | kidney changes |
| 2.5–5.0 grams | acute dose | death |

Source: Adapted from Newbrun, 1975.[2]
Note: The toxic effect may have been observed only in experimental animals; ppm = parts per million.

The mechanism of the lethal action of fluoride is not exactly known but is generally presumed to be the result of high concentrations of fluoride ion intracellularly that produce a profound inhibition of a wide variety of enzymes. Tissue respiration and energy production in general are depressed. Fluoride is known to complex with a number of divalent metal cations that are essential for certain enzymes to function. In fatal cases it is reported that the blood does not clot properly owing perhaps to fluoride interacting with the blood's calcium ions.

CHRONIC TOXICITY. Chronic toxicity refers to the nonbeneficial effects produced by small, moderate, or large exposure to the drug over a long period. There are several notable chronic toxic effects of fluoride.

During the time of tooth mineralization a concentration of fluoride ion in the drinking water of more than 2 ppm may lead to the production of dental fluorosis or mottled enamel. This is characterized clinically by white horizontal lines, brown discoloration of the tooth surface, and even enamel hypoplasia. It should be kept in mind by the dental hygienist that not all white opacities of the enamel are a direct result of too high an exposure of fluoride. There would appear to be a narrow dose-response relationship involved in that 10% of children drinking water with 1 ppm fluoride may develop mild dental fluorosis; and, it is estimated, at a level of 4 to 6 ppm fluoride in the drinking water over a period of time 100% of the children will demonstrate mottled enamel. This is one reason why the prescribing of daily fluoride doses must be carefully determined and based upon a knowledge of the usual daily ingestion of fluoride by the patient.

If an individual is exposed to 20 to 80 mg of fluoride ion per day for over a period of 10 to 20 years a condition known as crippling fluorosis may result. This is really a disease of the past, since industrial workers in plants and mines where such high concentrations of fluoride may exist are protected today by regulatory and safety codes. Crippling fluorosis is characterized by hypermineralization of bone, exostoses, and ligament calcification.

## FLUORIDE PREPARATIONS

It is possible to administer the correct amount of fluoride to every individual by utilizing the wide variety of fluoride preparations. The ideal situation is to make fluoride ion available in the community drinking water in a concentration of 1 ppm so that the individual from at least birth through 13 years of age will be exposed to this proper dietary level. If the community water supply does not contain 1 ppm fluoride ion naturally, the appropriate amount of fluoride should be added to bring the concentration to this optimum level. The fluoride level of public drinking water must be accurately regulated by engineering control. Although more and more communities throughout the world are actually attaining the ideal situation, there are many which fall short.

To keep all the fluoride preparations organized for better understanding it is helpful to classify the products into at least three groups: the professionally prescribed systemic supplements, the professionally applied topical products, and the self-applied topical products.

PROFESSIONALLY PRESCRIBED SYSTEMIC FLUORIDE SUPPLEMENTS. Because of the necessity of regulation of the daily dosage of fluoride ion, the supplemental products that are ingested are available only upon prescription by the dentist or the physician. It can only be hoped that in the not too distant future the responsibility for determining proper supplemental fluoride will be given to all dental hygienists. The supplemental fluoride product is the preparation of choice when the patient is in an area with less than 1 ppm fluoride ion in the drinking water and the patient is between 6 months and 13 years of age. The supplemental ingested fluoride shows beneficial reduction in tooth decay best when initiated early (reduction of decay by 50 to 75%) or when begun at 6 years of age (reduction of decay by 20 to 45%).

Two important factors are involved in this type of fluoride administration, the determination of the correct daily dose by knowing the patient's age and the concentration of fluoride ion in the drinking water. The relationship between these factors is expressed officially by the Council on Dental Therapeutics, but a slightly clearer expression of the same relationship as modified from Parkins[3] is shown in Table 6.2.

The choice of products includes the more convenient form for the very young as the appropriate number of drops placed directly in the mouth, as well as chewable tablets for the older youngsters. The daily dose appears to have best results when taken just before bedtime after brushing and flossing and swished in the mouth before swallowing, and when the user ingests nothing before going to sleep. The various accepted preparations by the Council on Dental Therapeutics are shown in Table 6.3. There is, of course, no justification for the prescribing of commercially available fluoride and vitamin combination products.

PROFESSIONALLY APPLIED TOPICAL FLUORIDES. In areas that do not have the benefit of 1 ppm fluoride ion in the drinking water the topical application of fluoride to the erupted crowns has been proven to produce a significant reduction in dental decay. Even in

### Table 6.2.   Determination of Supplemental Fluoride Dose

| Patient Age (Years) | Fluoride Ion Concentration In Drinking Water | | |
|---|---|---|---|
| | 0–0.3   ppm | 0.3–0.7   ppm | 0.7   ppm |
| 0.5–1 | 0.25   mg | 0   mg | 0   mg |
| 1–3 | 0.5   mg | 0.25   mg | 0   mg |
| 3–6 | 1.0   mg | 0.5   mg | 0.25   mg |

Source: Data adapted from Picozzi, 1975[4].
Note: ppm = parts per million.

those areas where the drinking water contains the optimal amount of fluoride, the scheduled topical application of fluoride is beneficial to the erupted crowns of individuals who show greater than normal susceptibility to caries.

The dental hygienist or the dentist applies the fluoride ion topically, using either solutions or gels that are commercially available. One of the first obvious differences between the fluoride preparations used as systemic supplements and those used for topical administration is the concentration of fluoride ion. The optimum fluoride ion concentration in drinking water is 1 ppm or 0.001 mg per ml fluoride; the usual 2.2 mg sodium fluoride tablet (as systemic supplement) represents approximately 1 mg of fluoride ion. For topical fluoride application the usual neutral 2% sodium fluoride solution contains approximately 9 mg per ml fluoride ion; the usual 8% stannous fluoride solution contains approximately 19 mg per ml fluoride ion; and the typical acidulated phosphate-fluoride preparations contain approximately 12 mg per ml fluoride ion. It would appear that to reduce dental decay a much higher concentration of fluoride is required for topical administration than is required to produce equivalent results via the systemic route of administration.

Studies have shown that the topical application of 12 mg per ml fluoride ion does not significantly increase fluoride concentration in surface enamel; at least the preapplication levels of enamel fluoride return to the same level in 5 to 8 weeks.[4] It is believed that in addition to fluoride uptake into the apatite crystal there must also be a formation of enamel films of protective insoluble salts such as calcium fluoride.

Sodium fluoride solutions are prepared as 2% aqueous preparations that are relatively stable so that a fresh solution does not need to be made daily. The solution has an agreeable taste, is nonirritating to soft tissue, and does not discolor the teeth or restorative materials. The optimum sodium fluoride concentration to be used topically is unknown. The procedure for application involves first an initial prophylaxis of the clinical crowns, isolation and air-drying of the teeth, and the application of fluoride solution for 3 minutes. The procedure is repeated at one week intervals for a total of four sessions. The complete series is carried out at ages 3, 7, 11, and 13. This technique has resulted in a reduction of 30 to 40% in the incidence of caries.

On the basis of experimental evidence, acidified solutions of sodium fluoride permit a greater uptake of fluoride ion by surface enamel when the fluoride is topically applied. The acid most commonly employed is orthophosphoric acid, and the fluoride ion is derived from both sodium fluoride and hydrofluoric acid. The pH of these solutions and gels is approximately 3. The Council on Dental Therapeutics has accepted 21 such preparations as shown in Table 6.4. As noted, all products are similar, with the major

**Table 6.3. Sodium Fluoride Preparations Accepted by Council on Dental Therapeutics for Dietary Supplementation[a]**

| Name of Manufacturer | Commercial Name of Product | Dosage Form and Strength | Dosage Unit |
|---|---|---|---|
| Fluoritab Corp. | Fluoritab | Liquid: 13 mg/ml | 0.17 ml (4 drops) |
| | | Tablets: 2.21 mg | 1 tablet |
| Kirkman Labs., Inc. | Flura-Drops | Liquid: 13 mg/ml | 0.18 ml (4 drops) |
| | Flura-Loz | Lozenge: 2.21 mg | 1 lozenge |
| | Flura-Tablets | Tablets: 2.21 mg | 1 tablet |
| Lorvic Corp. | Karidium | Liquid: 4.42 mg/ml | 0.5 ml (8 drops) |
| | | Tablets: 2.21 mg | 1 tablet |
| Hoyt Labs. | Luride Drops | Liquid: 0.22 mg/drop | 10 drops |
| | Luride Lozi-Tab | Tablets: 1.1 mg | 1 tablet |
| | | 2.2 mg | 1 tablet |
| Janar Co. | Nufluor Chewable Tablets | Tablets: 2.2 mg | 1 tablet |
| Pacemaker Corp. | Pacemaker Nafeen Solution | Liquid: 4.42 mg/ml | 0.5 ml (8 drops) |
| | Pacemaker Nafeen Tablets | Tablets: 2.2 mg | 1 tablet |
| Professional Pharmaceutical Products | So-Flo Tablets | Tablets: 2.21 mg | 1 tablet |

[a]Each dosage unit is said to deliver at minimum 2.2 mg sodium fluoride which is equivalent to 1 mg of fluoride ion.

## Table 6.4. Acidulated Phosphate-Fluoride Preparations
### Accepted by the Council on Dental Therapeutics for Topical Applications

| Commercial Name of Product | Dosage Form | Sodium Fluoride Concentration (%) | Hydrogen Fluoride Concentration (%) | Total Fluoride Concentration (mg/ml) | Orthophosphoric Acid Concentration (%) |
|---|---|---|---|---|---|
| Cavi-Trol Acidulated Phosphate Fluoride Topical Gel | Gel | 2 | 0.34 | 12.27 | 0.98 |
| Codesco Topical Fluoride Phosphate Anticaries Gel | Gel | 2 | 0.35 | 12.37 | 0.98 |
| Credo Topical Gel | Gel | 2 | 0.35 | 12.37 | 0.98 |
| Credo Topical Solution | Solution | 2 | 0.35 | 12.37 | 0.98 |
| Dental Hygiene Topical Fluoride Gel | Gel | 2.6 | 0.16 | 13.28 | 0.98 |
| Fluorident Liquid | Solution | 2 | 0.34 | 12.27 | 0.98 |
| Fluor-O-Kote Topical Fluoride Gel | Gel | 2 | 0.35 | 12.37 | 0.98 |
| Getz Oxyl Fluoride Gel | Gel | 2 | 0.35 | 12.37 | 0.98 |
| Karidium Phosphate Fluoride Topical Gel | Gel | 1.36 | 0.65 | 12.32 | 0.012 |
| Karidium Phosphate Fluoride Topical Solution | Solution | 2 | 0.34 | 12.27 | 0.98 |
| Kerr Topical Flura-Gel | Gel | 2. | 0.35 | 12.37 | 0.98 |
| Luride Phosphate Topical Gel | Gel | 2 | 0.35 | 12.37 | 1.2 |
| Luride Phosphate Topical Solution | Solution | 2 | 0.34 | 12.27 | 0.98 |

**Table 6.4. Continued**

| Commercial Name of Product | Dosage Form | Sodium Fluoride Concentration (%) | Hydrogen Fluoride Concentration (%) | Total Fluoride Concentration (mg/ml) | Orthophosphoric Acid Concentration (%) |
|---|---|---|---|---|---|
| Pacemaker Topical Fluoride Gel | Gel | 2.6 | 0.16 | 13.28 | 0.98 |
| Pacemaker Topical Fluoride Solution | Solution | 2.6 | 0.16 | 13.28 | 0.98 |
| Predent Topical Fluoride Treatment Gel | Gel | 2.6 | 0.16 | 13.28 | 0.98 |
| Rafluor Topical Gel | Gel | 2 | 0.35 | 12.37 | 1.05 |
| Rafluor Topical Solution | Solution | 2 | 0.34 | 12.27 | 0.98 |
| Rescue Squad Topical Gel | Gel | 2.6 | 0.16 | 13.28 | 0.98 |
| So-flo Phosphate Topical Gel | Gel | 2 | 0.35 | 12.37 | 0.98 |
| So-flo Phosphate Topical Solution | Solution | 2 | 0.34 | 12.27 | 0.98 |

difference being in the flavoring agents used by the manufac-turers. The procedure used involves prophylaxis, isolation and drying of the teeth, and then an application of the solution or the gel for 4 minutes. The single application is repeated at either 6 or 12 month intervals. The solutions and gels are stable when stored in plastic containers, are not irritating to soft tissue, do not discolor the teeth or restorative materials, and possess a slight astringency. The choice of solution or gel is according to the dental hygienist's personal preference. At the present time, the gels are more popular.

Stannous or tin fluoride in an 8%, freshly prepared aqueous solution is the third type of topical fluoride preparation. Although there is no doubt about the ability of stannous fluoride solutions to reduce the incidence of dental decay, there are several major disadvantages of stannous fluoride when compared with either neutral or acidified sodium fluoride preparations. The aqueous solution is not stable, since the stannous fluoride undergoes oxida-tion and hydrolysis which destroy the agent's anticaries activity; therefore, solutions must be made immediately before use. The 8% solution has a disagreeable taste, is quite astringent, produces gingival blanching, and, worst of all, will produce discoloration of teeth, especially those with areas of hypomineralization or carious lesions or around margins of restorations. The discoloration is due to the tin and not to the fluoride. More well-controlled studies are needed in an attempt to define the optimal dose of stannous fluoride to produce the anticaries action. It is possible that several of the stated disadvantages would disappear if a different concen-tration of stannous fluoride were employed.

Fluorides are also applied topically in the form of fluoride-containing prophylactic pastes used by the dental hygienist in cleaning the patient's teeth. Two new pastes are available, and the data accumulated thus far regarding their cariostatic properties are promising. The Council on Dental Therapeutics has not accepted any such preparation at the time of this writing. In no way should the use of a fluoride-containing prophylactic paste replace the use of a topical fluoride solution or gel. It has been demonstrated that a typical prophylaxis will remove a few microns of highly mineralized, fluoride-containing enamel; therefore, if the prophylaxis is not to be followed by topical fluoride application, the prophylaxis paste should contain fluoride.

PATIENT APPLIED FLUORIDE PREPARATIONS. For a number of good reasons it would be desirable to have fluoride preparations available that the patient can use himself; procedures are needed for the individual to employ at home. Since dentifrices are so widely used in the toothbrushing task in a large part of the world, it seems clear that fluoride should be incorporated into such excellent cleaning aids. Thus far the Council on Dental Therapeutics has accepted only two fluoride-containing dentifrices, Colgate with MFP Fluoride and Crest toothpaste. The former includes sodium monofluorophosphate (0.76%) and the latter contains stannous fluoride (0.4%). Both formulations have been clearly shown to reduce the incidence of dental decay when used daily. However, there has not yet been reported a definitive clinical study indicating whether one of these fluoro-dentifrices is superior to the other in anticariogenic activity.

At the present time a number of studies are being conducted to determine the value of fluoride-containing mouth rinses. In these studies the individual rinses his mouth daily with a dilute solution of neutral sodium fluoride, stannous fluoride, or acidulated phosphate-fluoride containing usually 0.02% fluoride ion. Preliminary results appear promising, but dental hygiene will need to await the final outcome.

### REFERENCES

1. Scopp, I.W.: Oral Medicine. 2nd Edition. Saint Louis, Mosby, 1973.
2. Newbrun, E.: Fluorides and Dental Caries. Springfield, Ill., Charles C Thomas, 1975.
3. Moss, S.J. (ed.): Fluorides: an Update for Dental Practice. New York, Medcom, 1976.
4. Picozzi, A., and Smudski, J. (eds.): Pharmacology of Fluorides. Symposium of the Pharmacology, Therapeutics and Toxicology Group, International Association for Dental Research. Atlanta, Georgia. March 21, 1974.
5. Wilkins, E.M.: Clinical Practice of the Dental Hygienist. 4th Edition. Philadelphia, Lea & Fegiber, 1976.
6. Brown, W.E., and Konig, K.G. (eds.): Cariostatic mechanisms of fluorides. Caries Res., 11:Suppl. 1, 1977.
7. Stiles, H.M., Loesche, W.J., and O'Brien, T.C. (eds.): Microbial Aspects of Dental Caries. Vol. 1-3. Washington, D.C., Information Retrieval, 1976.
8. Christensen, H.E. (ed.): The Toxic Substances List. 1973 Edition. Rockville, Maryland, U.S. Department of Health, Education and Welfare, 1973.

### SUPPLEMENTARY REFERENCES

Smith, Frank A. (ed.): Pharmacology of Fluorides. Handb. exp. Pharmak., Vol. 20/1 and 20/2. Berlin, Springer-Verlag, 1966.

# 7

## DESENSITIZING AGENTS

The drugs to be described in this chapter are unique to dentistry; they are one group of the dental specialty agents used by the dental hygienist. These drugs may be individually classified pharmacologically in a number of groups, but for our purposes they are known, correctly or incorrectly, throughout dental hygiene as desensitizing agents. Immediately the dental hygienist must understand that in medical and allergy circles, a desensitizing agent is one that produces a condition whereby the body no longer responds immunologically to a specific antigen. Of course, this is not the meaning given to a desensitizing agent in dentistry. Furthermore, to add to the confusion, a desensitizing agent in dentistry is said to be useful in treating hypersensitive teeth or, more specifically, hypersensitive dentin. Hypersensitivity also has a specific meaning in an immunological sense and should not be used to refer to the sensitivity of dentin to pain, heat, cold, and sweet substances; however, another name for the condition in which desensitizing agents are useful in dentistry does not exist in the dental literature. The condition, in reality, is best described as dentinal hyperalgesia, which may be further defined as the extreme sensibility or reactivity of the tooth to painful stimuli.

### DENTINAL HYPERALGESIA

The abnormal condition of tooth or dental hyperalgesia occurs when the vital dentin is exposed to the environment of the oral cavity. The oral cavity contains, continuously or periodically, a number of substances that qualify as adequate stimuli. The late periodontist, Professor Frank Everett, classified the various types of stimuli that produce this painful state.[1] Various mechanical stimuli from the dental instruments, toothbrushes, or oral habits (e.g., pipe smoking) are well known to produce such pain. Thermal stimuli, either hot or cold, will lead to pain. Chemical stimuli include either sweet or sour as well as food debris.

The primary tissue lesion of exposed vital dentin can occur in a number of ways. For instance, root surfaces may be exposed during periodontal instrumentation; dentin may be exposed under a crown preparation or under the restorative material filling a cavity. Even the best of restorative materials may allow marginal leakage and thereby painful stimuli to reach the dentin. Lastly, it is estimated that in approximately 10% of teeth no naturally occurring cementum covers the cervical portion of the root surface; the dentin is exposed.

It must be strongly emphasized that the proper, faithful procedures of normal oral hygiene go a long way in preventing the occurrence of this very discomforting situation.

Once the primary lesion is identified, then consideration can be given as to how the condition may be treated most effectively. There are a number of ways to relieve the pain. It can be masked by a variety of drugs, but the rational approach has always been to eliminate the cause of the pain. In the case of dentinal hyperalgesia the cause of pain is the abnormal exposure of vital dentin to the irritating oral environment. The treatment of choice would be, therefore, to reestablish an effective separation between the vital dentin and the oral cavity.

In accordance with the best of pharmacological principles and a knowledge of what a drug must do, then a desensitizing agent may be defined as a chemical or mixture of chemical substances which, when applied topically to the exposed dentin by the proper technique, causes the exposed dentinal tubules to be sealed. The effective sealing then prevents the irritants from inducing pain.

## CHARACTERISTICS OF PREPARATIONS

Over the last century dentists have introduced a countless number of empirical items that can be classified as desensitizing agents. When these substances are examined closely in terms of how they seal the exposed dentin, the following mechanisms emerge: (1) the denaturing of the superficial protein of the exposed dentinal tubular tissue to form the required barrier; (2) the depositing or precipitating of water-insoluble substances either on or in the exposed dentinal tubules; (3) the stimulation of the underlying odontoblasts to form secondary dentin (the natural barrier); and (4) a mechanism that does not involve the sealing of the dentinal tubules, but some action upon pulpal tissue to prevent its typical response to pain-producing irritants. With this background in mind a selected number of desensitizing agents in use today is presented. Remember that the procedure for the use of any desensitizing agent first requires that the exposed surface to which the drug is applied be clean (of debris and especially fatty material) and dry. How the exposed surface is cleaned and dried cannot but add to the condition's major symptom, pain.

FORMALIN, 40%. Formalin, 40%, is a saturated aqueous solution of formaldehyde gas. This preparation has been used with some reported success to desensitize exposed root surfaces. It is believed to act by a prompt denaturation or fixation of the protein with which it comes in contact. Formalin, 40%, certainly possesses at least these obvious disadvantages: a disagreeable odor and extreme irritation to all soft tissue to the extent of the production of a painful chemical burn wherever it touches the alveolar mucosa. Most clinical studies on formalin are old and testimonal in type. There are toothpastes available for home use which contain 1.4% formaldehyde as the desensitizing agent (e.g., Thermodent), but the effectiveness of such a preparation is still to be proven.

SILVER NITRATE SOLUTION, 10%. A 10% aqueous solution of silver nitrate or a 28% aqueous solution of silver ammonium nitrate has enjoyed some popularity in the past. The silver nitrate solution is first applied to the exposed dentin; then a solution containing a reducing agent such as sodium thiosulfate is applied with the resulting precipitation of insoluble elemental silver in the dentinal tubules. Silver nitrate has the disadvantages of not only being very caustic to soft tissue but also discolors practically everything it touches. It has been used most often on full crown preparations in an attempt to seal the exposed dentin. It was because of silver nitrate's discoloring properties that a zinc chloride and potassium ferrocyanide preparation was introduced.

ZINC CHLORIDE AND POTASSIUM FERROCYANIDE COMBINATION. Gottlieb's impregnation technique involves first the application of a 40% aqueous solution of zinc chloride to the exposed dentinal surface. This procedure produces some protein precipitation in the tubules. The zinc chloride solution must be kept away from the gingival margins. Then an aqueous 20% solution of potassium ferrocyanide is applied by rubbing to the same exposed surface. As the rubbing continues a white, curdlike, insoluble precipitation of zinc ferrocyanide seals the dentinal tubules. The entire procedure may be repeated a number of times. The Gottlieb technique has been used both on cavity preparations and on exposed root surfaces but is not too frequently employed today.

FLUORIDE DESENSITIZING PREPARATIONS. All fluoride-containing preparations are stored in plastic bottles. The oldest and still one of the most widely used fluoride preparations is Lukomsky's paste which consists of one-third sodium fluoride, one-third kaolin (hydrated aluminum silicate), and one-third glycerin. The combination makes a stiff, claylike paste which is rubbed into the exposed root surface with a porte-polisher, orangewood stick, or rubber cap for 1 to 5 minutes. Satisfactory results are claimed by both dentists and dental hygienists after several treatment sessions. There are no caustic effects on the gingiva or mucosa from contact with the paste. Remember that the paste contains 33.3% sodium fluoride and the patient should not be allowed to swallow the paste.

Another fluoride preparation consists of a saturated aqueous solution of sodium silicofluoride (approxmiately 0.7%) which is applied to the exposed dentinal surfaces. It is assumed that water-insoluble calcium fluoride forms in addition to a gel of silicic acid and calcium from the tooth. A modifiction of this procedure allows the sodium silicofluoride to stay in contact with the exposed surface for only 1 to 2 minutes; then the supernatant of a 5% aqueous suspension of calcium hydroxide is applied for a period of 1 minute. This modification allows for some (or it is hoped most) of the calcium ions to be supplied from the suspension and not from the tooth.

The sodium monofluorophosphate (0.76%) dentifrice has been shown clinically to possess desensitizing action when used regularly,[2] and it is presumed to be acting by precipitating calcium fluoride in the dentinal tubules.

The last fluoride preparation consists of a 1 or 2% aqueous solution of sodium fluoride, but a direct electric current (iontophoresis) is used to transport fluoride anions into the dentinal tubules. The exact mechanism of the iontophoretic application of fluoride is not known. It may involve a number of mechanisms. The procedure is currently one of the most popular, and it is being examined clinically and critically by Gangarosa.[3] The exact procedure to be used may be found in dental hygiene manuals.[4]

CORTICOSTEROID PREPARATIONS. The topical application of a number of commercially available corticosteroid preparations has had its consistent small group of supporters for almost 20 years. H.R. Stanley carried out extensive studies on the use of such agents, but the mechanism of action is still not clear.[5] Because the dentinal tubules would not seem to be sealed and the corticosteroid depresses secondary dentin formation, further research is necessary to elucidate a possible mechanism. The topical corticosteroid preparations are not recommended as desensitizing agents in dental hygiene.

## NONTREATABLE DENTINAL HYPERALGESIA

Lastly, it should be remembered that dentinal hyperalgesia may be due to (1) microscopic cracks in the tooth (or teeth), (2) exposed accessory root canals in the coronal part of the root, (3) occlusal trauma, or (4) long-term use of one of the oxygen-liberating agents for oral hygiene (surface decalcification). Any of these causes may be nontreatable.

## REFERENCES

1. Everett, F.G., Hall, W.B., and Phatak, N.M.: Treatment of hypersensitive dentin. J. Oral Thera. Pharm., 2:300, 1966.
2. Kanouse, M.C., and Ash, M.M.: The effectiveness of a sodium monofluorophosphate dentifrice on dental hypersensitivity. J. Peridontol., 40:38, 1969.
3. Gangarosa, L.: Personal communication.
4. Wilkins, E.M.: Clinical Practice of the Dental Hygienist. 4th Edition. Philadelphia, Lea & Febiger, 1976.
5. Kakehashi, S., Stanley, H.R., and Fitzgerald, R.: The exposed germ-free pulp: effects of topical corticosteroid medication and restoration. Oral Surg., 27:60, 1969.

PART **///**

# DRUGS USED BY THE DENTIST

# 8

## ANALGESICS

The drugs to be considered in this chapter have as their most important property the ability to relieve or obtund pain without producing a concomitant loss of consciousness or loss of any other modality of sensation. These agents are referred to as analgesics. They differ in chemical structure, in the kinds of pain they relieve, in potency, and in their ability to produce pharmacological effects other than analgesia. Some analgesics are so widely used that they are found in almost every family medicine cabinet; some analgesics are so widely misused that their handling must be supervised by federal law. These are the drugs that make the painfully diseased able to bear their suffering; these are the drugs that give those who are so inclined their escape from reality.

This large and important class of drugs has many facets. It is the purpose of this chapter on nonnarcotic and narcotic analgesics to clarify the actions and effects of these agents so that the rational basis for their therapeutic use in clinical practice is understood. The first task will be to review briefly some of the physiological mechanisms involved in analgesia and then consider some of the general principles of drug action involved in analgesia.

### THE PAIN EXPERIENCE

First, it is known that the pain experience includes several parts: (1) an initial stimulus, (2) the perception of the painful stimulus, and (3) the reactions to that painful stimulus. The reactions may be physical reactions or emotional reactions.[1] Secondly, it is known there are two general varieties of pain; each type appears to use different neuroanatomical pathways as shown schematically in Figure 8.1.[2,3]

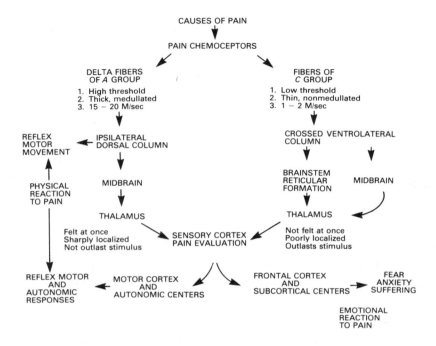

**Figure 8.1** The pain pathways. (Adapted and redrawn from Randall 1963.[3])

Integumental or cutaneous pain is characteristically bright or sharp, is felt at once, and is easily localized as to its origin. The afferent pathway carrying such a message includes mainly the large, myelinated, rapidly transmitting A fibers. The impulses do not outlast the painful stimulus. This type of pain may be considered as exciting (or at least provoking), and the individual prepares for fight or flight. You would experience this type of pain and utilize this particular pathway when the person sitting next to you stabs you with a sharp pin.

On the other hand, visceral pain is characteristically dull and aching, is not felt at once, and is not easy to localize as to its origin. The afferent pathway in this case includes mainly small, nonmyelinated, slowly transmitting C fibers. Impulses may long outlast the stimulus. The individual becomes immobile, depressed, very anxious, and usually nauseated and does not want to eat. One could experience such visceral pain several moments after being stabbed with the sharp pin when the entire arm begins to ache, or as a result of a spasm of the sphincter of Oddi.

The purpose in drawing attention to the two general varieties of pain is the fact that different analgesics are useful in treating or relieving the two different varieties.

## RATIONALE FOR PHARMACOTHERAPY OF PAIN

Where could or do drugs act in the scheme of the pain experience as depicted in Figure 8.1? Drugs are known to act at one or more sites in the pain pathways.

Drugs may eliminate the immediate cause of pain. If the immediate cause of pain is known, it would be rational to eliminate that cause if possible. Some drugs are used specifically in this way. In the acute attack of angina pectoris the patient experiences a severe, crushing pain in the chest which lasts several minutes. One of the most effective analgesics in this situation is nitroglycerin, which promptly relieves the pain. Although the exact mechanism of action of nitroglycerin is not known, rarely is nitroglycerin referred to as an analgesic.[4] Another example would be the patient who experiences an acute attack of glaucoma when there is a slight interference with the rate of drainage of fluid from the anterior chamber. The administration of pilocarpine contracts the sphincter muscle of the iris, which in turn opens the drainage canals, lowers the elevated intraocular pressure, and eliminates the pain.[5] Rarely is pilocarpine referred to, however, as an analgesic.

Drugs may interfere with the sensitivity of the pain chemoceptors. A drug could certainly produce analgesia if it could depress the sensitivity of the peripheral pain chemoceptors. Lim has shown these receptors to be sensitive to a number of the proposed naturally occurring pain-producing substances such as bradykinin.[6]

Drugs may block the afferent pain pathways. A drug would produce analgesia if it blocked the nerve fibers involved in transmitting the afferent pain impulses. An example of such a drug would be a local anesthetic.

Drugs may inhibit the cortical interpretation of pain. A drug could produce analgesia if it were able to depress the cortical mechanisms involved in perceiving the incoming impulses as painful.

Drugs may inhibit the reactions to pain. It is conceivable that drugs would produce an analgesic effect if they could block the emotional reaction to pain, i.e., the fear involved in the anticipation of pain. Autonomic agents that would block the reflex physiological reactions to pain would not serve as analgesics; nor would skeletal muscle relaxants that prevented physical or motor reactions to pain serve as effective analgesics.

## PHARMACOLOGICAL CLASSIFICATION

The analgesics are classified pharmacologically in a number of ways, but perhaps the simplest is as follows: (1) mild analgesics, whose standard is aspirin; (2) moderate analgesics, whose standard is codeine; and (3) strong analgesics, whose standard is morphine. A drug is placed into one of these groups in accordance with the agent's ceiling analgesic effect.

Another classification that requires some recognition is the older, less accurate grouping as nonnarcotic and narcotic analgesics. A drug is placed in one of these two categories depending upon how well it fits the established characteristics of the two groups.

Nonnarcotic analgesics are effective in relieving the integumental type of pain from a chemical stimulation or an inflammation (rheumatic pain, headaches of vascular or muscular origin, muscle pain, and the variety of "algias"). Pain relief occurs without cortical depression. The general site of analgesic action is considered to be a combination of blocking pain pathways centrally and blocking the pain chemoceptors located in the peripheral, local tissues. No serious drug dependence occurs with any nonnarcotic analgesic.

In contrast, narcotic analgesics are most effective in relieving the visceral type of pain (as experienced in myocardial infarction, crushed bone, and some forms of terminal cancer). Pain relief occurs usually with some degree of cortical depression. The general site of analgesic action is considered to be only central, i.e., within the central nervous system. Lastly, it is well known that a serious level of drug dependence can occur with a narcotic analgesic.

## THE CEILING CONCEPT

It has been found both experimentally and clinically that there is a certain dose or amount of an analgesic above which no further analgesia is obtained from the drug alone.[7] In other words, there is a dose for each analgesic which produces a maximum pain-relieving effect. For example, in an individual, 300 mg of aspirin will relieve a certain amount of pain; 600 mg will relieve more pain, but 1,000 mg will not relieve more than 600 mg, nor will 2,000 mg of aspirin. Thus, if 600 mg of aspirin, given at the appropriate time intervals, will not relieve the particular pain involved, then there is no rational basis for increasing the dose. This dose, approximately 600 mg for aspirin, is referred to as the drug's oral ceiling analgesic dose. There are also ceiling analgesic doses for all other mild and moderate analgesics; e.g., codeine's oral ceiling analgesic dose is approximately 60 mg. Until recently it was not thought that the strong narcotic analgesics had ceiling doses, but, in man at least, well-controlled clinical studies have shown that morphine has an oral ceiling analgesic dose of approximately 10 mg and meperidine has an oral ceiling analgesic dose of approximately 50 mg.[8] The ceiling effect is illustrated in Figure 8.2.

It must be clearly understood that the actual mg dosage used for an analgesic has nothing whatever to do with whether the drug is classified as a mild, moderate, or strong analgesic. In other words, aspirin (regardless of the dose) can never be the strong analgesic morphine is, nor is codeine capable of relieving the severity of pain that a strong analgesic can. Figure 8.3 summarizes this concept. An analgesic is placed in the mild, moderate, or strong category depending upon the degree of clinical or pathological pain it can relieve when the drug is given at its ceiling analgesic dose. Expressed another way, the maximum amount of pain which an analgesic can relieve when given in its ceiling analgesic dose is referred to as the drug's ceiling analgesic effect.

Previously it was pointed out that there were different types of pain, those of different severity, arising from different sites in the body or from different painful stimuli. Depicted in Figure 8.3 are three different pain-inducing situations: A, B, and C. Each induces a different severity of clinical pain. From this simple diagram, it can be perceived that some pain-inducing situations (e.g., situation A)

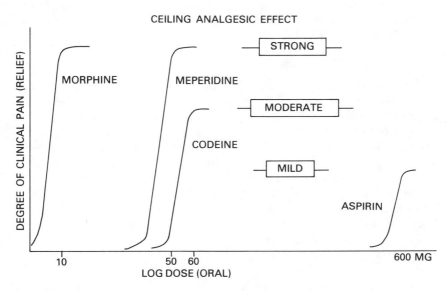

**Figure 8.2** Ceiling analgesic effect. See text for further details.

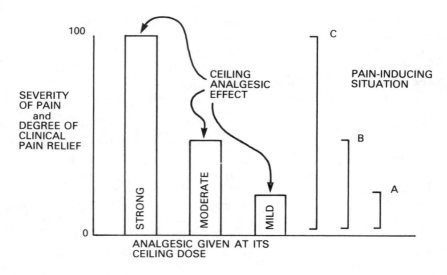

**Figure 8.3** The ceiling concept. See text for further details.

can be relieved by a mild analgesic alone. Needless to say, a moderate or strong analgesic would also relieve this same pain. Likewise there are some pain-inducing situations that only a strong analgesic can relieve. It is hoped that the dental hygienist will grow to understand why it is necessary to start with the mild analgesic and work up to the strong analgesic when it is not possible to identify the cause of the patient's pain.

## MILD ANALGESICS

The mild analgesics are also traditionally referred to as the analgesic-antipyretics or the nonnarcotic analgesics. Of the three drug class titles, certainly that of mild analgesics comes closest to the truth, i.e., all agents in this group are mild analgesics, not all possess both analgesic and antipyretic effects, and some may even possess narcotic properties if administered in the proper dose and under certain conditions. Although a number of different chemical classes of drugs are analgesic-antipyretics, there can be little doubt that the salicylates are by far the most important. If for no other reason, the salicylates are ingested in enormous amounts by Americans as shown in Table 8.1.

### Salicylates

The family of salicylate drugs includes in actuality few different chemical compounds. The chemical structures of the major salicylates are shown in Figure 8.4.

Salicylic acid (orthohydroxybenzoic acid) is the active form of the salicylates in the body. However, salicylic acid itself is never administered internally because it is extremely irritating. The drug is found in external preparations and is used for its keratolytic effect, i.e., it produces sloughing of the skin (e.g., in the removal of corns or warts).

Methyl salicylate, the methyl ester of salicylic acid, also known as Oil of Wintergreen, possesses the irritating properties of salicylic acid and is, therefore, used externally as a counterirritant, i.e., an agent which when applied locally increases the flow of blood through a limited area of the skin. Methyl salicylate is a popular flavoring agent and is used in small amounts as a pharmaceutical aid. It must not be overlooked that methyl salicylate is a toxic substance. Children who have been drawn to methyl salicylate by its pleasant characteristic odor have swallowed as little as one teaspoonful and died.[9] Methyl salicylate is so rapidly absorbed through the intact skin that within 5 minutes after its application, salicylate may be found in the urine.

Sodium salicylate, salicylamide, and especially acetylsalicylic acid or aspirin are all used for their systemic salicylate action.

The mild analgesics, as so well exemplified by acetylsalicylic acid, are not just weak analgesics, for they have other useful pharmacotherapeutic applications which cannot be overlooked. Aspirin produces no less than four distinguishable pharmacological effects. Besides its ability to obtund certain types of low intensity pain, aspirin is well known for its ability to lower an elevated body temperature (antipyretic effect), to suppress the inflammatory reaction (antiinflammatory effect), and to increase the renal elimination of uric acid (uricosuric effect).

**Table 8.1    Aspirin Consumption in the United States, 1973**

Estimated 35 million pounds

OR

17,500 tons

OR

15,900,000 kilograms

OR

in terms of 5 grain tablets (300 mg each)

53,000,000,000 tablets

OR

approximately 250 tablets for every citizen

SALICYLATE FAMILY

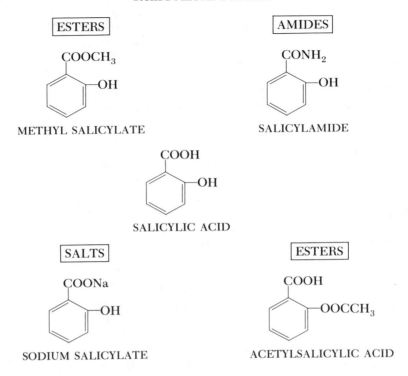

Figure 8.4   Chemical structures for members of salicylate family.

ANTIPYRETIC EFFECT. The antipyretic effect of aspirin results from an action of the drug at the hypothalamic level.[10] Aspirin produces increased heat loss in the fevered individual; it does not lower a normal body temperature.

Since the advent of the antibiotics, some may say there is little rationale for the continued use of drugs that only reduce the elevated body temperature without eliminating the cause of the fever. However, until antibiotics can lower a fever as quickly as aspirin, this drug will be used until the infecting, fever-producing organisms are controlled.

The regulation of the body's temperature occurs through a delicately balanced mechanism located in two regions of the hypothalamus.[11] The anterior region acts as a center for heat elimination, and the posterior region as a center for heat conservation. Thermodetectors located in the skin for external temperature sensing and others located in the hypothalamus for internal blood temperature sensing continuously send a flow of impulses to the centers for the initiation of the necessary changes. On the one hand, the skeletal muscle metabolic machinery stands ready to shiver to create heat when the temperature needs to be raised; on the other, the cutaneous vasculature and sweat glands stand ready to promote heat elimination when the temperature needs lowering. The hypothalamic centers act much like a thermostat. When a bacterial toxin is present, it has the ability, the mechanism as yet unknown, to set up the thermostat 3 to 4 degrees. The body's immediate response via its thermodetectors is that the body is 3 to 4 degrees too cold. The normal physiological machinery is called upon to increase heat production (shivering or cold chills). When temperature reaches the new setting, it is maintained as in health.

The salicylates have the ability to act directly upon the hypothalamic thermostat mechanism and reset it down to the normal body temperature but not lower. The body responds to the drug just as though it found itself 3 to 4 degrees too warm and proceeds to use its peripheral machinery to eliminate the excess heat. The cutaneous vessels dilate and cutaneous blood flow increases; there is a shift of water from the tissues into the circulation with hemodilution or an increase in blood volume and an outpour of sweat; the temperature falls rapidly. Salicylates act to increase heat elimination. As the effective concentration of the drug dissipates, the temperature begins to rise again. Aspirin lowers a slight fever much more rapidly than a high fever. The site of action for the antipyretic effect is definitely central.

ANALGESIC EFFECT. The remarkable mild analgesic activity of the salicylates, such as aspirin, was an enigma (and embarrassment) to pharmacologists for many years until less than a decade ago. It was thought that, because the antipyretic action of aspirin was so clearly occurring at the hypothalamic level, the analgesic action (it was assumed) must be blocking the afferent pain pathways at the thalamic level. It is difficult to demonstrate, however, that aspirin will elevate an animal's pain reaction threshold much higher than the 35 to 40% that can be equalled by sleep or a placebo.[7]

It was through the keen observations of Professor Lim and his colleagues that everyone realized that the salicylates were clinically predictable in relieving low intensity integumental pain, the well known "algias" such as myalgia, neuralgia, arthralgia, or cephalalgia. The salicylates are useless in relieving visceral pain. What the "algias" have in common is a disturbed tissue fluid component; localized edema is usually involved. Moreover, Lim well appreciated aspirin's antiinflammatory effect which includes a reduction in edema. It was first hypothesized, then proven in the laboratory, that aspirin's analgesic action was only partly central but that the larger part of the analgesic action took place at the local tissue level. Lim proceeded to identify the peripheral pain chemoceptors and showed conclusively that aspirin and the other mild analgesics have the ability to block the pain produced by a large number of the proposed pain mediators such as bradykinin.[12] Although much more is involved in aspirin's antiinflammatory effects, the compound's ability to inhibit or alter the firing of the afferent pain pathway at the local tissue chemoceptor level is a large part.

The ceiling analgesic dose orally for aspirin in man is approximately 600 mg every 4 hours. This is also the antipyretic dosage for adults. The antiinflammatory and uricosuric effects require a much larger dose orally or as much as 5 to 8 gm per day. With these higher doses, aspirin's side effects or early toxic effects are easily seen. At these levels salicylates begin to show their deadly effect upon the respiratory and electrolyte systems of man.

EFFECTS ON RESPIRATION AND ELECTROLYTE BALANCE. There is no better way to understand the effects of aspirin upon the respiration and on the electrolyte balance of the body than to be able to describe succinctly the sequence of events, which are so predictable, so rapid, and often so tragic, as they occur when a small child has ingested a toxic dose of aspirin.[9] These events are presented in the form of a flow sheet in Figure 8.5.

Salicylate ion directly stimulates the respiratory center itself. It does so in close correspondence with the blood salicylate level. The initial hyperpnea is seen as a rate increase.

Almost simultaneously, salicylates proceed to uncouple oxidative phosphorylation which leads immediately to an increase in both tissue oxygen consumption and carbon dioxide production. The increased carbon dioxide, also a well-known respiratory stimulant, adds to the breathing rate increase directly induced by the salicylate by augmenting the depth of respiration. The hyperventilation keeps just ahead of the rate of carbon dioxide production, and acidosis does not develop. Indeed, sufficient carbon dioxide is blown off so that the first clinical manifestation is respiratory alkalosis. Immediately the kidney is brought into action to excrete the excess amount of bicarbonate and fixed base cations, sodium and potasssium, in order to compensate for the alkalosis. Compensation is successful but at the cost of a greatly lowered blood buffer capacity.

As the hyperventilation persists with uncoupled oxidative phosphorylation, carbohydrate metabolism shifts to the glycolytic pathways and an increase in the circulating blood levels of lactic and

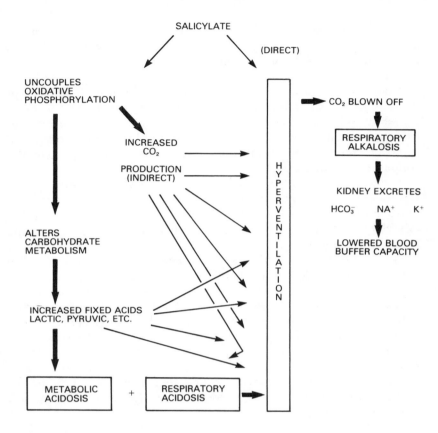

**Figure 8.5** Flow chart of salicylate-induced respiratory, metabolic, and electrolyte changes produced in man. See text for further details.

pyruvic acids which establishes metabolic acidosis. The carbon dioxide production begins to far outstrip the hyperpnea's ability to blow off carbon dioxide, and respiratory acidosis adds to the metabolic acidosis.

The child is usually first brought to the hospital in extremely acute acidosis and still severe hyperventilation. Unfortunately, it is often too late, and before much can be done the child suddenly ceases to breathe. Although such procedures as maintaining the child on prolonged artificial respiration and transfusing with whole blood are carried out, the fatigued respiratory center may not respond with an automatic rhytim and the child dies.

It is imperative that whenever a child shows hyperventilation he should be immediately taken to the hospital where intravenous infusions of the proper electrolyte and buffer systems can be started and blood tests for the salicylate level can be determined. It is critical to halt the hyperventilation by lowering of the salicylate blood level before the respiratory center fails.

The entire respiratory-electrolyte process described can take as little as 40 to 50 minutes between the time the drug has been ingested and death, depending upon the total dose absorbed and the general state of the child's health. Federal law now requires all aspirin to be sold in "childproof" containers. Table 8.2 shows the commercial availability of the toxic dose of aspirin.

EFFECTS ON CARDIOVASCULAR SYSTEM. Salicylates produce no significant effects upon the cardiovascular system when administered in therapeutic doses. However, it might be remembered that salicylates can increase the circulating blood volume in patients with an elevated body temperature.

EFFECTS ON GASTROINTESTINAL TRACT. As every television viewer knows, "Aspirin can upset your stomach." That is a true statement. Without question, the salicylates produce irritation of the gastric mucosa in therapeutic doses; and, upon chronic administration, salicylates have been shown to cause extensive ulceration in man. Any agent that causes gastric irritation may be expected to produce nausea and vomiting as well. In addition to stimulating the gastric reflexogenic zones to produce vomiting, the salicylates also stimulate the chemoreceptive trigger zone on the floor of the fourth ventricle to produce reflex, projectile vomiting when high blood levels are achieved.[13]

EFFECTS ON RENAL SYSTEM. The salicylates produce their uricosuric effects by their action upon the kidney. Their ability to increase the urinary excretion of uric acid is the basis for the therapeutic use of aspirin in the treatment of gouty arthritis.

In the metabolic disorder known as gout, there is a large increase in the body's production of uric acid, the normal end product of purine metabolism in man. The disease manifests itself as an arthritis due to the deposit of monosodium urate crystals in the joints. These deposits are known as tophi. Gout may take the form of an acute attack with a rapidly developed and severe synovitis or of a chronic ailment with periodic attacks. The salicylate uricosuric agents are far more effective in the treatment of chronic gout.

The salicylates can increase uric acid renal clearance by 100%. All available evidence indicates that the salicylates have a double effect on the kidneys' ability to handle uric acid (see Figure 8.6). When no salicylate is present, uric acid is filtered by the glomerulus, completely reabsorbed in the proximal convoluted tubules, and then actively secreted by the distal renal tubular cells

## Table 8.2. Commercial Availability
## of Acute Toxic Dose Acetylsalicylic Acid (aspirin)

Approximate Oral Toxic Dose (Man) = 20 gm per 150-pound adult
or about
130 mg per pound of body weight

| Adult Aspirin Tablets | Flavored Baby Aspirin Tablets |
|---|---|
| 100 tablets per bottle | 36 tablets per bottle |
| 5 grains or 325 mg per tablet | 1¼ grains or 81 mg per tablet |
| 32.5 grams of aspirin total | 2.9 grams of aspirin total |
| 62 tablets kill 150 pound adult | 36 tablets kill 22-pound child |
| 9 tablets kill 22-pound child | |

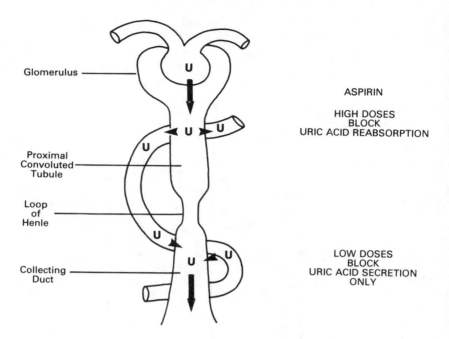

**Figure 8.6**   Effect of aspirin in low and high doses on renal excretion of uric acid (U).

into the urine. In low doses commonly used for mild analgesia, aspirin blocks the distal tubular secretion of uric acid, resulting in an increase in plasma uric acid levels.[14] For this reason, small doses of aspirin are absolutely contraindicated in the patient with a history of gout. However, in doses of 5 to 8 gm of aspirin per day, the drug not only blocks the distal secretion of uric acid, but also blocks the proximal reabsorption of uric acid. Thereby, aspirin can rid the plasma of uric acid and is most widely used in the treatment of chronic gout. The salicylates, in analgesic amounts, completely antagonize the uricosuric effects of the drug, probenecid (Benemid).

EFFECTS ON BLOOD. The salicylates alter the blood clotting mechanism. In therapeutic dosage levels, aspirin has been shown to interfere with the normal aggregation of platelets at the site of bleeding for as long as 7 days.[15] The salicylates are also known to produce hypoprothrombinemia. This effect occurs when large amounts of aspirin are taken over several days or when usual doses are taken regularly every day. Aspirin's action appears to resemble closely that of the coumarin anticoagulants in that aspirin prolongs prothrombin time by inhibiting prothrombin's biosynthesis in the liver (as well as factors VII, IX, and X). The anticoagulant effect can be reversed by the administration of vitamin K preparations.

An important and practical application to clinical dentistry and dental hygiene exists. The usual dental patient who seeks your services only when pain has gone on for some time may be expected to have taken a large amount of aspirin in the previous several days and is likely still to be taking aspirin. The patient should be expected to have a prolonged prothrombin time, and the practitioner must be prepared for prompt and effective control of local bleeding.

Another factor regarding aspirin and the blood must be remembered. Well-controlled studies in man show that when 3 gm aspirin are taken orally a day, 70% of the users lose an average of 2 to 6 ml of blood daily by way of the gastrointestinal tract.[13] In most instances, this degree of blood loss is insignificant, but over a prolonged period and with additional blood losses for other reasons, this side effect can become highly significant. It is now well confirmed that the mechanism of gastrointestinal bleeding is a result of the local irritating effects of particles of undissolved aspirin upon the gastric mucosa. These same undissolved aspirin particles no doubt play a role in the ulcerogenic effect of aspirin.

ABSORPTION FOLLOWING ORAL ADMINISTRATION. Aspirin is only taken orally. If the tablet disintegrates properly and dissolves in the gastric juice and if the stomach is empty, rapid absorption across the gastric mucosa could take place. Aspirin is a weak organic acid with a $pK_a$ of about 3.5. Aspirin is also rather insoluble in aqueous, acid solutions. The surface pH of the gastric mucosa (empty) is commonly found to be about 2. The aspirin is over 97% nonionized and in an absorbable form at this more acidic pH, but the drug comes out of soluiton as it is in the process of being absorbed. These undissolved aspirin particles irritate. Although at the duodenal pH the aspirin would be much more in the ionized form and thus less readily absorbed, the drug does stay in solution and is absorbed mainly from the duodenum owing no doubt to the enormous absorptive surface available (compared to that of the gastric mucosa).[16]

DISTRIBUTION. Once the aspirin is absorbed into the circulation, it is almost completely ionized as acetylsalicylate anion at blood pH of 7.3. There is little doubt that the acetylsalicylate exerts some of the analgesic-antipyretic effects, but because of the rather rapid hydrolysis of acetylsalicylate by esterases to acetate and salicylate, the salicylate ion also is active. This anion is highly bound to plasma albumin (up to 85%) and is known to displace several commonly used drugs from the plasma protein binding site.[9]

BIOTRANSFORMATION AND EXCRETION. Salicylate that is free in the circulation is filtered by the glomerulus, and its fate thereafter depends upon the pH of the urine that is being formed by the renal tubular cells. In the usual acidic urine that results from our American diets, practically all of the salicylate is reabsorbed passively across the proximal convoluted tubular cells. After being biotransformed to salicyluric acid and salicyl-glucuronide in the liver, salicylate is secreted along with its metabolites by the distal renal tubular cells (see Figure 8.7).

If the urine being formed is alkaline, e.g., pH 8, which can be fairly easily accomplished by ingesting sodium bicarbonate, then the fate of filtered salicylate is different. Under these conditions, there is so much more salicylate in the anion form that it is not significantly reabsorbed from the proximal renal lumen and it passes on into the bladder. The alkalinization of the urine is a critical part of the emergency treatment of salicylate acute poisoning, since the plasma drug level can be lowered quite quickly once the proximal tubular urine is alkaline.[17]

### Nonsalicylates

The other chemical classes of mild analgesics offer little if any advantage over aspirin as an analgesic-antipyretic. Therefore, the

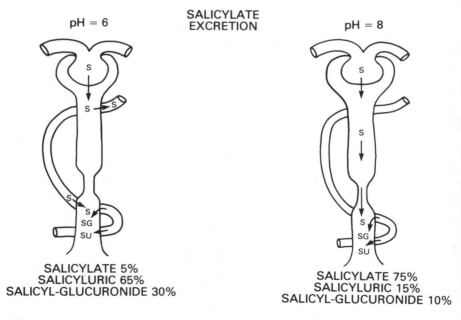

SALICYLATE EXCRETION

pH = 6

pH = 8

SALICYLATE 5%
SALICYLURIC 65%
SALICYL-GLUCURONIDE 30%

SALICYLATE 75%
SALICYLURIC 15%
SALICYL-GLUCURONIDE 10%

**Figure 8.7** Salicylate (S) excretion at pH 6 (shown on left) and at pH 8 (shown on right).

majority of these nonsalicylate mild analgesics are used clinically as a substitute for aspirin when the patient is known to be hypersensitive to salicylates or when aspirin is otherwise contraindicated or simply when a patient finds salicylate side effects too distressing. For an excellent review of these mild analgesics the reader is referred to the article by Beaver.[18]

PARAAMINOPHENOL DERIVATIVES. Both acetanilid and phenacetin (acetophenetidin) are biotransformed in the body to N-acetyl-p-aminophenol or acetaminophen, the active drug (see Figure 8.8). The metabolite, acetaminophen, is the drug of choice of the three, because both acetanilid and phenacetin are also converted in part to substances that cause methemoglobinemia. Acetaminophen (Tylenol) does not cause methemoglobinemia. Acetaminophen shares aspirin's mild analgesic and antipyretic properties at the same oral ceiling analgesic dose (approximately 600 mg), but differs in a number of ways from aspirin. Acetaminophen does not produce gastrointestinal ulcerations, nor does it possess antiinflammatory (antirheumatic) or uricosuric effects, nor does it produce an anticoagulant effect. There is no question in the minds of a growing number of clinicians that acetaminophen should perhaps be used as the first choice mild analgesic-antipyretic instead of aspirin. This is based more upon what acetaminophen does not do (when compared with aspirin) rather than upon what acetaminophen can do better than aspirin. Today the use of phenacetin has little justification, since it is converted to acetaminophen in the body and since its chronic use has been linked to the development of renal papillary necrosis.[19]

PYRAZOLON DERIVATIVES. A number of pyrazolon derivatives have come and gone over the years, and most of them have possessed to varying degrees the majority of the four major therapeutically useful effects of aspirin. Unfortunately, the pyrazolon agent's toxicity has eventually precluded its usefulness. These drugs may cause fatal agranulocytosis and, what is worse, they do so unrelated to the dose. Nonetheless, there are several pyrazolon derivatives still available, e.g., phenylbutazone (Butazolidin) and its active metabolite oxyphenbutazone (Tandearil). These two drugs are used primarily for their antiinflammatory and uricosuric effects and must not be considered as routine mild analgesics.

ANTHRANILIC ACID DERIVATIVES. The prototype for this newer class of nonsalicylate mild analgesics is the drug mefenamic acid (Ponstel). Like the pyrazolon derivatives, these drugs must not be considered as routine mild analgesics. They find their primary therapeutic use in the symptomatic treatment of the various inflammatory diseases. Mefenamic acid is relatively new, but already it is known to be more toxic than aspirin. It may produce diarrhea and

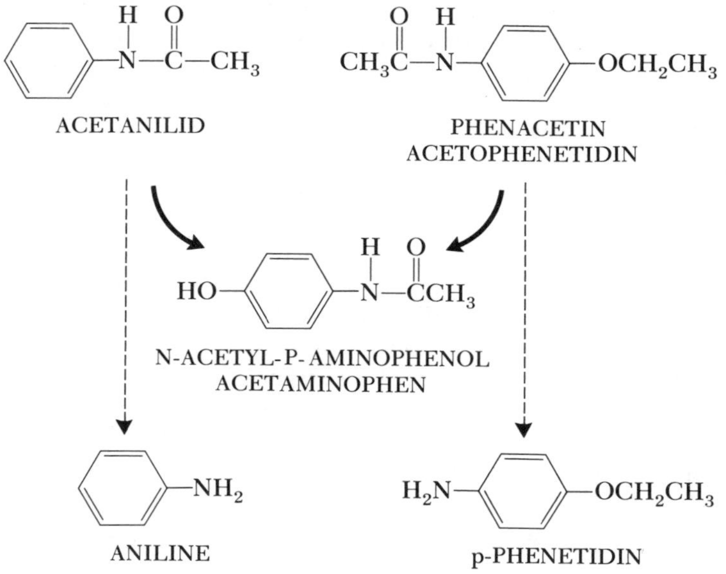

**Figure 8.8** Nonsalicylate mild analgesics. Acetaminophen is one of the metabolites produced by body from either acetanilid or phenacetin.

severe gastrointestinal bleeding; it is relatively contraindicated in asthmatics and should not be given to women of child-bearing age or to children under 14 years old. If the drug is prescribed at all, it should not be used for longer than 7 days. All in all, mefenamic acid really has little practical use in modern dentistry as a mild analgesic.

### Analgesic Combinations

If you have been raised in the United States of America, you already know that there is much ballyhoo over the relative effectiveness of aspirin alone versus the combination products containing two or more mild analgesics. The original rationale for the combination of two mild analgesics (one from one chemical class and another from another chemical class) was no doubt purely empirical, but over the years it has been repeatedly confirmed that the mild analgesic effects of the different drugs are additive, whereas their individual toxicities are not additive.[9] In other words, one can use a smaller dose of aspirin combined with a smaller dose of phenacetin and achieve the same mild analgesia as a larger dose of either used alone. Since each type of mild analgesic produces a different type of toxicity, the smaller amounts of each type mean a lower incidence of toxic effects. Different commercial products do differ and must be compared carefully.[20]

The mild analgesics show additive analgesic effects with the moderate analgesics as exemplified by codeine. Since it is now known the two analgesics (aspirin and codeine) act at different sites, there could be an advantage of prescribing the combination.

### Precautions and Contraindications

Over the years it has been learned that even for a drug as widely used without professional supervision as aspirin there are certain definite precautions to be recognized.

DISEASE STATES. Patients with existing or with a recent history of gastrointestinal ulceration should not be given aspirin; nor should a patient with a history of hypersensitivity reactions to salicylates be given any salicylates. Aspirin is known to have a mild antidiabetic action of its own which results in the promoting of tissue utilization of glucose.[21] Therefore, aspirin must be used with care in diabetics. The mild analgesic substitute of choice in each of these situations is acetaminophen.

DRUG-DRUG INTERACTIONS. As the reader will see when Table 8.3 is examined, the salicylates are capable of interacting unfavorably with a number of drugs that the patient may be taking; the practitioner must be aware of these specific salicylate interactions at least. In each case in which salicylate would be contraindicated because of a potentially harmful drug interaction, the mild analgesic, acetaminophen, may be substituted. The dentist and dental hygienist need to have a reference in the office to all the commercial drugs that contain aspirin, such as that found in the article by Leist and Banwell.[23]

### STRONG AND MODERATE ANALGESICS

In contrast to the nonnarcotic, mild analgesics, the narcotic, strong analgesics are drugs that can relieve almost any kind of pain without producing at the same time a complete loss of consciousness or loss of any other modality of sensation. To be consistent, we will refer to these drugs as the strong or moderate analgesics rather than the narcotic analgesics. All narcotics are not either moderate or strong analgesics; however, all strong and moderate analgesics, when given in the appropriate dose, may produce narcosis.

Analgesia and analgesic have been defined and now the term *narcotic* needs a definition. Literally a narcotic is a drug that produces narcosis, which is a state of impaired consciousness from which the patient can be aroused but to which he immediately

## Table 8.3.    Salicylate Drug Interactions

It is assumed that the dental patient is taking the usual therapeutic dose of one of the drugs listed in the INTERACTANT column in this table. Should the general dental practitioner give his patient aspirin, the patient's response is listed in the column labeled POSSIBLE INTERACTION. Each response refers to man.

| INTERACTANT | POSSIBLE INTERACTION |
|---|---|
| 1. Urinary acidifiers | Urinary acidifiers decrease the urinary excretion rate of salicylates and thus potentiate them. Salicylism may result from small decreases in pH. |
| 2. Alcohol (ethyl) | Alcohol increases the incidence and intensity of gastric hemorrhage caused by salicylates (aspirin). Buffering reduces the probability of hemorrhage. |
| 3. Urinary alkalinizers | Urinary alkalinizers increase the urinary excretion rate of salicylates and thus inhibit them. Increase of pH of less than one unit (5.8 to 6.5) may decrease plasma levels by 50%. |
| 4. Antacids | Antacids inhibit salicylates by decreasing their absorption. |
| 5. Anticoagulants, oral (coumarin derivatives, e.g.) | Salicylates in large doses potentiate the anticoagulants by depressing prothrombin formation in liver and displace anticoagulant from their secondary binding sites. This may lead to severe hemorrhage in presence of anticoagulant unless dosage is reduced. |
| 6. Antidepressants, tricyclic | Death has occurred with this combination. Mechanism not well understood. |
| 7. Antidiabetics, oral | *See* sulfonylureas, below. |
| 8. Ascorbic acid (vitamin C) | Salicylates increase the rate of urinary excretion of ascorbic acid (inhibits vitamin). Vitamin C, by lowering urinary pH, decreases urinary excretion of salicylates (augments). |
| 9. Chlorpropamide (Diabinese) | In large doses salicylates have an additive effect and further lower blood glucose levels. |
| 10. Corticosteroids | Both salicylates and corticosteroids have an ulcerogenic effect on gastrointestinal mucosa (increase danger of perforation of ulcer.). |

## Table 8.3. Continued

| INTERACTANT | POSSIBLE INTERACTION |
|---|---|
| | Corticosteroids may increase the clearance rate of salicylates, and steroid withdrawal with continued ingestion of aspirin may lead to aspirin poisoning. Aspirin augments anti-inflammatory effect of the steroid owing to its ability to displace steroid from its plasma protein binding sites and thus allow more to reach the tissues. |
| 11. Phenytoin (Dilantin) | Large doses of aspirin have been reported to augment the effect of Dilantin perhaps by displacing the antiepileptic from its secondary binding sites. |
| 12. Indomethacin (Indocin) | Both salicylates and indomethacin have an ulcerogenic effect on gastrointestinal mucosa, and their combined effect may be especially dangerous, even fatal. Aspirin decreases the antiinflammatory action of indomethacin by promoting its excretion. |
| 13. Insulin | Salicylates enhance the hypoglycemic effect. |
| 14. Penicillins | Salicylates potentiate the antibacterial effect of the penicillins. |
| 15. Phenobarbital (Luminal) | Phenobarbital inhibits the analgesic effect of aspirin owing to enzyme induction. |
| 16. Probenecid (Benemid) | Probenecid potentiates salicylates by inhibiting their renal tubular transport, but salicylates are contraindicated with this drug because aspirin inhibits its uricosuric action. |
| 17. Propranolol (Inderal) | $\beta$-adrenergic blockers such as Inderal inhibit the antiinflammatory action of aspirin. |
| 18. Reserpine (Serpasil) | Reserpine inhibits the analgesic action of aspirin. |
| 19. Sulfonamides | Salicylates enhance the antibacterial action of sulfonamides and increase sulfonamide toxicity. Salicylates displace sulfonamides from plasma protein binding sites. |
| 20. Sulfonylureas (Diabinese, Dymelor, Orinase) | Salicylates potentiate sulfonylureas by displacing them from their plasma protein binding sites and by an additive hypoglycemic effect. |

Source: Data adapted and selected from Martin, 1971.[22]

returns. The mildest form of narcosis is characterized by stupor or lethargy. The limbs feel heavy and the body feels warm; laziness, drowsiness, a clouding of the mental processes, and a disinterest in the surroundings are common. The sudden appearance of the state of narcosis can be perceived as pleasant or uncomfortable and frustrating, depending upon the state of the individual.

Narcotic analgesics are capable of producing this semiaware level of consciousness, but long before they produce narcosis or in doses lower than those that cause narcosis, these agents can establish an indifference to painful stimuli.

The word *narcotic* also has a legal definition, i.e., a specific type of chemical compound that falls under the jurisdiction of the Comprehensive Drug Abuse Prevention and Control Act of 1970.[24] Not all drugs legally called narcotics can produce the drug-induced state of narcosis.

In contrast to the mild analgesics, the strong and moderate analgesics are particularly useful in relieving the visceral type of pain or that characterized by pain perception far outlasting the stimulus. However, drugs cannot be placed into neat little categories of unique characteristics. The strong analgesics can relieve or suppress any kind of pain when given in sufficient dosage. Their unusual trait is that they can do this without making the patient completely unconscious.

## General Classification

All strong and moderate analgesics are further classified into one of two general groups, opiates or opioids, according to their origin.

OPIATES. A strong or moderate analgesic is called an opiate if it is any one of the following: (1) opium, the crude drug, which is defined as the dried, milky exudate of the unripe seed pod of the plant *Papaver somniferum* (the sleep-bearing poppy); (2) a galenical preparation of opium, e.g., a tincture, powder, or crude extract of opium; (3) a naturally occurring alkaloid or active principle of opium, e.g., morphine and codeine; or (4) a semisynthetic derivative of an opium alkaloid, e.g., a chemical modification of morphine or codeine, such as heroin.

OPIOIDS. A strong or moderate analgesic is called an opioid if it is a completely synthetic compound that mimics the pharmacological actions of morphine.

The drug opium has been in recorded use since at least 4000 B.C., but it was not until about 1807 that its major alkaloid, morphine, was isolated by the German pharmacist Friedrick W.A. Serturner. Morphine's total laboratory synthesis was accomplished in 1952,[25] but because the cost of synthesis is prohibitively high morphine is still obtained from *Papaver somniferum*.

Two chemically different types of alkaloids are found in opium, the phenanthrenes and the benzylisoquinolines (see Figure 8.9). The analgesic action is the characteristic property of the phenanthrenes, morphine and codeine. The isoquinolines, papaverine and noscapine, are not strong or moderate analgesics but possess other useful therapeutic properties.

### Morphine

For the sake of brevity and particularly for what will be a simpler way of understanding the pharmacological effects of these

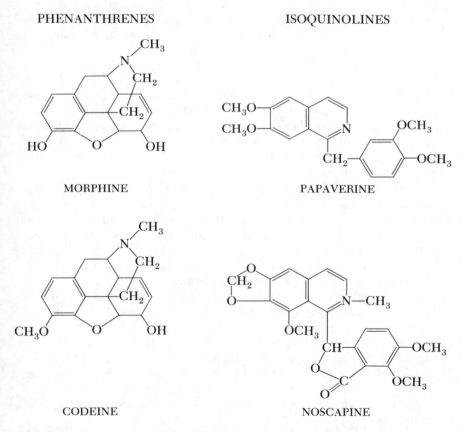

**Figure 8.9** Two major chemical groups of opium alkaloids—the phenanthrenes and the isoquinolines.

analgesics, the fairly detailed actions of morphine on the various organ systems of man will be presented because morphine is the standard or prototype of all strong analgesics. Then, since the actions of the morphone derivatives and substitutes are actually only a variation on the morphine theme, only such variations will be emphasized in the discussions of these agents. The moderate analgesics, the prototype of which is codeine, will be included in the discussion.

The most prominent action of morphine is its potent or strong analgesic action exerted on the central nervous system. Starting at the highest levels and working down to the spinal cord, let us consider the important actions of morphine at each level.

EFFECTS ON CEREBRAL CORTEX. Early in this chapter it was explained that the pain experience could be divided into several parts: the perception of the painful stimulus and the response or reactions to the painful stimulus—both physical and emotional reactions to pain.

Morphine is known to produce analgesia in at least three ways (1) Morphine raises both the "pain reaction threshold" and the "pain perception threshold" to some degree, that is, morphine must depress the afferent pain pathways. (2) Morphine reduces or eliminates the emotional reaction to pain, that is, morphine must act on the central component where the impulses are interpreted. (3) Morphine promotes both sedation and sleep. It is well known that sleep, itself, facilitates both (1) and (2).[26]

The best of experimental evidence clearly shows that the important factor in the analgesic action of these drugs is their ability to reduce or eliminate the emotional reaction to pain, that is, the anxiety induced by the anticipation of pain. In fact, the patient under morphine is not physiologically free of pain; he is inattentive or is unaware of the pain. The analgesic action of morphine is intimately connected with, but independent of, the drug-induced unrealistic false state of personal well-being, known as euphoria. The euphoric effect is definitely not experienced by all who are given morphine, although analgesia is manifested. The patient who is in severe pain is the one who most probably may experience euphoria. It is now known that the administration of morphine to a person who is healthy and free of any pain may even produce the opposite of euphoria—namely, dysphoria. The patient panics and has hysteria, visual and auditory hallucinations, and great psychic discomfort.

There is one other cortical effect of morphine to be mentioned. Morphine is known to depress certain areas in the cortex that normally send inhibitory impulses to subcortical centers or nuclei.

When the drug inhibits the inhibitory input to an area, the drug is said to "release" the area from the inhibitory control. Perhaps one of morphine's best known peripheral responses is due in part to the cortical release of the subcortical Edinger-Westphal nucleus. As a result of an increase in the outflow of pupillary constrictor tone, "pinpoint" pupils or miosis is experienced as shown diagrammatically in Figure 8.10.

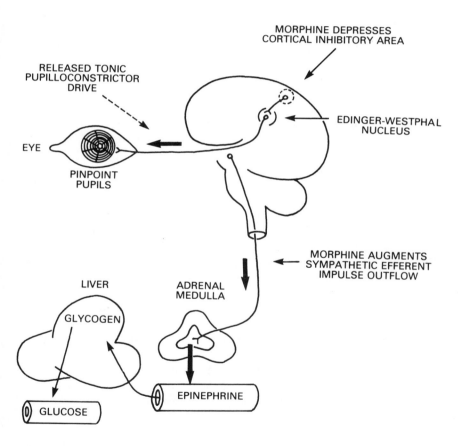

MORPHINE

MORPHINE DEPRESSES
CORTICAL INHIBITORY AREA

RELEASED TONIC
PUPILLOCONSTRICTOR
DRIVE

EDINGER-WESTPHAL
NUCLEUS

EYE

PINPOINT
PUPILS

MORPHINE AUGMENTS
SYMPATHETIC EFFERENT
IMPULSE OUTFLOW

LIVER        ADRENAL
MEDULLA

GLYCOGEN

GLUCOSE      EPINEPHRINE

HYPERGLYCEMIA

**Figure 8.10** Morphine-induced miosis and transient hyperglycemia. See text for further details.

EFFECTS ON HYPOTHALAMUS. At the level of the hypothalamus, morphine can be observed to produce a dual action, i.e., it stimulates some functional areas and inhibits others to result in a number of its notable clinical effects.

It has been confirmed repeatedly that morphine produces a transient hyperglycemia in man,[27] which is the basis for the drug's relative contraindication in the diabetic patient. Because morphine excites the foramen of Munro, an increased flow of impulses goes out over the sympathetic nervous system, one result of which is the outpour of adrenal medullary epinephrine. The catecholamine, in turn, initiates a breakdown of liver glycogen which is the source of the increased circulating blood glucose (see Figure 8.10).

Morphine and its derivatives are also well-known stimulants of the supraoptic nuclei which lead ultimately to a release into the circulation of the antidiuretic hormone from the posterior pituitary.[28] This is an example of morphine's ability to excite and depress simultaneously at the hypothalamic level (see Figure 8.11).[29]

EFFECTS ON BRAIN STEM (ESPECIALLY MEDULLA OBLONGATA). At this level of the central nervous system some of morphine's most undesirable effects are observed. Here two of morphine's most predictable actions are exerted on living tissue; these are respiratory depression and vomiting.

Morphine produces a primary depression of respiration in man, i.e., even in the smallest active doses, these drugs slow the respiratory rate and to some extent increase the depth of respiration.[30] The opiates and opioids, as shown in Figure 8.12, have a dual action upon the respiratory machinery: they reduce the sensitivity of the respiratory center to carbon dioxide, and at the same time they enhance the flow of afferent impulses to the respiratory center from the stretch receptors in the lungs as well as from the chemoreceptors of the carotid body.

Perhaps this dual effect of depressing and enhancing at the same time is best observed, concerning respiration, in the victim of an acute overdose whose breathing is very slow and barely discernable. The administration of oxygen alone to the patient may be expected to cause only a further respiratory depression or even to produce apnea. In the patient under morphine the respiration may be driven only by the chemoreceptor reflex mechanisms for which hypoxia is the adequate stimulus. If the hypoxia is eliminated, the stimulus is removed. What must be done is to give oxygen, surely, but also to plan to breathe for the patient.

Although the specific location of man's coughing center has not been identified, it is agreed at least that it is in the medulla oblongata. The narcotic analgesics profoundly depress this center

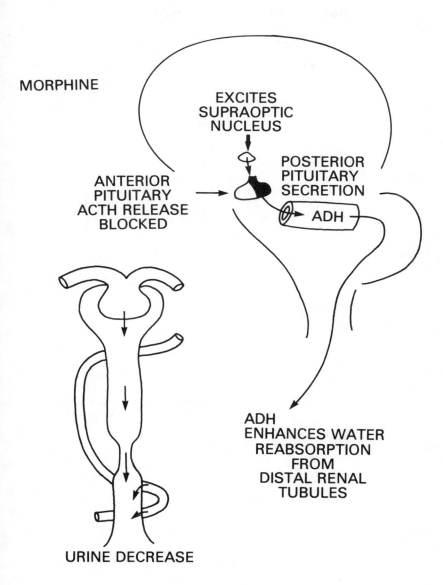

**Figure 8.11** Morphine-induced release of antidiuretic hormone (ADH) which acts upon renal mechanisms to reduce formation of urine. Morphine also inhibits release of adrenocorticotropin (ACTH).

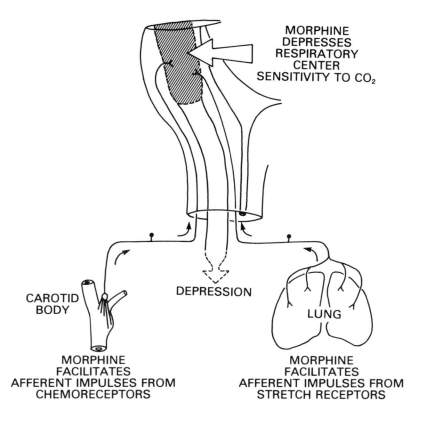

MORPHINE
RESPIRATORY DEPRESSION

MORPHINE
DEPRESSES
RESPIRATORY
CENTER
SENSITIVITY TO $CO_2$

DEPRESSION

CAROTID
BODY

LUNG

MORPHINE
FACILITATES
AFFERENT IMPULSES FROM
CHEMORECEPTORS

MORPHINE
FACILITATES
AFFERENT IMPULSES FROM
STRETCH RECEPTORS

**Figure 8.12**   Morphine-induced effects upon respiratory system.

which is the rational basis for the second most frequent therapeutic use of these drugs, i.e., their antitussive action. Of the group, codeine, rather than morphine, is the standard to which all antitussive agents are compared.

There can be no questions but that one of morphine's definite drawbacks is its emetic action. As shown in Figure 8.13 the drug stimulates directly a small reflexogenic zone located in the area postrema on the floor of the fourth ventricle. The zone is called the chemoreceptive trigger zone (CTZ).[31] When this zone is excited, impulses are sent a short distance to the vomiting center located in the reticular formation. Morphine does not directly stimulate the vomiting center itself. In addition, morphine facilitates the flow of afferent impulses to the vomiting center from other reflexogenic zones such as the utricular maculae of the labyrinthine apparatus. Thus, morphine is more apt to produce vomiting in the ambulatory patient.[32] Paradoxically, morphine is also an antiemetic, for once it stimulates the CTZ it blocks the mechanism. Afferent impulses from the gastric mucosal reflexogenic zone are also facilitated.

EFFECTS ON SPINAL CORD. Lastly, in the central nervous system, morphine can be seen to produce dual effects, even at the spinal level. The drug enhances the monosynaptic reflexes (e.g., the knee jerk) and depresses the polysynaptic reflexes (e.g., flexor and crossed-extension).[33]

In large overdose morphine is known to produce strychninelike convulsions in man.[34] The site of this action is diffused throughout

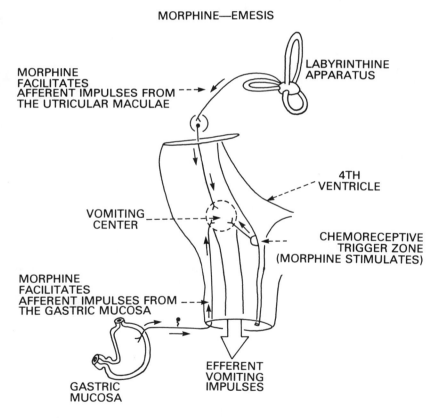

**MORPHINE—EMESIS**

LABYRINTHINE APPARATUS

MORPHINE FACILITATES AFFERENT IMPULSES FROM THE UTRICULAR MACULAE

4TH VENTRICLE

VOMITING CENTER

CHEMORECEPTIVE TRIGGER ZONE (MORPHINE STIMULATES)

MORPHINE FACILITATES AFFERENT IMPULSES FROM THE GASTRIC MUCOSA

EFFERENT VOMITING IMPULSES

GASTRIC MUCOSA

**Figure 8.13**  Morphine-induced effects upon vomiting mechanism.

the entire neural axis. In the use of these morphinelike analgesics there is exerted a dual effect, both inhibition and excitement.

Lurking below those overt symptoms of general depression are the excitatory phenomena. These phenomena are the basis for the contraindication of administering central nervous system stimulants to a patient who is manifesting a hyperreactive response to morphine or to those who are acutely poisoned and comatose. Given even small doses of the stimulant, the patient may be carried from coma to convulsions. In such a situation the antidote of high specificity is a drug categorized as a narcotic antagonist.

CARDIOVASCULAR EFFECTS. In usual doses for the patient in pain, morphine produces few obvious observable changes in the cardiovascular system,[35] but extensive clinical experience with morphine warns against making any unwarranted conclusions just because there are few observable changes. Perhaps it is more accurate to say that the usual therapeutic doses of morphine may predispose the patient to cardiovascular collapse.

If the patient happens to be a hyperreactor or suffers from untreated hypothyroidism, then depression of the vasomotor center, enhanced bradycardia, and general vasodilation with peripheral pooling of blood may result.[36] The untreated hypothyroid patient is sensitive to all the effects of morphine. This patient must not be confused with the patient who is being given thyroid hormone as replacement therapy. The latter may be receiving more thyroid than he needs and actually responds as if he were hyperthyroid. In this case, the patient would be less sensitive to the usual doses of morphine.

It can be demonstrated that morphine is able to produce peripheral vasodilation.[30] The mechanism for this vascular smooth muscle relaxation is complex and would appear to include the following: (1) morphine is known to release histamine which is a strong vasodilator;[37] (2) morphine-induced respiratory depression causes generalized local tissue hypoxia, buildup of hydrogen ions and carbon dioxide, all of which are strong vasodilators; and (3) morphine may directly relax vascular smooth muscle.

Although the cardiovascular effects of morphine are not significant when therapeutic amounts are administered, these effects can become a potential problem when the patient is already taking another drug that is acting upon the cardiovascular system (e.g., one of the antihypertensive agents).

GASTROINTESTINAL EFFECTS. The most spectacular effects of morphine outside the central nervous system are those exerted upon the gastrointestinal tract. If the action had to be described in one word, that word would be spasmogenesis. As shown in Figure

8.14, all sphincters, as well as the intestinal wall, contract.[38] Propulsive waves cease, whereas the nonpropulsive waves increase. The overall effect is constipation, which can be allowed to become as serious a condition as the one for which the morphine was administered in the first place. The problem, of course, is magnified by the patient's inattentiveness to the call to defecate.

It is obvious that with the pyloric sphincter in spasm, stomach emptying time is prolonged.

The spasm of the sphincter of Oddi can cause a considerable rise in biliary intraductal pressure which can result in the painful condition of biliary colic. Even in usual therapeutic doses, morphine may cause biliary pain temporarily in certain patients before the drug reaches an effective analgesic concentration. Thus, morphine's analgesic effects will mask pain that the drug is causing.

URINARY EFFECTS. In the urinary system, as in the gastrointesti-

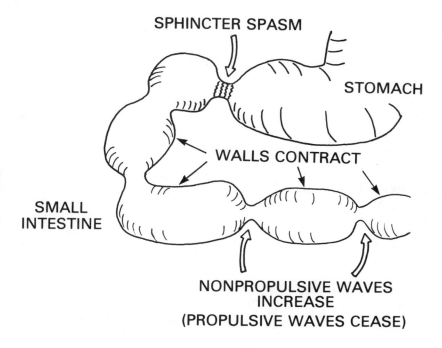

SPHINCTER SPASM

STOMACH

WALLS CONTRACT

SMALL INTESTINE

NONPROPULSIVE WAVES INCREASE
(PROPULSIVE WAVES CEASE)

CONSTIPATION

**Figure 8.14**  Morphine-induced effects upon sphincters and walls of intestines lead to constipation.

nal system, morphine causes smooth muscle contraction. As depicted in Figure 8.15, the spasms of ureteral smooth muscle walls can so elevate renal pelvic pressure as to cause severely painful renal colic. Once again, however, morphine's strong analgesic effects mask this drug-induced pain.

In the urinary bladder, morphine produces contraction of the detrusor muscles, which causes urinary urgency, but the drug also

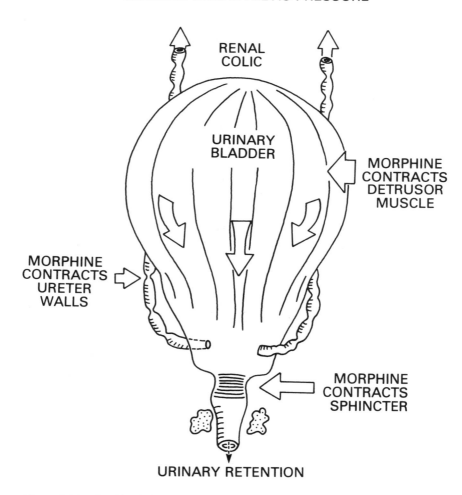

**Figure 8.15** Morphine-induced effects upon urinary system.

contracts the vesicle sphincter, which makes emptying of the bladder impossible. The overall effect is urinary retention.

### Comparative Features

It now becomes necessary to consider a selected number of derivatives and substitutes of opium. There is no question but that the dentist and dental hygienist should be aware of the large number of strong and moderate analgesics available. There are so many different drugs and drug products and thousands of facts that could be learned at this point. Nonetheless, the essential factual information about each of the strong and moderate analgesics may be obtained from various accurate drug information resources. What is needed when one is first confronted with the task of making rhyme and reason of all the opiates and opioids is a simplified classification and a few examples. A complete comparison of their chemical structures and effects to morphine's may be found in any drug encyclopedia reference.[39] The number of different examples to follow has been kept to a minimum.

The opium derivatives and substitutes can be subdivided into six subgroups or classes for the sake of convenience: the morphines, the morphinones, the morphinans, the methadones, the meperidines, and miscellaneous. The highly selected information about each of the example drugs is considered important specifically for the purposes of this text.

MORPHINES. These opiates include the major analgesic alkaloids of opium, as well as several other drug products. Morphine is a naturally occurring alkaloid of opium and is the standard to which all other strong analgesics are compared. The general effects of morphine have been presented earlier in this chapter. Next to morphine, methylmorphine or codeine is the most important alkaloid of opium. It is the standard moderate analgesic and antitussive agent. Codeine may be considered as being able to produce the same effect as morphine, but not as well. Codeine, of course, has a lower ceiling analgesic effect. Codeine produces less sedation owing to its greater central excitatory properties. For this and other reasons, codeine is rarely if ever administered intravenously, and the oral route of administration is the most common for this drug. Codeine is definitely not the opiate drug abuser's choice, and there is a low incidence of actual codeine drug dependence. It is thought that codeine is partly converted to morphine in man.[40]

Diacetylmorphine (heroin) is an opiate of this group which on a mg basis is more potent than morphine, but it bears the same efficacy in all respects.[41] Heroin is not used therapeutically in the United States. It is the drug of choice for many opiate abusers.

Camphorated Tincture of Opium (paregoric) is a galenical preparation that is not used in dentistry as an analgesic. It is a hydroalcoholic preparation containing camphor and opium which is used rationally only in the treatment of diarrhea.[42] It is not unusual to find paregoric still prescribed by older medical practitioners for a mother to rub on her teething child's gingiva, supposedly to relieve the pain locally. If it does relieve the pain, it is because the 0.4 mg/ml of morphine found in paregoric is absorbed.

MORPHINONES. These analgesics are also opiates and are semisynthetic derivatives of morphine and codeine. Two, hydromorphone and oxymorphone, were obtained by a chemical modification of morphine.

Hydromorphone (Dilaudid) is a strong analgesic that resembles morphine in every way except that it is more potent on a mg for mg basis.[43] Oxymorphone (Numorphan) is the most potent of all the opium-derived strong analgesics considered in this chapter. Each of these morphine derivatives has sister codeine derivatives, which like codeine are moderate analgesics only and, as may be expected, are both more potent on a mg basis than codeine. These drugs are hydrocodone (Dicodid) and oxycodone, which is the analgesic found in the commercial product Percodan.

MORPHINANS. The third large subgroup of analgesics introduces the opioids or the completely synthetic morphine and codeine substitutes. Levorphanol (Levo-dromoran) is a strong analgesic that is also more potent mg for mg than is morphine. Its existence proved man could fully synthesize a morphinelike strong analgesic without having to begin with morphine. When the equivalent codeine substitute is sought, the interesting drug dextromethorphan (Romilar) is found. This drug is devoid of all analgesic properties but still retains the strong antitussive action of codeine. It is one of the most popular nonnarcotic antitussives on the market.

METHADONES. These opioids are a definite structure change from the morphine structure. Methadone (Dolophine) is equivalent to morphine mg for mg but possesses several significant differences. Methadone has a longer duration of action and definitely fewer sedative properties than morphine.[43] In addition, methadone has a less severe abstinence syndrome than does morphine or heroin; therefore, such drug abusers may be converted to methadone-dependent persons and then later withdrawn from methadone.[44] No equivalent codeine substitute exists, but instead there is the drug propoxyphene (Darvon) which has a mild analgesic ceiling effect only. It is not a moderate but mild analgesic.[18] Propoxyphene is not classified legally as a controlled substance as of this writing; however, individuals have been reported to become dependent upon it and show an abstinence syndrome when the drug is abruptly withdrawn.[45] It is predicted that this drug will be a controlled substance by 1978.

MEPERIDINES. The fifth subgroup of analgesics is made up of opioids and here meperidine is found. Meperidine (Demerol) is one of the most commonly administered and prescribed strong analgesics by physicians and dentists in the United States. On a mg for mg basis meperidine is about five to ten times less potent than morphine, but it still possesses, in the appropriate doses, the same ceiling analgesic effect. Meperidine differs in a number of significant ways from morphine. Some of the more important differences include less spasmogenic effect on the lower gastrointestinal tract, less urinary retention, and less pupillary constrictor effect. The drug, in contrast to morphine, possesses some atropinelike properties.[46] It is said to lead to a more dangerous abstinence syndrome, and its effects are more difficult to antagonize.

A true codeine substitute does not exist in the meperidine subgroup as a moderate analgesic, but there is a weak, mild nonnarcotic analgesic known as ethoheptazine (Zactane). There is really no indication for this drug in dentistry.

PENTAZOCINE. This recently introduced opioid is certainly different, very interesting, and probably a glimpse of what can be expected in the future. The effects of pentazocine (Talwin) will be easier to understand after the reader examines the material on narcotic antagonists. For now, it can be stated that pentazocine when given by the intravenous route produces a strong analgesic ceiling effect. However, when administered orally, pentazocine is at best only a moderate analgesic. Pentazocine's most unusual property is that it is a weak narcotic antagonist.

### Therapeutic Use in Dentistry

Morphine, codeine, and their derivatives or substitutes are used in dentistry. In most circumstances regarding dental disease, dental treatment, and dental pain, the mild, aspirin type of analgesic is the most helpful. In this respect dentistry is most fortunate in that most pain that is to be dealt with is of the integumental type. However, certain types of oral disease or treatment involve more severe pain, and in these instances it will be necessary to prescribe a moderate or strong analgesic.

A general rule regarding analgesics, which has developed over the years, is quite simple but difficult to follow. In the treatment of any pain for which an analgesic is indicated, always begin with the mildest analgesic; then if it does not afford relief, prescribe a combination of mild and moderate analgesics; then and only then move up to the single strong analgesic such as meperidine.

## Precautions

There are several precautions regarding the use of strong and moderate analgesics in addition to those already mentioned. Some patients may have diseases that are known to interact unfavorably with the strong analgesics. The patient with hypertension has his arterial blood pressure held in delicate balance usually by one or more drugs and a diet. Morphine depresses the central regulatory mechanisms for the cardiovascular system just enough to produce augmented hypotension. The patient with diabetes mellitus has his circulating blood sugar held in a delicate balance; morphine produces hyperglycemia. The patient with an acute or chronic respiratory disease such as emphysema is always a high risk for giving morphine; primarily, morphine's respiratory depressant effects must be remembered, and secondly, the ability of these agents to release histamine in the patient with bronchial asthma may precipitate an acute bronchospasm. Patients with a current history of gall bladder disease should be given opiates with due caution. Patients who are hypothyroid are extremely sensitive to all the effects of morphine, and the dose of any opiate or opioid must be reduced. The opposite is true for the hyperthyroid patient who requires usually a larger dose to achieve a strong analgesic effect. Dental patients with concurrent convulsant disorders may be give strong analgesics but only with extreme caution, since these drugs do possess excitatory effects. Finally, patients with a history of drug dependence may be given one of these drugs but only after careful consideration. You are doing them no favor by broadening their drug experience.

Another similar but different type of precaution involves the unfavorable interaction between the strong analgesics and certain other drugs the patient may be taking. A general rule would be that the combination of depressant effects of the strong analgesics with the depressant effects of any other central nervous system depressant can lead quickly to overdepresssion. A significant potentiation of central nervous system depression is seen with some of the phenothiazine derivatives that are used for their antipsychotic and antihistaminic effects.[47]

Lastly, serious attention must be given to the interaction between narcotic analgesics and monoamine oxidase inhibitors (MAOI). There are at least seven MAOI on the market today, and if the patient is taking one of these, a strong analgesic is not prescribed unless the patient is in the hospital and can be treated immediately should the interaction occur. Many deaths from this combination of drugs have been reported in the literature. Meperidine is especially prone to cause the interaction and is absolutely contraindicated. The other opiates and opioids produce a less severe reaction and are relatively contraindicated. The mechanism of the interaction is not fully understood.[48]

## NARCOTIC ANTAGONISTS

We are indeed fortunate to have available drugs known as narcotic antagonists. Some years ago it was noted that the replacement of a methyl group with an allyl group on the nitrogen atom of morphine gave a compound whose spectrum of action included reversal of the effects of morphinelike analgesics.[49, 50]

There are now two types of narcotic antagonists, the partial agonist and the "true" antagonists. The partial agonists are the older of the two groups. The prototype is nalorphine (Nalline) or N-allylnormorphine. To appreciate this type of antagonist, one must consider what nalorphine will do in three types of patients.

What happens when nalorphine is administered to a patient who has no circulating narcotic analgesic in the body? The effects look almost like those caused by morphine in man, such as the same degree of analgesia and smooth muscle response. There is a noteworthy exception: nalorphine is much more likely to produce severe dysphoria, which is most unpleasant. For this reason, no narcotic-dependent person or drug abuser would pick nalorphine. It is not a drug of abuse. Unfortunately, the dysphoric effect keeps it from being used as an analgesic.[51]

What happens when nalorphine is administered to a patient who has circulating narcotic analgesic in the body? Within about 15 minutes or sooner an almost complete reversal of all the narcotic analgesic's effects occurs.[52]

What happens when nalorphine is administered to a currently dependent narcotic abuser? The full-blown withdrawal or abstinence syndrome is precipitated almost immediately and can be very dangerous.[53]

Of great importance is the specificity of the partial agonist type of narcotic antagonist. These antagonists are specific for opiates and opioids only. They reverse neither the central nervous system depressant effects of the barbiturate and nonbarbiturate sedative-hypnotics nor the depression caused by the psychopharmacological agents, the antihistamines, general anesthetics, or alcohol. In fact, the partial agonists potentiate the respiratory depression caused by these drugs.[54]

Pentazocine is a partial agonist type of antagonist and is the result of the long search for a strong analgesic that is not subject to drug abuse. Knowing that nalorphine produces strong analgesia in man and is not abused led to the further modification of nalorphine's structure in an attempt to get rid of the undesired dysphoric properties. Pentazocine is the result. It is a weak partial agonist with relatively good analgesic properties and with a low incidence of dysphoria.[55] Because of its partial agonist properties, it cannot be given to a patient already under the influence of an opiate or opioid either therapeutically or as a drug abuser. Should a patient be given pentazocine and he hyperreacts, what is used as an antagonist? If another partial agonist such as nalorphine is tried, the patient will probably die in further depression. The antidote is the "true" narcotic antagonist naloxone (Narcan).[56]

Naloxone possesses no agonist properties; therefore, when given to the patient without circulating narcotic analgesic it produces little if any effect. In the patient under the influence of narcotic analgesic, naloxone produces a prompt reversal of all effects in much the same way as seen with nalorphine. Naloxone will also precipitate the abstinence syndrome. One of naloxone's benefits is the fact that, although it specifically reverses only the effects of the opiates and opioids, it will not further add to the respiratory and circulatory depression produced by the sedative-hypnotics, antianxiety agents, general anesthetics, or alcohol.[57] No drug dependence has yet been reported. The narcotic antagonist finds its major usefulness in dentistry in the emergency treatment of the hyper-reactor to strong or moderate analgesics.

## REFERENCES

1. Beecher, H.K.: The measurement of pain. Pharmacol. Rev., 9:59, 1957.
2. Gerard, R.W.: The physiology of pain. Ann. N.Y. Acad. Sci., 86:6, 1960.
3. Randall, L.O.: Non-narcotic analgesics. In Physiological Pharmacology. Edited by W.S. Root and F.G. Hofmann. New York, Academic Press, 1963, Vol. 1.
4. Aronow, W.S.: Management of stable angina. N. Engl. J. Med., 289:516, 1973.
5. Grant, W.M.: Physiological and pharmacological influences upon intraocular pressure. Pharmacol. Rev., 7:143, 1955.
6. Lim, R.K.S.: Pain. Annu. Rev. Physiol., 32:269, 1970.
7. Beecher, H.K.: Measurement of Subjective Responses. New York, Oxford, 1959.
8. Lasagna, L., and Beecher, H.K.: The analgesic effectiveness of codeine and meperidine (Demerol). J. Pharmacol. Exp. Ther., 112:306, 1954.
9. Woodbury, D.M.: Analgesic-antipyretics, antiinflammatory agents, and inhibitors of uric acid synthesis. In The Pharmacological Basis of Therapeutics. 5th Edition. Edited by L.S. Goodman and A. Gilman. New York, Macmillan, 1975.
10. Wit, A., and Wang, S.C.: Temperature-sensitive neurons in preoptic/anterior hypothalamic region: action of pyrogen and acetylsalicylate. Am. J. Physiol., 215:1160, 1968.
11. Euler, C. von: Physiology and pharmacology of temperature regulation. Pharmacol. Rev., 13:361, 1961.

12. Lim, R.K.S.: Neuropharmacology of pain and analgesia. *In* Pharmacology of Pain. Proceedings of the Third International Pharmacological Meeting. Edited by R.K.S. Lim, D. Armstrong, and E.G. Pardo. New York, Pergamon Press, 1968. Vol. 9.

13. Salter, R.H.: Aspirin and gastrointestinal bleeding. Am. J. Dig. Dis., *13*:38, 1968.

14. Yu, T., and Gutman, A.B.: Study of paradoxical effects of salicylate in low, intermediate and high dosage on the renal mechanisms for excretion of urate in man. J Clin. Invest., *38*:1298, 1959.

15. Evans, G., Packham, M.A., Nishizawa, E.E., Mustard, J.F., and Murphy, E.A.: The effect of acetylsalicylic acid on platelet function. J. Exp. Med., *128*:877, 1968.

16. Barr, W.H., and Penna, R.P.: Internal analgesics. *In* Handbook of Non-Prescription Drugs. Co-edited by G.B. Griffenhagen and L.L. Hawkins. Washington, D.C., American Pharmaceutical Association, 1973.

17. Smith, M.J.H., and Smith, P.K.: The Salicylates: a Critical Bibliographic Review. New York, John Wiley & Sons, 1966.

18. Beaver, W.T.: Mild analgesics: a review of their clinical pharmacology. Am. J. Med. Sci., *250*:577, 1965.

19. Gilman, A.: Analgesic nephrotoxicity: a pharmacological analysis. Am. J. Med., *36*:167, 1964.

20. Is all aspirin alike? Med. Lett. Drugs Ther., *16*:57, 1974.

21. Whitehouse, M.W.: Some biochemical and pharmacological properties of anti-inflammatory drugs. Prog. Drug Res., 8:301, 1965.

22. Martin, E.W.: Hazards of Medication. Philadelphia, Lippincott, 1971.

23. Leist, E.R., and Banwell, J.G.: Products containing aspirin. N. Engl. J. Med., *291*:710, 1974.

24. Comprehensive Drug Abuse Prevention and Control Act of 1970. Public Law 91-513. 91st Congress, October 27, 1970.

25. Gates, M. and Tschudi, G.: The synthesis of morphine. J. Am. Chem. Soc., *74*:1109, 1952 and 78:1380, 1956.

26. Keele, C.A.: The assay of analgesic drugs on man. Analyst, 77:111, 1952.

27. Campos, H.A.: Role of central nervous system catecholamines in morphine hyperglycemia. Fed. Proc., *19*:272, 1960.

28. Giarman, N.J., and Condouris, G.A.: The antidiuretic action of morphine and some of its analogs. Arch. Int. Pharmacodyn. Ther., 97:28, 1954.

29. Briggs, F.N., and Munson, P.L.: Studies on mechanism of stimulation of ACTH secretion with aid of morphine as blocking agent. J. Clin. Endocrinol. Metab., *57*:205, 1955.

30. Eckenhoff, J.E., and Oech, S.R.: The effects of narcotics and antagonists upon respiration and circulation in man. Clin. Pharmacol. Ther., *1*:483, 1960.

31. Wang, S.C., and Glaviano, V.V.: Locus of emetic action of morphine and Hydergine in dogs. J. Pharmacol. Exp. Ther., *111*:329, 1954.

32. Comroe, J.H., and Dripps, R.D.: Reactions to morphine in ambulatory and bed patients. Surg. Gynecol. Obstet., 87:221, 1948.

33. Wikler, A., and Frank, K.: Hindlimb reflexes of chronic spinal dogs during cycles of addiction to morphine and methadon. J. Pharmacol. Exp. Ther., 94:382, 1948.

34. Wikler, A.: Sites and mechanisms of action of morphine and related drugs in the central nervous system. Pharmacol. Rev., 2:435, 1950.

35. Papper, E.M., and Bradley, S.E.: Hemodynamic effects of intravenous morphine and Pentothal sodium. J. Pharmacol. Exp. Ther., 74:37, 1942.

36. Lowenstein, E.: Cardiovascular response to large doses of intravenous morphine in man. N. Engl. J. Med., *281*:1389, 1969.

37. Feldberg, W., and Paton, W.D.M.: Release of histamine from skin and muscle in the cat by opium alkaloids and other histamine liberators. J. Physiol. (Lond.), *114*:490, 1951.

38. Chapman, W.P., Rowlands, E.N., and Jones, C.M.: Multiple-baloon kymographic recording of the comparative action of DEMEROL, morphine and placebos on the motility of the upper small intestine in man. N. Engl. J. Med., *243*:171, 1950.

39. Jaffe, J.H., and Martin, W.R.: Narcotic analgesics and antagonists. *In* The Pharmacological Basis of Therapeutics. 5th Edition. Edited by L.S. Goodman and A. Gilman. New York, Macmillan, 1975.
40. Way, E.L., and Adler, T.K.: The Biological Disposition of Morphine and its Surrogates. Geneva, World Health Organization, 1962.
41. Martin, W.R., and Fraser, H.F.: A comparative study of physiological and subjective effects of heroin and morphine administered intravenously in addicts. J. Pharmacol. Exp. Ther., *133*:388,1961.
42. Aviado, D.M.: Krantz and Carr's Pharmacologic Principles of Medical Practice. 8th Edition. Baltimore, Williams & Wilkins, 1972.
43. Eddy, N.B., Halbach, H., and Braenden, O.J.: Synthetic substances with morphine-like effect. Bull. WHO, *17*:569, 1957.
44. Isbell, H., Wikler, A., and Eisenman, A.J.: Liability of addiction to 6-dimethylamino-4-4-diphenyl-3-heptanone (methadone "amidone" or "10820") in man. Arch. Intern. Med., *82*:362, 1948.
45. Darvon and Darvon-N. Med. Lett. Drugs Ther., *14*:37, 1972.
46. Murphree, H.B.: Clinical pharmacology of potent analgesics. Clin. Pharmacol. Ther., *3*:473, 1962.
47. Lambertsen, D.J., Wendel, H., and Longenhangen, J.B.: The separate and combined respiratory effects of chlorpromazine and meperidine in normal men controlled at 46 mmHg alveolar pCO$_2$. J. Pharmacol. Exp. Ther., *131*:381, 1961.
48. Goldberg, L.I.: Monoamine oxidase inhibitors. J.A.M.A., *190*:456, 1964.
49. Weijlard, J., and Erickson, A.E.: N-Allylnormorphine. J. Am. Chem. Soc., *64*:869, 1942.
50. Hart, E.R., and McCawley, E.L.: The pharmacology of N-allylnormorphine as compared with morphine. J. Pharmacol. Exp. Ther., 82:339, 1944.
51. Lasagna, L., and Beecher, H.K.: The analgesic effectiveness of nalorphine and nalorphine-morphine combinations in man. J. Pharmacol. Exp. Ther., *112*:356, 1954.
52. Eckenhoff, J.E., Elder, J.D., and King, B.D.: The effect of N-allyl-normorphine in treatment of opiate overdosage. Am. J. Med. Sci., *222*:115, 1951.
53. Wikler, A., Fraser, H.F., and Isbell, H.: N-allylnormorphine: effects of single doses and precipitation of acute "abstinence syndromes" during addiction to morphine, methadone, or heroin in man (postaddicts). J. Pharmacol. Exp. Ther., *109*:8, 1953.
54. Martin, W.R.: Opioid antagonists. Pharmacol. Rev., *19*:463, 1967.
55. Paddock, R., Beer, E.G., Bellville, J.W., Ciliberti, B.J., Forrest, W.H., Jr., and Miller, E.V.: Analgesic and side effects of pentazocine and morphine in a large population of postoperative patients. Clin. Pharmacol. Ther., *10*:355, 1969.
56. Kallos, T., and Smith, T.C.: Naloxone reversal of pentazocine-induced respiratory depression (Letter) J.A.M.A., *204*:932, 1968.
57. Jasinski, D.R., Martin, W.R., and Hoeldtke, R.D.: Effects of short- and long-term administration of pentazocine in man. Clin. Pharmacol. Ther., *11*:385, 1970.

## SUPPLEMENTARY REFERENCE

Brecher, E.M. (ed.): Licit and Illicit Drugs. Boston, Little, Brown, 1972.

# *9*

## SEDATIVES

The allaying of the dental patient's anxiety regarding treatment is a challenge which the modern dentist gladly accepts. A wide variety of drugs and routes of administration are available to assist the nondrug, educational methodology in patient management. In this chapter the following drug groups will be considered: the classical sedative-hypnotics, the antianxiety agents, and the inhalational sedatives.

### SEDATIVE-HYPNOTICS

The drugs traditionally classified as sedative-hypnotics are non-selective, general depressants of the central nervous system. These widely prescribed agents depress the excitability or function of all cells. Under appropriately selected conditions, a sedative-hypnotic is capable of producing any degree of central nervous system depression with resulting behavioral response ranging from a slight reduction in attentiveness to loss of consciousness, coma, and death.

Without intending to be facetious, and so that the specific pharmacological properties of the sedative-hypnotics, as they are presented, may be more meaningful, some practical understanding of their desirable effects in man is worthwhile. One has to observe only the name given to this major class of therapeutic agents to deduce the two important desired conditions that can result following their administration to man. Although every dental hygienist has some conception of the terms *sedation* and *hypnosis*, the following working definitions are presented.

When the patient's general condition is compared before and after the administration of a sedative (a drug which produces sedation), the effects of the drug can be observed to include (1) a state of calmness, (2) a lessened degree of motor excitability, and (3) a lessened degree of apprehension or anxiety (behavioral excitability). This drug-induced state is manifested without the patient going to sleep or losing consciousness. The ideal sedative would be expected to produce this wakeful and serene condition without simultaneously causing any other effects, especially those that might be harmful to the patient's general health.

Pharmacologically speaking a hypnotic is a drug which, when administered under the appropriate conditions, causes the patient to go to sleep. When the drug's effects pass, the patient would awaken just as he would after a period of natural sleep.

It is to be emphasized that, clinically, any one particular sedative-hypnotic is capable of producing either sedation alone or sedation and drug-induced sleep. Smaller doses of the same drug are utilized when only sedation is desired. Larger doses, obviously, sedate the patient prior to compelling him to go to sleep.

The foregoing may be considered the classical introductory description of this group of popular therapeutic agents and can be found in almost every textbook of pharmacology. Although it does not consist of untrue statements, it is certainly misleading for the novice in the light of modern clinical pharmacology.

The sedative-hypnotics might well be discussed only as hypnotics, agents used specifically in the symptomatic treatment of insomnia. This is the one most useful property that every sedative-hypnotic drug possesses. Since the rapid development of the field of psychopharmacology, the continued practice of a separate presentation of the sedative properties of these agents has a tendency to make one believe that there must be a number of definable pharmacological differences between the effects produced by sedatives and the effects produced by the antianxiety agents. Although there is little question that the mechanisms of action, as currently understood, are not the same for the two groups of compounds, the clinical effects produced by each and the basic reason for which the practitioner would prescribe such drugs are similar, if not identical. Perhaps, it would be less confusing from a clinical point of view to present the sedative characteristics of these drugs at the same time the antianxiety agents are considered. Indeed, such a comparison will be made later in this chapter.

One reason for enthusiastic support of the development of the antianxiety agent was that the available drugs (the sedative barbiturates) were not accomplishing the effect desired by the dentist. The sedative-hypnotics in general are prone to produce considerable drowsiness and some degree of motor incoordination while allaying the patient's hyperexcitable state or anxiety. The more desired condition, in many instances, is one in which the patient's apprehensions and anxieties are relieved while at the same time allowing him to continue at his vocational endeavor as a contributing member of society.

Lastly, it is true that in amounts less than those required to put the patient to sleep, the majority of the sedative-hypnotics have a calming effect. Unfortunately, the dose required to produce satisfactory daytime sedation is close to that which causes drowsiness; this is not the case with many of the antianxiety agents now available.

The sedative-hypnotics, for our purposes, may be divided into two arbitrary groupings: the barbiturates and the nonbarbiturates. Since the barbiturates are considered the prototype of all the sedative-hypnotics, the barbiturates will be presented in appropriate detail. Then, a selected number of nonbarbiturate sedative hypnotics will be considered, only in respect to their differences as compared to the prototype. The entire subject of sedative-hypnotics has been reviewed.[1]

### Barbiturates

The most often prescribed sedative-hypnotic today is a barbiturate. The barbiturates, first introduced into therapeutics at the turn of the century, are a highly versatile group of agents despite the fact that their depressant activity is nonselective. Not only are they effective as sedatives and hypnotics but also some are useful in producing a rapid induction to general anesthesia, which is then maintained by one or more of the general inhalational anesthetics. In addition, several barbiturates are well-established clinically in the continuous control of specific forms of epilepsy. Certain barbiturates are the drugs of choice in halting generalized convulsions.

It should be mentioned that these same sedative-hypnotic barbiturates are the object of abuse or misuse. Their ability to cloud man's mind and thereby remove him for a period of time from the realities of the environment no doubt plays a primary role in their abuse liability.

The barbiturates are condensation products of various substituted malonic acids and urea. Malonic acid condenses with urea to form barbituric acid and water as shown in Figure 9.1. Barbituric acid itself is devoid of sedative or hypnotic properties. However, when the two hydrogen atoms attached to carbon-5 are replaced by a variety of alkyl or aralkyl groups (some 1,222 different combinations of five or less carbon atoms for each group are possible), there results a host of pharmacologically active barbiturates. These di-

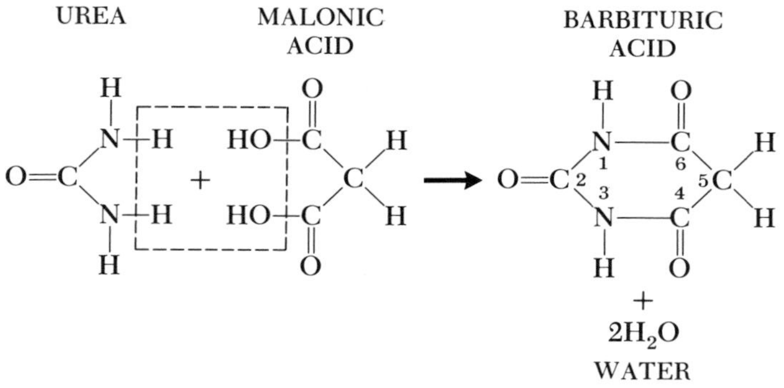

UREA            MALONIC            BARBITURIC
                  ACID                 ACID

**Figure 9.1**  Barbituric acid synthesis.

substituted barbituric acids are only slightly water soluble and possess $pK_a$'s between 7.3 and 8.4. The sodium salts of the barbiturates are readily soluble in water and form alkaline solutions. These solutions are not uniform in their stability at room temperature, and expiration dates can be found on the labels of the commercial barbiturate solutions.

In recent years, condensation products of a number of 5,5-disubstituted malonic acid compounds and thiourea have been produced and made commercially available. These agents are referred to as thiobarbiturates to distinguish them from the oxybarbiturates. Table 9.1 lists the structures of selected popular barbiturates.

CENTRAL NERVOUS SYSTEM EFFECTS. The barbiturate brings about both sedation and sleep through its depressant action (prolongation of neuronal recovery time following passage of an impulse) on the neurons in the central nervous system. Two significant questions as yet do not have complete answers. As general neuronal depressants, why do barbiturates depress the various functional components to varying degrees, when given in small doses; and how do the barbiturates interact with living tissue at the molecular level so as to bring about their well-known effects?

Since the outstanding work of Moruzzi and Magoun in 1949,[2] the functions of the brain stem reticular formation and its role in the phenomena of man's conscious and unconscious states have been described and corroborated by many investigations. In general terms, all the evidence thus far accumulated would indicate that the barbiturates produce an imbalance between the brain's inhibitory and facilitory mechanisms. The clinical effects of barbiturates are not due to the progressive, uniform depression of all centrally

# Table 9.1. Names, Structures, Doses of Selected Barbiturates

| Barbiturate | Commercial Name | R | $R_1$ | $R_2$ | X | Hypnotic Dose[a] (grams) |
|---|---|---|---|---|---|---|
| **LONG-ACTING** | | | | | | |
| Barbital | Veronal | ethyl | ethyl | H | O | 0.3–0.5 |
| Mephobarbital | Mebaral | ethyl | phenyl | CH₃ | O | (b) |
| Metharbital | Gemonil | ethyl | ethyl | CH₃ | O | (b) |
| Phenobarbital | Luminal | ethyl | phenyl | H | O | 0.1–0.2 |
| **SHORT- TO INTERMEDIATE-ACTING** | | | | | | |
| Amobarbital | Amytal | ethyl | isoamyl | H | O | 0.1–0.2 |
| Butabarbital | Butisol | ethyl | sec-butyl | H | O | 0.1 |
| Pentobarbital | Nembutal | ethyl | 1-methylbutyl | H | O | 0.1 |
| Secobarbital | Seconal | allyl | 1-methylbutyl | H | O | 0.1 |
| Vinbarbital | Delvinal | ethyl | 1-methyl-1-butenyl | H | O | 0.1–0.2 |
| **ULTRASHORT-ACTING** | | | | | | |
| Hexobarbital | Evipal | methyl | cyclohexenyl | CH₃ | O | (c) |
| Methohexital | Brevital | allyl | 1-methyl-2-pentynyl | CH₃ | O | (c) |
| Thiamylal | Surital | allyl | 1-methylbutyl | H | S | (c) |
| Thiopental | Pentothal | ethyl | 1-methylbutyl | H | S | (c) |

a = Oral adult hypnotic dose in grams; (b) = used as antiepileptic agent only; (c) = used as intravenous anesthetic.

located neurons. Indeed, under the influence of barbiturates, the excitability of certain neuronal pathways is greatly enhanced. Thus inhibition or depression of the central nervous system is not simply the reduction or lack of excitability, but to the contrary an active process.

Barbiturates depress the neuronal activity of the brain stem reticular formation. With the exception of several barbiturates, this action is observed under experimental conditions at a time when the drug directly depresses cortical cells. The brain stem reticular formation receives collaterals from the major afferent sensory pathways and sends facilitory impulses (the ascending reticular activating system) to the cortex to produce behavioral arousal or an increase in attentiveness. The brain stem reticular formation also sends inhibitory impulses to the cortex.

Under the proper conditions, the barbiturates appear to have the greatest affinity for those ascending brain stem reticular processes that send inhibitory impulses to the cortex. Such drug-induced depression causes a "release" phenomenon with the overall clinical picture of excitement. This may well explain the phase of delirium or stage of excitement patients are observed to pass through when slow intravenous infusions of a barbiturate are being given. In addition, it is tempting to suggest (i.e., definitive evidence is still required) that this indirect excitatory action of the barbiturate underlies the reason why small children may respond to the pedodontist's use of barbiturate premedication by becoming more highly excited than before they received the barbiturate.

The most commonly observed and clinically desirable effects of barbiturates on the central nervous system, i.e., sedation or hypnosis, result from the appropriate depression of both the ascending inhibitory and ascending facilitory impulses from the brain stem reticular formation plus their ability to depress directly cortical neuronal activity almost simultaneously with their depression of the subcortical reticular formation. The fact that the sleeping patient as a result of a barbiturate can be awakened by external stimuli would indicate that the major lemniscal afferent sensory pathways, as well as the Betz cells of the motor cortex, are not so depressed during barbiturate hypnosis that they are unable to function.

As the amount of administered barbiturate is increased above hypnotic doses, more generalized central nervous system depression occurs almost identical to that observed during general anesthesia. The most resistant functional area of the central nervous system to the barbiturates is that of the vital centers located in the medulla oblongata. With a sufficient dose, however, the barbiturates rapidly lead to fatal depression of the central respiratory mechanisms. The recorded barbiturate preference of those who have successfully committed suicide bears silent testimony to the drug's ability to depress acutely and permanently the vital centers of the central nervous system.

The sedative-hypnotic effects of the barbiturates may be explained in the following grossly oversimplified manner. The cortical cells' response to incoming excitatory impulses depends to a large extent upon their background level of excitability at the moment. This level of excitability is determined by the balance of facilitory and inhibitory impulses that are impinging upon the cortical cells at this time. The rostral portion of the brain stem reticular formation includes the ascending reticular activating system which, when appropriately excited by afferent sensory impulses, produces behavioral arousal or awakening. The activating system via the diffuse projecting system increases the background level of excitability of the cortical cells.

Afferent sensory impulses bearing the characteristics, instant by instant, of our internal and external environment are continuously arriving at the cells of the sensory cortex via the major lemniscal pathway. How these impulses are subsequently interpreted and what our behavioral response to them will be as a result depends upon the background level of excitability of the cortical cells.

In therapeutic doses the barbiturates depress neuronal activity of the ascending reticular activating system of the brain stem as well as directly depress the excitability of the cortical cells. Under the influence of a barbiturate, the afferent sensory impulses upon arrival find the cortical cells depressed, and the impulses no longer are interpreted as something to be apprehensive about. The person's level of awareness to his surroundings is reduced by the drug. The degree of this drug-induced reduction in awareness is referred to as sedation when the patient is awake but a little drowsy so that he no longer appears too concerned with his internal or external surroundings. Exposing the sedated patient to sufficiently intense stimuli can override the drug-elevated threshold, and behavioral arousal can result.

When the hypnotic dose of barbiturate has been administered, the usual incoming afferent sensory impulses are no longer sufficient to excite the ascending reticular activating system of the brain stem, and the patient falls asleep. When the tissue concentration of barbiturate decreases or the natural level of environmental stimuli increases, the patient again awakens to a state of drowsiness.

In anesthetic doses, the barbiturates so depress the central nervous system in general that the patient no longer can be aroused by the application of external stimuli. In this event, a return to consciousness is dependent more upon the rate at which the tissue concentration of barbiturate decreases.

ANALGESIC EFFECT. Perhaps some practitioners remember only that when a barbiturate is administered as a general intravenous anesthetic, one of the drug's noted effects is some degree of analgesia. Therefore, it is believed incorrectly that when a barbiturate is administered orally in sedative or hypnotic doses, the barbiturate will also manifest analgesic effects. In reality, just the opposite occurs. Patients in moderate to severe pain are not sedated nor do they go to sleep if given only a barbiturate. Such patients are apt to become confused and hysterical because they can no longer control their posture with accuracy or respond in terms of time and spacial discriminations with the same precision as they could before the barbiturate was given, and yet at the same time pain perception has not been significantly altered.

When given alone, barbiturates are not analgesics. It has been demonstrated that even in doses that almost produce a loss of consciousness, the barbiturate can produce only a slight (20%) increase in the cutaneous pain threshold.

ANTICONVULSANT EFFECTS. When barbiturates are administered in doses sufficient to produce general anesthesia, they are capable of counteracting an existing generalized seizure or convulsions as well as preventing the clinical manifestations of convulsions induced either electrically or chemically. This anticonvulsant property is common to all nonselective central nervous system depressants that are sufficiently potent to produce a state of general anesthesia. Although this type of depressant activity is not unique to the barbiturates, their anticonvulsant action, from a practical, clinical point of view, is one of the barbiturates major attributes.

It is true that all hypnotic barbiturates are anticonvulsants, but it is not correct to state that all barbiturates are clinically effective antiepileptic agents. Although the difference may not be appreciated by the nonepileptic, it is by the epileptic patient. The goal of antiepileptic pharmacotherapeutics is not only to keep the patient seizure free but also to allow him to remain a functional member of society. In the anticonvulsant-induced state of central nervous system depression the former is certainly accomplished, but the latter is not. Only a few barbiturates possess antiepileptic properties (e.g., phenobarbital, mephobarbital, and metharbital) because of their more selective depression of the central nervous system.

RESPIRATORY EFFECTS. The barbiturates depress respiration. However, in the doses utilized clinically for sedation or hypnosis, the barbiturates cause no greater reduction in man's respiratory exchange than does natural sleep, but patients who are taking other central nervous system depressants at the time a barbiturate is given readily exhibit a decrease in respiration to the point of hypoxia. Dental patients who have pulmonary emphysema are unusually sensitive to the respiratory depressant effects of barbiturates.

The barbiturates have been demonstrated to depress directly the sensitivity of the medullary respiratory center to its natural stimulus, carbon dioxide. When the patient's respiration is profoundly depressed by a barbiturate, it is the patient's hypoxic condition that then maintains the respiration, shallow though it is. In such a situation the administration of oxygen alone may produce apnea because the carotid body chemoreceptor mechanism will no longer drive the respiration. The patient must be given oxygen and, in addition, respiration must be maintained artificially. Adequate tissue oxygenation can be maintained for some time by this procedure, even though the patient will not breathe on his own owing to the barbiturate. Barbiturates cross the placental barrier and depress the respiration of the fetus even in small oral doses that may not greatly depress the mother's gaseous exchange.

VASOMOTOR CENTER EFFECTS. Barbiturates, when given orally, alone and in sedative or hypnotic amounts, rarely cause a significant alteration in the arterial blood pressure, cardiac rate, rhythm, or minute output in man. Any alteration in these circulatory parameters may be accredited to the patient's reduced physical activity or state of sleep. This does not mean, however, that the barbiturates have no effect upon the circulation. They do depress neuronal activity in the medullary vasomotor center, but this depression is usually adequately compensated for by a readjustment peripherally.

It would be well advised for the dental practitioner to be cautious in his administration of barbiturates to patients with either untreated arterial hypertension or with drug-controlled hypertensive disease. In the former patient the depressant effect of barbiturates on the central vasomotor area is greatly exaggerated, leading to a transient but precipitous fall in blood pressure. In the latter patient, the barbiturate action when added to that of the various antihypertensive agents often results in syncope due to an acute transient hypotensive episode.

AUTONOMIC NERVOUS SYSTEM EFFECTS. Once again in the dosage usually prescribed for either sedation or hypnosis, the barbiturates produce few clinical manifestations in man as a result of interference with normal autonomic functions. When administered intravenously too rapidly, the barbiturate produces a transient blockade of autonomic ganglia. This action most assuredly would result in a fall in mean arterial blood pressure, and this must be carefully considered by the dental practitioner who, in the emergency situation, might administer a barbiturate as an anticonvulsant. Not all barbiturates are equally effective in inhibiting ganglionic transmission; the most effective in this regard is amobarbital, and the least effective is thiopental.

OTHER EFFECTS. In the usual oral sedative or hypnotic doses prescribed for adults, the barbiturates produce few effects that cannot be attributed to the patient's drug-induced reduction in physical activity. There has been no confirmed, clinical evidence reported that the barbiturates, in the usual adult dosages, cause directly any significant irreversible change in skeletal muscle activity, renal function, liver function, metabolism, or the normal functions of the gastrointestinal tract. Evidence has been reported, however, that hypnotic doses of phenobarbital in children lead to a considerable reduction in the renal elimination of potasssium.[3] In addition, two of the antiepilpetic barbiturates, phenobarbital and mephobarbital, can produce a megaloblastic anemia upon prolonged daily use. Fortunately, this drug-induced disease responds favorably to folic acid.

ABSORPTION. The barbiturates can be administered in the form of their water-soluble sodium salts or as the almost water-insoluble acid. Aqueous solutions of the sodium salts are alkaline (e.g., the pH of a phenobarbital sodium aqueous solution is 9.3). Most often the barbiturates are administered orally, rectally, intravenously, or intramuscularly. These weak organic acids in aqueous solution with a pH of 1 to 2 (gastric contents) are almost totally in their nonionized, lipid-soluble form which readily crosses the lipoid membrane of the gastric mucosa. Therefore, the barbiturates are rapidly absorbed into the circulation following oral ingestion. In the aqueous, less acidic solution of the upper small intestine (pH 6.7) more of the barbiturate is in its charged or ionized, less absorbable form. However, with the pH of the intestinal contents at 6.7, still over 50% of the barbiturate in solution would be in the nonionized, lipid-soluble form that readily crosses into the circulation. The oral route of administration is the most frequently used clinically unless the barbiturate is to be given for its general anesthetic or anticonvulsant properties in which case it is the sodium salt of the barbiturate in aqueous solution that is injected intravenously.

DISTRIBUTION. Like most drugs, a barbiturate must be transported via the circulation to its site of action where the drug must reach a certain concentration in order to be effective. Many factors influence the barbiturate's distribution. One of the important influences is the binding of barbiturates to plasma proteins. In this reversibly bound form, the barbiturate is not all free to diffuse into the various tissues as the drug initially flows through. Each barbiturate is bound to plasma protein to a different extent. Thiopental appears to be bound to the extent of 90% of the drug's circulating concentration, whereas barbital is bound to plasma protein to the extent of approximately 15% of its circulating concentration. In general terms, the order of increasing percentage bound to plasma protein from 15% to 90% is as follows: barbital, phenobarbital, pentobarbital, secobarbital, and thiopental.

As the barbiturates diffuse out of the circulation and into the various tissues (down their concentration gradient), the rate of their penetration is determined to a large extent by the lipid solubility of their nonionized form. The relative order of lipid solubility for the aforementioned barbiturates in terms of lowest solubility to highest lipid solubility is barbital, phenobarbital, pentobarbital, secobarbital, and thiopental. Therefore, although there is much more nonplasma protein-bound barbital that could penetrate into tissue from the circulation, its diffusion into the tissue is relatively slow owing to the low lipid solubility of nonionized barbital. This information can be correlated with the clinical evidence that even following intravenous administration there is a considerable lag in the onset of barbital's action because of its low lipid solubility and slow diffusion into its brain site of action.

In most cases a drug's duration of action is determined mainly by the rate at which it is inactivated by metabolism or is physically eliminated by excretion. Considerable evidence now shows that such is not the case for the highly lipid-soluble barbiturate thiopental. The brief duration of action of the thiopental following intravenous administration is due to the drug's high lipid solubility and its redistribution from tissue to tissue according to the individual tissue's blood flow, amount of cardiac output received, and mass. Because the brain receives such a large percentage of the cardiac output, the initial high concentration of thiopental that can diffuse from the circulation does so first in the brain (thus, an immediate onset of action). In not too many circulation times or passes through the brain tissue, however, the plasma concentration of thiopental becomes much lower than that of the brain, and the effective concentration of thiopental rapidly falls at its site of action (thus, a very short duration of action). Because of its high lipid solubility, the drug eventually is accumulated in the adipose tissue (which receives a relatively poor blood supply) from which it is slowly released and metabolized.

METABOLISM. The major site for barbiturate metabolism in man is the liver. The enzymes of the microsomal fraction catalyze the oxidative dealkylation of the carbon-5 substituted side chain. More polar and thus more rapidly excreted metabolites are formed.

One of the available barbiturates, barbital, is not metabolized by the body and is excreted essentially unchanged in the urine. Two other barbiturates, phenobarbital and aprobarbital, have approximately 20 to 25% of a single dose unchanged by metabolic processes. For the remaining barbiturates, including thiopental, extensive metabolic alterations of structure occur in the liver, bringing about their inactivation. In general terms, side chain oxidation is rapid for the long, unsaturated, branched chains and is progressively slower as the side chain is shorter and saturated. The thiobarbiturates are desulfurated, and those nitrogen-substituted barbiturates (e.g., mephobarbital) are N-dealkylated.

There is difference of opinion recently regarding the durations of actions of the various clinically available barbiturates.[4] For many years the barbiturates have been classified according to their relative duration of action into usually four groups; the long-acting, the intermediate-acting, the short-acting, and the ultrashort-acting. Such a categorization was based upon animal studies and not upon clinical investigations. There would not be any great dilemma if it were not for the fact that the young dental school graduate actually uses such a classification in the selection of a barbiturate for a particular patient. There is no problem regarding the barbiturates of choice as general anesthetics. It is also apparent that the usual sedative doses of the various barbiturates used for this purpose all show a clinical duration of action between 6 and 8 hours. The controversy involves the duration of action of the usual hypnotic doses in man. It would appear that barbiturates traditionally classed as long-acting produce a period of sleep lasting 6 to 8 hours, and the intermediate-acting and short-acting hypnotic barbiturates induce sleep lasting between 3 and 8 hours. It is also believed that a period of 6 to 8 hours of drug-induced sedation follows the hypnotic effect of all barbiturates. Perhaps the differences in actual duration of hypnotic effect are clinically insignificant, but since the classification is a relative matter in the first place, it should be maintained if for no other reason than general simplicity.

EXCRETION. The major pathway of excretion of the barbiturates is the kidney. The drugs or their metabolites go into the urine. Only barbital and, to a much lesser degree, phenobarbital are excreted in the urine in an unchanged form.

CAUTIONS, SIDE EFFECTS, AND CONTRAINDICATIONS. The cautions to be remembered prior to prescribing a sedative or hypnotic drug may be considered in general terms, as well as in specific terms, depending upon the effects desired and the particular agent to be used.

The nature of the actions of these agents requires the practitioner to consider how active the patient intends to be while taking the drug. The patient must be warned that even in sedative amounts these agents may subtly so impair his spatial judgment that the driving of an automobile or the working with or around machinery with exposed moving parts may be extremely hazardous and should therefore be avoided. It may be wise for the dental practitioner to make a general office rule that whenever a patient is to take a drug of this class, a responsible adult must accompany the patient to the dentist's office and be nearby at home.

The nonselective central nervous system depressants can be expected to interact with many other drugs. The sedative-hypnotic action is increased in degree and duration by other nonselective central nervous system depressants, such as ethyl alcohol, the intake of which by the patient is not of course under the practitioner's control, but the patient should be warned about the hazards. Of the selective central nervous system depressants the phenothiazine antipsychotic agents greatly augment the depressant action of the sedative-hypnotics. The antidepressant monoamine oxidase inhibitors as well as the narcotic analgesics similarly increase these drugs' effects. The practitioner must also keep in mind that many other types of compounds, such as a number of the antihistamines, have a central nervous system depressant activity, and these also potentiate the sedative-hypnotics.

The patient whose arterial blood pressure is under the control of an antihypertensive agent may experience a precipitous fall in blood pressure when given a barbiturate, owing to the depressant effect upon the vasomotor center. Since the sedative-hypnotics possess some degree of respiratory depressant activity, their administration to patients with various pulmonary insufficiency disorders (e.g., emphysema) is definitely contraindicated.

The practitioner must become far more aware in the future of the many detrimental drug interactions that he can unwittingly precipitate. The barbiturates (especially phenobarbital) have been shown to induce the formation of microsomal enzymes which normally metabolize other drugs, such as the coumarin anticoagulants. Under the influence of the sedative-hypnotic, the coumarin's effectiveness may disappear unless its dosage is increased. Of course, the anticoagulant dosage must be reduced when the barbiturate is no longer taken, or the symptoms of anticoagulant overdosage will occur. The metabolism of phenytoin is also agumented by phenobarbital.

When the dental practitioner's patient happens to be a drug-controlled epileptic who may require some further form of sedation before dental treatment, it is mandatory for the practitioner to work closely with the patient's neurologist in the selection and administration of the appropriate agent.

The barbiturates are absolutely contraindicated in patients with acute intermittent porphyria, as well as in those who have manifested previous allergic reactions to one of the barbiturates.[5] Hypersensitivity reactions to the barbiturates are well known and usually involve the skin. These reactions include generalized morbilliform type of rash, urticaria, bullous erythema multiforme, and angioneurotic edema. Fortunately, such drug-induced conditions usually are reversed by the withdrawal of the drug.

When it comes to untoward side effects, the barbiturates have not spared the dental profession. It took only two years after the introduction of the barbiturates at the turn of the last century before stomatitis medicamentosa due to barbital was reported in the literature.[6] For further references and a review of this condition, the reader is referred to the work of Kennett.[7]

The sedative-hypnotics have been known to induce a variety of unexpected or idiosyncratic reactions. Perhaps the most often observed and distressing to patient and practitioner alike is the opposite response to what the sedative-hypnotic is expected to produce, i.e., excitement. Although the clinical data are convincing only in respect to establishing that this paradoxical reaction does occur, many suggest that young children and the elderly show the highest incidence.

ACUTE AND CHRONIC INTOXICATION. An adequate review of acute and chronic barbiturate intoxication is beyond the scope of this chapter. The reader is referred to several excellent discussions in this most important area.[8, 9]

There is no question but that tolerance develops to some of the effects of barbiturates, but it must be clearly understood that little tolerance develops to the lethal dose of the barbiturates; this is in contrast to the development of a high grade tolerance to the narcotic analgesics. Whereas the heroin abuser may easily develop (and with some rapidity) tolerance to ten lethal doses of the drug, the barbiturate abuser must ever be watchful of his dosage because, if he exceeds his maximally tolerated dose by as little as 100 mg, he may find himself in profound coma. It almost goes without saying that because of the barbiturate abuser's mentally confused state his continued existence day to day is most difficult to predict.

### Nonbarbiturates

Prior to the introduction of the barbiturates, three nonbarbiturate sedative-hypnotics, in particular, had enjoyed widespread use. There were the inorganic bromide salts, chloral hydrate and paraldehyde. In the general practice of dentistry today there would be no reason to use any of the bromides or paraldehyde as sedative-hypnotics. The same can be said for the practice of medicine.

Chloral hydrate and its several derivatives are enjoying a comeback in therapeutics, and their use in dentistry is well known.

During the 1950's a number of nonbarbiturate sedative-hypnotics were introduced, and most are still available. In general, none of these newer agents has offered any superior properties or fewer toxic side effects than those already possessed by the barbiturates. Perhaps the only justification for these newer agents is the occasional patient who cannot tolerate a barbiturate for a variety of reasons and who requires a sedative-hypnotic. Even in these instances, chloral hydrate could be prescribed. All of the nonbarbiturate sedative-hypnotics have been reported to induce drug dependence.

CHLORAL HYDRATE (NOCTEC). Chloral hydrate was first synthesized in 1832 but was not introduced as a hypnotic until 1869. It was originally thought that chloral hydrate was slowly converted to chloroform by the body because of in vitro evidence that chloral hydrate reacted with alkali to form chloroform. It was later learned that chloral hydrate was reduced in the body to another compound that was responsible for its sedative-hypnotic activity.[10] That compound is trichloroethanol.

The nonselective central nervous system depressant action of chloral hydrate does not differ significantly from that of the barbiturates when both are administered orally. Chloral hydrate possesses little, if any, analgesic activity other than that which would normally be observed by sleep alone. Indeed, chloral hydrate has been reported to produce excitement and confusion in the patient who is in pain.

Chloral hydrate is an effective anticonvulsant, but a barbiturate or diazepam is definitely the drug of choice in the emergency control of acute convulsions. Like the barbiturates, chloral hydrate when given in sufficient amounts can produce general anesthesia, but the barbiturates are preferred.

It is often stated in texts that chloral hydrate causes a much lower incidence of excitement or delirium in children and the elderly in contrast to the barbiturates. Indeed, chloral hydrate is currently widely used as a premedication in pedodontics in preference to barbiturates assumedly because of this property of the nonbarbiturate. There is a definite paucity of well-controlled clinical studies to prove or disprove this belief.

Chloral hydrate in therapeutic amounts has little effect upon respiration or the cardiovascular system. At least the drug causes no greater alteration in these systems than nondrug-induced sleep.

Unfortunately, chloral hydrate is a highly irritating substance to both skin and mucous membranes. If the drug is ingested orally without properly diluting it with water or if it is given on a empty stomach, chloral hydrate causes a high incidence of gastric irritation with its normal sequelae of nausea and vomiting. These irritating effects have now been mostly avoided by the use of derivative compounds that slowly release chloral hydrate into the gastric contents. Such drugs include petrichloral (Perichlor) and chloral betaine (Betachlor).

Chloral hydrate is readily absorbed from the gastrointestinal tract and converted mainly in the liver to trichlorethanol, the active sedative-hypnotic metabolite, and to a smaller extent to tricholoracetic acid. The major end product excreted in the urine is the glucuronide of trichloroethanol known as urochloralic acid. Some urochloralic acid is also secreted in bile.

Both acute and chronic intoxication to chloral hydrate are known in man. Acute intoxication closely resembles that of barbiturate overdosage with the additional hazard that liver damage is likely following huge accidental overdosages of the drug (certainly not unusual for a halogenated hydrocarbon). The average adult lethal dose is estimated to be approximately 10 gm.

Chloral hydrate should not be given as such to patients with a history of gastrointestinal ulcerations. Nor is it wise to administer the agent in the presence of either cardiac, renal, or liver insufficiency. Dermatitis has also been reported following this hynotic's ingestion.

ETHCHLORVYNOL (PLACIDYL). Ethchlorvynol is a sedative-hypnotic which is a liquid at room temperature and is administered orally in the form of liquid-filled capsules. The compound is rapidly absorbed and best given with milk or with meals. This precaution eliminates much of the giddiness and ataxia observed if the drug is taken on an empty stomach.

Ethchlorvynol would appear to produce less respiratory depression than an equivalent amount of barbiturate. An interesting feature of this sedative-hypnotic is the difficulty with which general anesthesia is obtained in experimental animals. Ethchlorvynol does possess some skeletal muscle-relaxing properties as well as anticonvulsant activity. It has been utilized on a limited scale in the treatment of epilepsy in man. The agent is not an analgesic and is of little, if any, value as a sedative for patients who are seriously disturbed or who are in pain. Dependence has been reported with the drug's use.

METHYPRYLON (NOLUDAR). This nonbarbiturate sedative-hypnotic shows its major usefulness as a daytime sedative. Methyprylon does not possess significant analgesic, muscle relaxant, anticonvulsant, antiemetic, or antipyretic properties; it is also not useful as a general anesthetic agent. Methyprylon depresses respiration to a lesser extent than do the barbiturates. Its side effects are similar to those of the barbiturates with the additional problem that methyprylon is converted in the body to tetrahydropyridine (up to 3% found in urine following methyprylon administration). Although direct evidence has not been given for methyprylon, it is known that its metabolite has been implicated in causing agranulocytosis. In therapeutic dosage there is as yet no evidence that the drug is toxic to the kidneys, liver, or bone marrow.

METHAQUALONE (QUAALUDE). The most recent nonbarbiturate sedative-hypnotic agent to become available is methaqualone. It would appear to offer absolutely nothing more, and maybe less, than what the barbiturates can do so well. In reality, it is unfair to make any judgment regarding methaqualone since it is so new. It is used both as a sedative and as a hypnotic, but paresthesias of the extremities have been reported to occur prior to the onset of sleep, especially if the patient is prevented from going to sleep once having taken the drug.

Methaqualone dependence is known. Perhaps the most serious early problem associated with this agent is the report of one case of aplastic anemia that is related to this drug. It should not be prescribed for those with liver or renal damage, nor to children under 14 years of age nor to pregnant women or even those who might become pregnant.

## ANTIANXIETY AGENTS

The group of psychopharmacological agents known officially as the antianxiety agents used to be called the minor tranquilizers, minor ataractics, and even anxiolytic sedatives. The antianxiety agents are used to treat symptomatically the fears, apprehensions, and tensions in patients with neuroses and depressive states. These drugs are also used in those who are mentally normal but who react adversely to unusual environmental stress. These drugs are also grossly misused today for masking every little stress of life.

There are three groups of antianxiety agents classified by their chemical structures: (1) the substituted diols (glycerols or carbamates), (2) the benzodiazepines, and (3) the diphenylmethanes. Although each group consists of a number of derivatives commercially available, only the prototypes of each group will be considered, i.e., meprobamate (Equanil; Miltown), diazepam (Valium), and hydroxyzine (Atarax), respectively. There are many different, effective ways of approaching the learning of the pharmacology of any particular drug class. The antianxiety agents are best learned by comparisons of their effects and will be presented in that manner. First, the antianxiety agents as a group will be compared with the antipsychotic agents; then, meprobamate as the oldest member of the antianxiety agents will be compared with the sedative barbiturates; and, lastly, one antianxiety prototype will be compared with another.

COMPARISON WITH ANTIPSYCHOTIC AGENTS. Table 9.2 compares the general effects of the antianxiety agents and the antipsychotic agents. It will be noted that both groups produce emotional calmness and mental relaxation. However, these important effects are shown by the antipsychotic agents primarily in a patient who has schizophrenia and not in the patient who is experiencing neurosis or some form of situational anxiety. If the selected antipsychotic agent does show some effectiveness in the treatment of pretreatment apprehension, it is due to the drug's ability to produce some sedation as a side effect. The antianxiety agents, on the other hand, best demonstrate their ability to produce emotional calmness and mental relaxation in the patient with neuroses or situational anxiety and are practically useless in the patient with schizophrenia. The other similarities and differences shown in Table 9.2 are self-explanatory.

MEPROBAMATE COMPARED WITH BARBITURATES. The antianxiety agents, as exemplified by meprobamate, are continuously compared in the clinical literature with the sedative barbiturates, such as phenobarbital. Since the sedation-producing barbiturates have been used so much longer and so much is known about their desired and undesired effects, it only seems natural to compare the newer antianxiety agents with these effects. In man, phenobarbital and meprobamate produce a number of similar effects. Both drugs may be shown to produce at a lower dose an antianxiety effect and at a higher dose a sedative effect. This may be referred to as the drug's antianxiety-sedative ratio. Meprobamate demonstrates a higher ratio at the therapeutic dose levels than does phenobarbital.

## Table 9.2. Comparison of Antipsychotic and Antianxiety Agents

EFFECTS OF ANTIPSYCHOTIC AGENTS

1. Produce emotional calmness and mental relaxation.
2. Only some agents possess sedative side effects.
3. Highly effective in controlling symptoms of acutely and chronically disturbed, especially schizophrenia.
4. Cause reversible extrapyramidal symptoms in susceptible patients.
5. Little to no tendency to produce physical dependence or habituation.
6. In usual doses do not depress cortex.
7. Possess varying degrees of autonomic effects.

EFFECTS OF ANTIANXIETY AGENTS

1. Produce emotional calmness and mental relaxation but not of the same quality as that induced by antipschotic agents.
2. Do not possess antipsychotic activity.
3. Particularly effective in treatment of common psychoneurotic states such as nervous tension, mild depression, psychosomatic disorders.
4. Do not produce extrapyramidal symptoms and have relatively low incidence of annoying side effects.
5. Some physical dependence may occur, depending on dose taken and duration of therapy.
6. May have some degree of cortical depression activity, especially in higher doses.
7. Generally less effect on peripheral autonomic nervous system.
8. Some anticonvulsant properties.
9. Depressant activity on spinal reflex activity (polysynaptic reflexes).

The actual difference between the antianxiety effect and the sedative effect is difficult to define, indeed, if there is any valid difference. In both conditions the patient experiences quietening of mental processes and lessening of muscle tension, but sedation also includes a greater degree of drowsiness, a greater lack of spatial judgment, and a greater degree of possible euphoria. Generally speaking, Americans tend to prefer the sedative type of effect for their anxiety because the sedative effect can be felt and related to the effects produced by ethyl alcohol in low doses.

Neither meprobamate nor phenobarbital is effective in the treatment of the more serious mental illnesses (psychoses). They possess no antipsychotic properties and, moreover, may even worsen the psychotic state. As may be expected, neither drug produces extrapyramidal or parkinsonian side effects that are so frequently observed in the patient taking antipsychotic agents, such as chlorpromazine (Thorazine).

Both meprobamate and phenobarbital lead to tolerance development, psychological dependence (habituation), and physical dependence, but in each of these parameters meprobamate exceeds phenobarbital. Much more severe dependence develops to meprobamate than to phenobarbital. The withdrawal symptoms caused by the separation of the physically dependent person from either drug produces a similar pattern in type, severity, and duration. Grand mal type of seizures is common to both, and death during withdrawal has been reported for both drugs.

Unlike the antipsychotic agents, both meprobamate and phenobarbital depress both conditioned and unconditioned responses in experimental animals as well as in man.

Meprobamate and phenobarbital are both anticonvulsants. Indeed, phenobarbital has been used clinically as an effective antiepileptic agent for many years. Although meprobamate has enjoyed some service as an antiepileptic agent, its effectiveness cannot really compare with that of phenobarbital. Both drugs cause cortical depression at higher doses, but this is seen much more readily with any barbiturate. Both drugs are alike in that neither possesses any antihistaminic or antiemetic effects, which are common to many antipsychotic agents. Neither meprobamate nor phenobarbital affects the autonomic nervous system or the endocrine systems at sedative doses. Lastly, these two agents depress the spinal polysynaptic pathways, an effect which contributes to their ability to relax skeletal muscle (or more accurately, relieve muscle tension). There is little doubt that, at therapeutic dose levels, this central muscle relaxing property is more characteristic of meprobamate.

MEPROBAMATE AND PHENOBARBITAL. Some noteworthy differences between meprobamate and phenobarbital bear mentioning in addition to those suggested above. For example, the two drugs certainly have different sites of major action in the central nervous system. Meprobamate's activity is mainly limited to the subcortical levels of the thalamus and limbic systems, whereas phenobarbital's sites of action most importantly include the cortex.

On a pharmacolgical basis the most striking difference between meprobamate and phenobarbital is their dose-response curves. Meprobamate possesses a shallow dose-response curve, whereas that of phenobarbital is much steeper. What this means clinically is that a small quantitative change in the dose will give a much greater change in response for phenobarbital than for meprobamate.

Other minor differences, at comparable doses, would include that meprobamate produces less respiratory depression, less sleepiness, more muscle relaxation, a longer onset but shorter duration of withdrawal effects, a lower overall acute toxicity and incidence of side effects, less depression of performance ability (e.g., auto driving), and a lower incidence of initial central nervous system excitation or confusion in the very young and the elderly.

MEPROBAMATE AND DIAZEPAM (VALIUM). In general terms, diazepam possesses all the similarities and differences in relation to phenobarbital as discussed for meprobamate, but there are some important or significant differences between diazepam and meprobamate which are shown in Table 9.3.

In addition to the differences listed in the table, and perhaps to explain some of those differences, the following may be mentioned. Diazepam and meprobamate do not share the same major sites of action in the central nervous system. Although both drugs exert their beneficial antianxiety action at subcortical levels, diazepam's action would appear to be limited to the limbic system (at equal antianxiety doses). Diazepam would also appear to possess an even more shallow dose-response curve than meprobamate.

HYDROXYZINE (ATARAX). The third group of antianxiety agents is the diphenylmethane subclass, which is exemplified by its prototype hydroxyzine (Atarax). This antianxiety agent is rarely used in adults in dentistry but widely used by the oral route in pedodontics. Hydroxyzine differs from both diazepam and meprobamate primarily in the range of undesired side effects. For example, hydroxyzine possesses more extensive effects on the peripheral autonomic nervous system. In striking contrast to diazepam, hydroxyzine actually increases skeletal muscle tone, lowers the convulsive threshold, and apparently lacks any potential for drug

### Table 9.3. Comparison of Two Antianxiety Agents (at Therapeutic Doses)

| | Diazepam | Meprobamate |
|---|---|---|
| Antianxiety action | Strong | Moderate |
| Sedation (drowsiness) | Weak | Moderate |
| "Taming" | Strong | Weak |
| Anticonvulsant | Strong | Moderate |
| Skeletal muscle relaxant | Strong–Moderate | Weak–Moderate |
| Impairment of performance | Weak–Moderate | Moderate–Strong |
| Block of aggressive behavior | Strong | Weak (without sedation) Moderate (with sedation) |
| Peripheral autonomic effects | Weak (anticholinergic) | None |
| Overall toxicity | Moderate | Strong |
| Tolerance and psychological dependence | Weak | Strong |

Drugs Used by the Dentist

dependence. These same characteristics apply to the other antihistamines with strong sedative effects, namely, diphenhydramine (Benadryl) and promethazine (Phenergan). Hydroxyzine is more likely to produce some feeling of inner restlessness or mental fuzziness rather than the well-known, slightly inebriated effect. This drug's effects are not liked by adults, which is no doubt the major reason no drug abuse has been reported for hydroxyzine (see Table 9.4).

## Use in Dentistry

Antianxiety agents are more and more widely used in general dentistry, as well as in the specialties. There are several important uses. The antianxiety agents are used in carefully selected patients who are unable to handle the emotional stress engendered by the situation of dental treatment. In other words, the drugs could be utilized in otherwise normal individuals who react adversely to this specific stress with situational anxiety. This becomes a form of patient management much like the use of a local anesthetic as in a special form of patient management.

It must be kept in mind there is nothing really so special about the antianxiety agents in terms of allaying patient anxiety in the dental office. For postpuberty and preelderly patients a 100 mg oral dose of secobarbital after the patient reaches the office will with great predictability relieve all nervousness.

### Table 9.4.  Selected Antianxiety Agents

| Generic Name | Trade Name | Adult Antianxiety Dose[a] | Onset of Action | Duration of Action |
|---|---|---|---|---|
| GLYCEROL DERIVATIVES | | | | |
| Meprobamate | Equanil | 400–800 mg | 60–120 min | 6–8 hr |
| Tybamate | Solacen | 250–500 mg | 60 min | 4–6 hr |
| Carisoprodol | Soma | 200–350 mg | 60–120 min | 4–6 hr |
| BENZODIAZEPINE DERIVATIVES | | | | |
| Chlordiazepoxide | Librium | 5–25 mg | 6–8 hr | 24 hr |
| Diazepam | Valium | 2–10 mg | 30–60 min | 12 hr |
| Oxazepam | Serax | 10–15 mg | 30–60 min | 6 hr |
| ANTIHISTAMINE DERIVATIVES | | | | |
| Hydroxyzine | Atarax | 25–100 mg | 60 min | 4–6 hr |
| Promethazine | Phenergan | 25–50  mg | 60 min | 4–6 hr |

a = All doses are to be given orally.

It has been suggested only recently that the antianxiety agents be used for the actual symptomatic (or masking) treatment of dental patients who manifest oral soft tissue lesions, e.g., lichen planus, which are believed to be a result, partially perhaps, of mild to moderate neurotic states. Let it be understood that only certain instances of oral soft tissue lesions appear to have an affective component; therefore, use of these agents in a dental patient for these reasons should be in consultation with the patient's physician.

## Cautions, Side Effects, and Contraindications

Quite obviously the antianxiety agents possess adverse as well as beneficial effects. The Medical Letter almost annually publishes an updated listing of the adverse effects of these agents.[11] The most commonly seen side effect with all the antianxiety agents is drowsiness (the same may be said for the sedative barbiturates). There are, in addition, a number of specific, straightforward precautions to consider prior to the administration of the agent. Care must be exercised in elderly and especially debilitated patients, since these individuals give the highest incidence of hyperreactions. The glaucomatous patient must not receive diazepam or hydroxyzine because of their anticholinergic side effects. Since physical and psychomotor performance is affected, all patients must be warned not to operate an automobile or to work around open machinery. Both diazepam and meprobamate have recently been identified as teratogenic agents.[12] Therefore, these drugs are not to be administered to patients of child-bearing age or in the first trimester of pregnancy.

The antianxiety agents interact unfavorably with a number of other drugs the patient may be taking. For instance, ethyl alcohol greatly potentiates the effects of diazepam;[13] therefore, the dental patient who receives diazepam must be warned to abstain from ethyl alcohol for at least 24 hours.

The antianxiety agents synergize with the central nervous system depressant effects of the barbiturate and nonbarbiturate sedative-hypnotics, the narcotic analgesics (caution in posttreatment analgesic prescribing!), the antipsychotic agents, and the antidepressant monoamine oxidase inhibitors.

Lastly, it must be noted that the cost to the patient for oral sedatives varies widely, with the lowest for a barbiturate and the highest for an antianxiety agent.[13]

## INHALATIONAL SEDATIVES

Nitrous oxide has a long history, often involving controversy, and the mention of the drug's name can still polarize almost any gathering of the dental profession. Nitrous oxide is enjoying at the present time another cycle of popularity in dentistry.

Let it be clearly understood from the outset that nitrous oxide is *not* used today in clinical outpatient dentistry as a general anesthetic agent; nitrous oxide is *not* used today in clinical outpatient dentistry as an analgesic; nitrous oxide *is* used today in clinical outpatient dentistry as an inhalational sedative (i.e., a sedative administered by the inhalation route)—nothing more, nothing less. Nitrous oxide certainly does not replace the local anesthetic.

It has been a little over 200 years since man first synthesized nitrous oxide, although it has made up a small part of our atmosphere for millions of years. Nitrous oxide is still prepared commercially today by heating ammonium nitrate to about 260°C

$$NH_4NO_3 - - - - - - - \rightarrow N_2O + 2H_2O$$
$$\text{heat} -260°C$$

In this process nitrous oxide and water are not the only products. Once nitrous oxide is made, the drug-gas must be carefully washed and separated from both water and a number of impurities, all of which are hazardous to human health. The drug-gas is then subjected to many atmospheres of pressure, whereupon the colorless gas is compressed to a clear, colorless liquid with a specific gravity less than that of water. The liquid which boils at $-88.4°C$ is stored in familiar regulation size, color-coded metal tanks or cylinders. Selected physicochemical properties of nitrous oxide are shown in Table 9.5.

In the tank you would find nitrous oxide liquid, and above the liquid, nitrous oxide vapor—all absolutely water free. When the valve is opened, the gauge will show steadily a certain pressure between 700 and 800 pounds per square inch throughout most of the use of the gas from the cylinder. Each time the valve is opened and some of the gas escapes, the released gas is instantly replaced in the tank by an equal amount of gas from the vaporization of the liquid. For the liquid to vaporize requires a large amount of heat which comes from the metal tank walls. Vaporization greatly cools the tank, and if humidity in the room is high or the tank's outside surface is wettened, ice forms on the tank walls. As soon as the liquid is all converted to vapor and allowed to escape via the valve, the gauge pressure will fall to zero.

As shown in Table 9.5, nitrous oxide is not explosive or flammable but will support combustion, even in the absence of oxygen, because nitrous oxide, when heated to 450°C breaks down to nitrogen and oxygen. The latter allows for combustion to occur.

## Table 9.5. Selected Physicochemical Properties of Nitrous Oxide

A. Chemical structure $\quad N\!=\!N$ with $O$

B. Molecular weight = 44.01

C. Slightly sweet-smelling, colorless gas at room temperature and one atmosphere of barometric pressure

D. Specific gravity of gas at $25°C = 1.53$ (Air = 1.00)

E. Under 50 atmospheres pressure, gas is compressed to a clear, colorless liquid
   1. Specific gravity of liquid at $15°C = 0.8$ (water = 1.0)
   2. Boiling point = $-88.4°C$

F. Neither the gaseous nor liquid forms are flammable, but the gas will support combustion

$$2\ N_2O \xrightarrow{\text{heat at } 450°C} 2\ N_2 + O_2$$

G. Selected partition coefficients
   1. Water/gas    = 0.43
   2. Blood/gas    = 0.47
   3. Oil/gas      = 1.4
   4. Oil/water    = 3.2
   5. Tissue/blood
      a. Vessel-rich  = 1.06
      b. Muscle-skin  = 1.13
      c. Fat          = 2.3
      d. Vessel-poor  = 1.0

ABSORPTION. Nitrous oxide is rapidly absorbed from the pulmonary alveoli into the circulation. There are factors, of course, that modify the rate of absorption. The most important principle involved is that of the influence of the concentration gradient. Any substance (nitrous oxide included) actually moves continually from an area where the substance is in higher concentration to an area where the substance is in lower concentration. The greater the difference in concentrations between two areas, the faster the movement of the substance to the lesser concentrated area. Essentially no one has nitrous oxide in his body at the moment; there is zero concentration in the respiratory alveoli. If the patient is required to breathe a mixture of gases containing nitrous oxide, the nitrous oxide would move rapidly from the mask to the alveoli down its concentration gradient. The higher the concentration at the mask, the more rapid the same concentration will develop in the alveoli.

Secondly, the patient's ventilation efficiency will determine how fast the nitrous oxide can reach the alveoli. Patients with an obstructed airway or various respiratory diseases (e.g., emphysema) can sharply alter the rate of absorption.

Thirdly, the higher the drug-gas's concentration in the alveoli, the higher the gradient from alveoli to blood and the faster the transfer.

SOLUBILITY IN BLOOD. The next major factor in getting the drug-gas absorbed is the solubility of the gas in blood. Nitrous oxide is relatively insoluble in blood, but contrary to what might appear on the surface to be logical, nitrous oxide's low blood solubility is a desirable property. A brief explanation is in order: when a gas dissolves in a liquid it does so in two different ways. The gas can *chemically* combine with some substance in the liquid and may be bound loosely or tightly. Secondly, the gas can *physically* dissolve as a gas separate from other chemicals in the liquid. It becomes an added, separate entity in the liquid; it remains as minute gas bubbles dispersed in the liquid. It is the physically dissolved gas that exerts the drug effects in the body.

Under normal conditions 100 ml of blood will carry about 45 ml of the gas in physical solution. To our knowledge nitrous oxide remains in the form of nitrous oxide throughout its sojourn in the body. It is not altered chemically in the body.

EXCRETION. The elimination of nitrous oxide from the body is relatively straightforward. When the high concentration at the mask is removed, the concentration gradient shifts in the opposite direction, and the nitrous oxide leaves the body in the expired air. Some small amounts of the drug-gas may be excreted by a number of other pathways.

EFFECTS. Nitrous oxide is known to produce predictable, dose-related effects upon the various organs and tissues of the body, such as the central and autonomic nervous systems, the respiratory system, the cardiovascular system, and the gastrointestinal system. On other systems and tissues of the body there is little evidence that nitrous oxide has any significant effect.

CENTRAL NERVOUS SYSTEM EFFECTS. Nitrous oxide, obviously, exerts its desirable effects upon the central nervous system. The drug-gas was actually used for over one hundred years before good quantitative data were obtained in man to show that nitrous oxide does alter processes in the central nervous system. By correlating clinical symptoms and electroencephalographic tracings, nitrous oxide was shown to be able to cause a range of effects from sedation at low concentrations to light general surgical anesthesia at high concentrations, and most importantly, nitrous oxide was able to bring about these effects without simultaneously producing hypoxia.[14]

By comparing the effects produced by nitrous oxide to those produced by other drugs, it is known that nitrous oxide is a member of a group of drugs known as the nonselective central nervous system depressants. These agents all produce the same type of effects, but to varying degrees at different concentrations. Other well known members of this group include the general inhalational anesthetics, the barbiturate and nonbarbiturate sedative-hypnotics (discussed at the beginning of this chapter) and ethyl alcohol. When the common central nervous system effects to all these agents are compared, it is found that nitrous oxide is the weakest, even when it is administered in its maximum safe dose (i.e., at 80% or a little less of the inspired air mixture). The drug-gas lacks intrinsic activity at its site of desirable action. It perhaps even has a low affinity for its receptor sites as well, but this is not really known.

It is currently widely accepted that nitrous oxide acts upon brain cells to cause depression. All sensations are affected: hearing, vision, taste, smell, as well as the abilities to concentrate or to calculate simple math problems. In addition, cerebellar functions are depressed with the patient showing motor incoordination, ataxia, and nystagmus.

As discussed for the barbiturates, nitrous oxide is known to alter first the activity in the ascending reticular activating system of the rostral portion of the midbrain reticular formation, and then almost immediately the drug depresses the neocortex. The limbic system is less depressed than the cortex.

SEDATIVE EFFECT. The cellular mechanism of nitrous oxide action is not known. As a result of slowly increasing drug concentrations, the overt clinical effects shown in Table 9.6 occur with a considerable variability from patient to patient. Fortunately, for our purposes in dentistry it is the very earliest effects of nitrous oxide, those seen at the lower concentrations, that are desired clinically, namely, light sedation in the conscious patient who is relaxed and free of apparent anxiety but who is perfectly capable of responding to verbal commands.

Nitrous oxide has no reported effect on peripheral afferent sensory impulse transmission, i.e., it is not a local anesthetic.

AUTONOMIC NERVOUS SYSTEM EFFECTS. There are few data available on nitrous oxide's effects on the autonomic nervous system. Like all nonselective central nervous system depressants, however, nitrous oxide will carry a patient to and through the second stage, or delirium stage, of general anesthesia. There would be an expected outpour of adrenal medullary epinephrine with

## Table 9.6.　Responses to Nitrous Oxide and Oxygen Mixtures

| Concentration of Nitrous Oxide in Oxygen | Response |
|---|---|
| 10% to 20% | Body warmth |
|  | Tingling of hands and feet |
| 20% to 30% | Circumoral numbness |
|  | Numbness of thighs |
| 20% to 40% | Numbness of tongue |
|  | Numbness of hands and feet |
|  | Droning sounds present |
|  | Hearing distinct but distant |
|  | Dissociation begins and reaches peak |
|  | Mild sleepiness |
|  | Some analgesia |
|  | Euphoria (depends upon patient) |
|  | Feeling of heaviness or lightness of body |
| 30% to 50% | Sweating |
|  | Nausea |
|  | Amnesia |
|  | Increased sleepiness |
| 40% to 60% | Dreaming, laughing, giddiness |
|  | Further increased sleepiness, tending toward unconsciousness |
|  | Increased nausea and possible vomiting |

Source: Modified from Bennett, 1974.[17]

typical sympathetic responses. In anesthetic concentrations of nitrous oxide it is known that under the best conditions, norepinephrine's effects are slightly augmented; however, there is no evidence that nitrous oxide alters the autonomic nervous system when administered in sedative concentrations.

CARDIOVASCULAR EFFECTS. On the cardiovascular system little effect has been seen, at least in man when hypoxia is absent. There is some suggestion that nitrous oxide may depress the mycocardium, but in man this effect is debatable. In most instances, any changes seen in this system may be accredited usually to the stage of delirium or to the large fluctuations in the arterial blood oxygen tension.

The only real, definitely proven detrimental effect upon human tissues produced by nitrous oxide is that seen following continuous use for 24 hours or longer. Patients who are suffering from tetanus may be so treated with nitrous oxide. Under these conditions a serious, even fatal, bone marrow depression may develop. This response to the drug is reversible by halting any further administration of nitrous oxide. It is of interest that this bone marrow depressing effect of nitrous oxide has been utilized clinically to produce symptomatic remission of leukemia. At this time, there is a growing interest in what possible effect nitrous oxide concentrations in the dental office atmosphere may be having on dental office personnel who may be inhaling up to 1 to 2% concentrations several hours per day over long time periods.[15]

RESPIRATORY EFFECTS. The effects of nitrous oxide itself on respiration are apparently not available. There is, however, no end to the respiratory studies showing nitrous oxide in combination with other general anesthetics. Used alone, it is suggested to increase respiration as stage two is approached, and combined with any other type of central nervous system depressant, nitrous oxide assuredly augments the respiratory depression.

GASTROINTESTINAL EFFECTS. On the gastrointestinal tract only insignificant effects are observed. Although the literature has widely differing reports upon the incidence of vomiting caused by nitrous oxide, it can be stated safely that the drug-gas can produce nausea and vomiting. The higher incidence thus far would seem to be associated primarily with the use of higher concentrations of nitrous oxide when proper oxygenation may be jeopardized. It is strongly recommended that any change in nitrous oxide concentration in the inspired gas mixture be brought about slowly and in steps; rapid raising or lowering of the drug-gas's concentration tends to produce a higher chance of nausea.

CAUTIONS, SIDE EFFECTS, AND CONTRAINDICATIONS. There are, nonetheless, two unwanted effects of nitrous oxide about which all who use it should be keenly aware. Both of these effects are based upon the comparative physicochemical properties of nitrous oxide and nitrogen. Nitrous oxide happens to be 34 times more soluble in blood than is nitrogen.

When a patient has been breathing high concentrations of nitrous oxide for a brief period (e.g., 5 minutes or longer), and is suddenly switched to breathing room air, the nitrous oxide rushes out of blood into the alveoli much faster than nitrogen can move from the alveoli into the blood. As a result the mixture of alveolar gases is diluted with nitrous oxide. This means that even though the patient is breathing room air with adequate oxygen in the room air, the oxygen concentration in the alveoli is less than what is required. The patient experiences what is referred to as diffusion hypoxia. The simple way to avoid this situation altogether is always to allow the patient to breathe 100% oxygen for several minutes after nitrous oxide use before permitting the patient to breathe room air.

Because nitrous oxide is 34 times more soluble in blood than is nitrogen, there is another possible clinical problem. Nitrous oxide will, as it is administered, diffuse into all the air-filled cavities of the body. Because nitrous oxide diffuses faster into the gas-filled cavity than nitrogen diffuses out of the same cavity, the cavity size may increase. Therefore, patients with middle ear disorders or those with recent tympanic membrane surgery should not be given the inhalational sedative nitrous oxide.

Over its long history of clinical use, many toxicities have been accredited to nitrous oxide, but few are actually due to the drug nitrous oxide itself. A large majority of these toxicities are due to hypoxia because the practitioner failed to understand how to administer the drug. At another time in nitrous oxide's past, there was a high incidence of toxic impurities in the preparations owing to our ignorance of the proper manufacturing procedures, but these problems have been resolved. One of the two direct tissue effects of nitrous oxide has been mentioned, namely, the ability of nitrous oxide to depress the bone marrow when the patient must breathe the drug-gas over prolonged time periods. Another potentially serious toxicity regarding nitrous oxide is not mentioned often enough. Nitrous oxide is a drug of abuse. As yet it is not adequately abused to be labeled as a controlled substance under the federal law. However, it must be recognized that as a nonselective depres-

**Table 9.7.  Inhalational Sedation ($N_2O$)**

| Relative Advantages | Relative Disadvantages |
|---|---|
| 1. Nonallergenic drug | 1. Cannot be used in certain patients<br>a. who fear losing consciousness<br>b. who are nonverbal<br>c. who have nasal obstruction |
| 2. Body does not have to metabolize the drug | 2. Always possible to have fire or explosion although drug is nonexplosive or flammable itself |
| 3. Less likely to interact unfavorably with other drugs patient is taking; or can reverse interaction quickly | 3. Adds to office expense |
| 4. Sedation level can be controlled almost from moment to moment | 4. Requires learning and keeping up with an additional skill |
| 5. Prompt recovery time allows patient to leave office without escort | 5. Cannot be used if other central nervous system depressants must be given prior to treatment, e.g., narcotic analgesics or antiemetics, because the added depression will allow the nitrous oxide to carry patient into excitement stage or general anesthesia |
| 6. After effects, e.g., headache or hangover, lower in incidence | |

## Table 9.8. Suggested Agents for Sedation Only of Dental Outpatients*

| Sedative Route | Children (Prepuberty) | Adults (14–65 years old) | Elderly (>65–70 years old) |
|---|---|---|---|
| Oral | Hydroxyzine Promethazine | Pentobarbital | Chloral hydrate |
| (before procedure) | Chloral hydrate (or combinations) | 100 mg | 500 mg |
| | 30–60 min BEFORE | 30–45 min BEFORE | 30–60 min BEFORE |
| Inhalation (before & during) | $N_2O$ | $N_2O$ | $N_2O$ |
| Intravenous | Not often used for children unless | Diazepam | Still looking for the best agent |
| (just before) | handicapped | titrated dose | |

* = Regular use of local anesthetic agent controls pain during the procedure.

sant of the central nervous system it has the same potential as the barbiturates and ethyl alcohol to become a dependence-producing agent. It is commonly known that nitrous oxide is used illicitly at parties when the tanks are not kept under close security by hospitals, clinics, or the manufacturer. Nitrous oxide may have some opiate characteristics as well.[16]

The most serious problem with nitrous oxide in terms of drug-drug interactions is its ability to potentiate profoundly the effects of every other known depressant of the central nervous system. Caution is always required in the planned use of nitrous oxide in the dental office where it must be determined with absolute accuracy what drugs the patient is currently taking. If the patient has circulating central nervous system depressant and nitrous oxide is administered in usual sedative concentrations, it is not difficult at all to carry the patient promptly into the second or third stage of general anesthesia.

It is of interest that the above caution prevails in the individual who has acutely ingested ethyl alcohol. However, the chronic alcoholic may demonstrate considerable tolerance to the effects of nitrous oxide. This is due to the cross-tolerance which develops between nonselective central nervous system depressants.

Some relative advantages and disadvantages of the inhalational sedative nitrous oxide are shown in Table 9.7. A comparison of suggested sedatives for outpatient dentistry is presented in Table 9.8.

## REFERENCES

1. Shideman, F.E.: Clinical pharmacology of hypnotics and sedatives. Clin. Pharmacol. Ther., 2:313-344, 1961.
2. Moruzzi, G., and Magoun, H.W.: Brain stem reticular formation and activation of the EEG. Electroencephalogr. Clin. Neurophysiol., 1:455, 1949.
3. Hill, L.L., Daeschner, C.W., and Moyer, J.L.: The influence of sedative agents upon renal hemodynamics. J. Lab. Clin. Med., 52:125-128, 1958.
4. Mark, L.C.: Archaic classification of barbiturates. Clin. Pharmacol. Ther., 10:287-291, 1969.
5. Weatherall, M.: Drugs and porphyrin metabolism. Pharmacol. Rev., 6:133, 1954.
6. Kress, L.: Veronalism. Br. Med. J. Epitome, 2:72, 1905.
7. Kennett, S.: Stomatitis medicamentosa due to barbiturates. Oral Surg., 25:351-356, 1968.
8. Koppanyi, T., and Richards, R.K.: The treatment of barbiturate poisoning with or without analeptics. Anesth. Analg., 37:182-186, 1958.
9. Clemmesen, C., and Nilsson, E.: Therapeutic trends in the treatment of barbiturate poisoning: The Scandinavian method. Clin. Pharmacol. Ther., 2:220-229, 1961.
10. Mackay, F.J., and Cooper, J.R.: A study on the hypnotic activity of chloral hydrate. J. Pharmacol. Exp. Ther., 135:271-274, 1962.
11. Reference Handbook. Med. Lett. Drugs Ther. New York, The Medical Letter, 1975.
12. Aarskog, D.: Association between maternal intake of diazepam and oral clefts. Lancet, 2:921, 1975.
13. Reference Handbook. Med. Lett. Drugs Ther. New York, The Medical Letter, 1973.
14. Faulconer, A. J., Pender, J.W., and Bickford, R.G.: The influence of partial pressure of nitrous oxide on the depth of anesthesia and the electrocephalogram in man. Anesthesiology, 10:601, 1949.
15. Cleaton-Jones, P., Austin, J.C., Banks, D., Vieira, E., and Kagan, E.: Does nitrous oxide harm the dentist? Lancet, 2:931, 1975.
16. Berkowitz, B.A., Ngai, S.H., and Finck, A.D.: Nitrous oxide "analgesia": resemblance to opiate action. Science, 194:967, 1976.
17. Bennett, C.R.: Conscious-Sedation in Dental Practice. St. Louis, Mosby, 1974.

## SUPPLEMENTARY REFERENCES

Brazier, M.A.B.: Sedatives and hypnotics 2, effects upon physiological systems. a. The electrophysiological effects of barbiturates on the brain. In Physiological Pharmacology Vol. 1, The Nervous System: Part A: Central Nervous System Drugs. Edited by W.S. Root and F.G. Hofmann. New York, Academic Press, 1963.
Isaacson, R.L.: The Limbic System. New York, Plenum Press, 1974.
Killam, E.K.: Drug action on the brain stem reticular formation. Pharmacol. Rev., 14:175, 1962.
Magoun, H.W.: The Walking Brain. 2nd Edition. Springfield, Ill., Charles C Thomas, 1963.
Moruzzi, G.: Active processes in the brain stem during sleep. Harvey Lect., 58:233, 1963.
Omura, T., Kuriyama, Y., Siekevitz, P., and Palade, G.E.: Effect of phenobarbital on the turnover of microsomal enzymes. In Microsomes and Drug Oxidations. Edited by J.R. Gillette, A.H. Conney, G.J. Cosmides, R.W. Estabrook, J.R. Fonts, and G.J. Mannering. New York, Academic Press, 1969.
Williams, R.L., and Karacan, I.: Pharmacology of Sleep. New York, John Wiley & Sons, 1976.

# 10

## CHEMOTHERAPEUTIC AGENTS

At the present time no dental hygienist in the United States is allowed by law to prescribe or administer an antibiotic to the patient. The dental hygienist does not determine through the process of oral diagnosis that a patient is in need of an antibiotic for the treatment of a specific oral infection. Nevertheless, the dental hygienist does have reason to know more about antibiotics than simply that this class of drugs is prescribed and administered by the dentist to the patient. The dental hygienist may be found in an awkward position, for example, when the patient gives a medical history of chronic ingestion of high doses of a corticosteroid. The dental hygienist may correctly suggest to the dentist that the patient should receive chemoprophylaxis for the dental hygiene procedure to be performed. When the dentist tells the dental hygienist that (for reasons known only to that dentist) the patient does not need chemoprophylaxis, what does the dental hygienist do in such a situation?

Furthermore, the dental hygienist must know those circumstances from the patient's history that require chemoprophylaxis. Someday in the not too distant future the dental hygienist will no doubt not only determine the patient's need for chemoprophylaxis (as is now the practice), but also prescribe the appropriate antibiotic for the patient.

Certainly the chemotherapeutic agents are some of the most important drugs prescribed by dentists. Indeed, competent modern dental therapeutics could not exist without the antibiotics.

## PHARMACOLOGICAL BASIS OF CHEMOTHERAPY

The type of drug most often administered in dentistry for therapeutic reasons is a chemotherapeutic agent. Furthermore, the chemotherapeutic agents are the most often prescribed drugs in both dentistry and medicine. For these reasons, if no other, an appropriate amount of time should be devoted to the pharmacodynamics of this important group of drugs with a special emphasis given to those agents so widely used in dentistry.

Before focusing attention upon several very selected groups of chemotherapeutic agents, it is essential to examine the more important basic concepts that have developed regarding these drugs over the last half century. One thing is certain, no other group of drugs has contributed more to the reduction of human suffering in the history of man.

### Definitions

Chemotherapy has come to mean a branch of pharmacotherapeutics in which drugs are used specifically to inhibit or destroy invading, infecting organisms with a minimal effect upon the host's tissues. This would include the drugs used to treat the infectious diseases caused by bacteria, fungi, viruses, spirochetes, rickettsiae, and mycoplasmas, as well as the drugs known as antimalarials, anthelmintics, trypanosomicides, schistosomicides, and many others. Chemotherapy also includes the use of drugs in the treatment of cancer, i.e., the antineoplastic agents. Chemotherapy, obviously then, involves an enormous number of drugs, parasites, and diseases.

A chemotherapeutic agent is a drug used either systemically or topically specifically to inhibit or kill an invading, infecting organism.

An antibiotic is a special type of chemotherapeutic agent, whose definition has been expanded recently. Originally an antiobiotic was a chemical substance produced by various species of microorganisms (usually bacteria, fungi, or actinomycetes) that suppresses the growth of other microorganisms and may eventually destroy them. In other words antibiotics originally included only naturally occurring agents, but now an antibiotic includes both the naturally occurring as well as the semisynthetic and fully synthetic agents.

### Selective Toxicity

One of the most fundamental concepts or principles in the realm of rational pharmacotherapeutics is that known as selective toxicity. In reality all effective, successful, and safe use of any drug, it could be argued, exemplifies the principle of selective toxicity. No better place is this seen, however, than in the proper use of antibiotics, for the primary pharmacological characteristic which antibiotics share is their selective toxicity for some invading organism rather than the host's cells.

How can a drug intermingle with all the host's living cells and have little if any effect upon them and at the same time inhibit the bacterial cells' growth or even kill the bacteria that are existing in juxtaposition to the host's cells? Such ways have been found to exploit the differences in biochemistry between the infecting organism and the host. Several examples of known mechanisms are described in general terms.

In the first place an antibiotic could inhibit a reaction that is vital to the parasite but not to the host's cells. Perhaps the reaction in question would not even occur in the host. Or the specific, vital reaction may occur in both host and parasite, but different precursor pathways are used in each and the antibiotic would inhibit only that pathway in the invading organism. The host's cells would not be affected by such an antibiotic.

Yet a more subtle way would be for the same vital reaction to occur in the cells of both host and parasite and for the antibiotic to inhibit both, but the sensitive site in the host cells is inaccessible or more resistant to the antibiotic. The reaction may occur much more slowly in the host's cells than in the parasite. That is to say, the rapidly growing micoorganism may be far more sensitive to the drug's inhibiting effect than the slowly changing host's cell.

The parasite and the host's cells could both possess the specific reaction that the antibiotic inhibits, but perhaps the host's cells can rapidly inactivate the antibiotic before it can accumulate in an effective concentration, whereas the parasite cannot inactivate the antibiotic. The host's cells may also have another pathway ready to be used to produce the very substance whose production the antibiotic is preventing.

As we understand antibiotic mechanisms of action today, it is observed that the mechanisms are directed against the invading, infecting organism and not directed toward enhancing the defense mechanisms of the host's cells. In regard to an antibiotic's selective toxicity for bacteria, the descriptive terms of *bactericidal* and *bacteriostatic* are used widely. This antibiotic is bactericidal or that antibiotic is bacteriostatic. It is known that the same antibiotic may be bactericidal in one situation and bacteriostatic in another. In the simplest of terms it can be demonstrated in vitro whether an antibiotic is bactericidal or bacteriostatic. Susceptible microorganisms, when exposed to a bactericidal drug, die even if they are transferred to a fresh, drug-free medium. Bacteriostatic antibiotics inhibit the growth of susceptible bacteria, but when the bacteria are transferred to a fresh drug-free medium growth begins again.

Figure 10.1 shows diagrammatically a plot of bacterial log growth against time. The colony of bacteria begins to grow rapidly and multiply after a resting or lag phase. Without adding anything to the culture medium, the organisms continue to multiply until food begins to grow and/or waste products accumulate; the rate of growth then reaches a plateau. If a bacteriostatic agent is added to the culture medium during the rapidly growing phase, the growth rate will plateau. If a bactericidal agent is added at the same point, the number of organisms would decline in time.

It can be readily appreciated that clinically (i.e., in vivo) it is often difficult to say actually whether a particular drug is bactericidal or only bacteriostatic. Weinstein points out correctly that the principal antimicrobial action is to retard bacterial growth, but

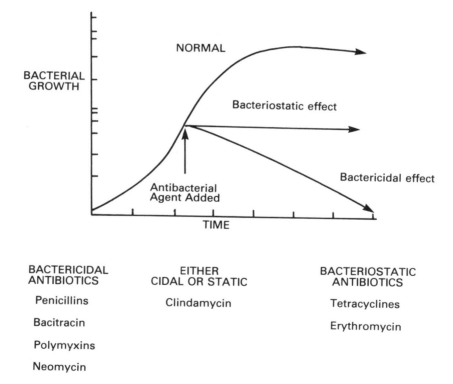

**Figure 10.1** Bactericidal or bacteriostatic antibiotics. There are many other antibiotics in each category but only these will be emphasized in this chapter.

some antibiotics in sufficient concentration certainly can kill bacteria both in vitro and in vivo.[1] The important thing to realize is that even the most effective antibiotics do not, except in unusual circumstances, cure an infection simply by virtue of their action on the offending organism. The patient's body is required to do its part as well. It is now widely accepted that even the bactericidal antibiotics require the effective intervention of the various defense mechanisms of the host in order to bring about the cure. The antibiotics, remember, act upon the invading organism and do not produce their antimicrobial effect by enhancing the host's natural defense mechanisms. The bactericidal agents, perhaps, depend less upon the defense mechanisms than the bacteriostatic agents which surely do.

## General Mechanisms of Antibiotic Action

For a group of drugs only 50 years old, a great deal is known about their sites and mechanisms of action. Thus far, the antibiotics inhibit or interfere with the susceptible organisms's biosynthetic mechanisms or metabolic processes.

There are really three general sites of action and four general mechanisms by which antibiotics affect the microbe. As shown in Figure 10.2 some antibiotics act upon the bacterial cell wall to inhibit the biosynthesis of new cell wall. The classic agents in this group are the penicillins.

Some antibiotics act on cytoplasmic components and inhibit the microorganisms's cellular mechanisms for protein synthesis. These can be further subdivided into those which bind with the ribosome 50S subunit (e.g., erythromycin and clindamycin) or with the 30S subunit (e.g., tetracyclines and neomycin).

Other antimicrobial drugs act on cytoplasmic components to affect intermediary metabolism (act as antimetabolites). The sulfonamides are such agents.

Lastly, a number of antibiotics act on the microorganisms's cytoplasmic membrane and interfere with the membrane's protective function and permeability characteristics. Examples are the polymyxins and the antifungal agents.

## Factors Influencing the Effectiveness of Antibiotics

Numerous factors influence the effectiveness of antibiotics in man. Although obvious, one of the most often overlooked factors is the individual antibiotic's scope of inhibitory activity. How widespread is the drug's antibacterial effects? Does it, for example, act upon only the gram-positive staphylococci or does it affect both gram-positive and gram-negative microorganisms as well as rickett-

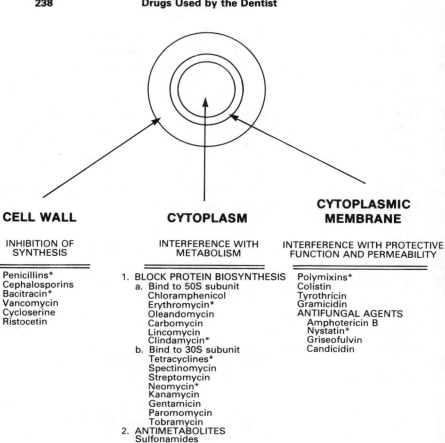

**CELL WALL**

INHIBITION OF
SYNTHESIS

Penicillins*
Cephalosporins
Bacitracin*
Vancomycin
Cycloserine
Ristocetin

**CYTOPLASM**

INTERFERENCE WITH
METABOLISM

1. BLOCK PROTEIN BIOSYNTHESIS
   a. Bind to 50S subunit
      Chloramphenicol
      Erythromycin*
      Oleandomycin
      Carbomycin
      Lincomycin
      Clindamycin*
   b. Bind to 30S subunit
      Tetracyclines*
      Spectinomycin
      Streptomycin
      Neomycin*
      Kanamycin
      Gentamicin
      Paromomycin
      Tobramycin
2. ANTIMETABOLITES
   Sulfonamides
   Sulfones

**CYTOPLASMIC
MEMBRANE**

INTERFERENCE WITH PROTECTIVE
FUNCTION AND PERMEABILITY

Polymixins*
Colistin
Tyrothricin
Gramicidin
ANTIFUNGAL AGENTS
   Amphotericin B
   Nystatin*
   Griseofulvin
   Candicidin

**Figure 10.2** Sites and mechanisms of action of antibiotics. Only those named antibiotics marked with (*) will be considered in this chapter.

sia? There is no way by which a specific antibiotic can become an effective antibacterial agent if the bacteria causing an infection are not susceptible to the antibiotic. Yet some clinicians each day prescribe antibiotics for patients with infectious diseases, and the clinician has no idea whether the causative organism is sensitive to the antibiotic prescribed. Such a practice is just silly.

The antibiotics are classified as narrow spectrum or broad spectrum as suggested in Figure 10.3. The spectrum refers to the relative range of the drug's antimicrobial action. If the antibiotic affects only gram-negative or only gram-positive bacteria it may be categorized as narrow spectrum. However, if the antibiotic in safe

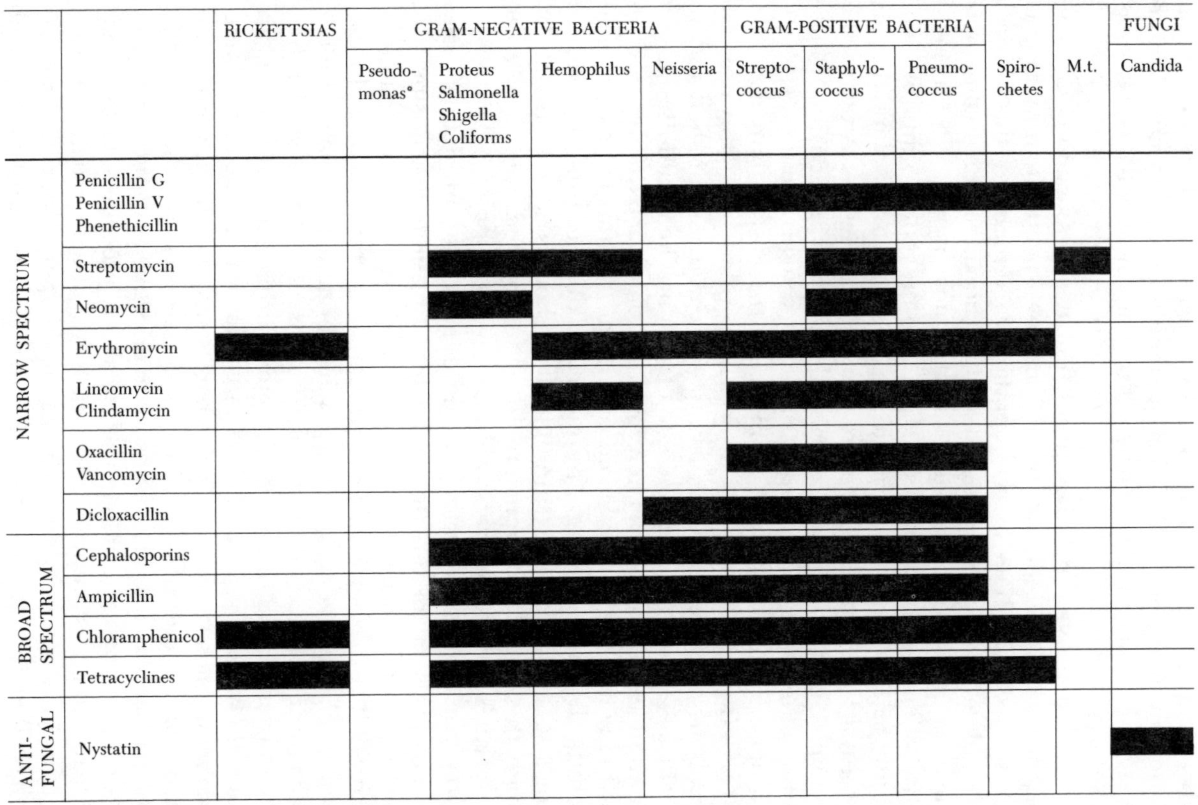

**Figure 10.3** Relative spectra of antimicrobial action for selected antibiotics: M.t. = *Mycobacterium tuberculosis*; (*) = none of the drugs listed are effective clinically against pseudomonas infections (carbenicillin or gentamicin are drugs of choice).

doses can adversely affect both gram-positive and gram-negative bacteria and possibly also act upon rickettsiae or viruses, it may be categorized as broad spectrum. A number of authorities consider only chloramphenicol and the tetracyclines as truly broad spectrum in their antimicrobial action. Yet other authorities may not be quite so rigid and may include ampicillin and the cephalosporins as broad in spectrum.

The dental hygienist should not find it necessary to commit to memory exactly which antibiotic is narrow spectrum and which is broad spectrum. It is more important to remember the clinical principle: use the antibiotic to which the infecting organism is sensitive, and the one which has the most narrow spectrum of activity. The reason behind this rule is to prevent the inhibition or killing of any more bacteria of the body's natural flora than is absolutely necessary. There are practitioners who disregard the principle, find it easy to prescribe the broadest spectrum of antibiotic when the invading organism is not known, and then sit back and hope for the best. Such a practice is to be condemmed.

The effectiveness of any drug will depend upon the ease by which the drug's effective concentration can be established and, in most cases, maintained at the site of action. The antibiotics are no different in this respect. Therefore, the pharmacokinetics of each antibiotic must be given due consideration. Factors to be discussed include the proper dosage, frequency of dosage, route to use, the drug's ability to distribute throughout the body's tissues, the rate by which the drug is biotransformed or inactivated, and finally the antibiotic's route of excretion.

Another important factor that influences the antibiotic's effectiveness is a characteristic of the infecting microorganisms, i.e., how old is the infection and how big is the infecting bacterial culture? The earlier antibiotic treatment is started, the better its chances of effectiveness, because when organisms are permitted to reach their stationary growing phase in tissues they become refractory to bactericidal drugs. Furthermore, drug-resistant mutants are more likely to arise in older and larger lesions owing to the larger number of bacteria present.[2] In other words, the older an infection, the higher the antibiotic dose probably required and the longer the time probably needed for exposure to effective concentrations. The older the culture, the slower the metabolic processes. Growth rate plateaus and most antibiotics are far more effective against young, rapidly growing cultures than against larger, older and usually well-walled infections (abscesses) that will require incision and drainage for cure.

As has been pointed out, for any antibiotic to be its most effective there must exist functioning, normal host defense mechanisms. As one may imagine, these defense mechanisms can definitely be impaired by a number of diseases. The number of functioning phagocytes at the infection site are reduced in conditions such as agranulocytosis or radiation injury. Diseases such as agamma-globulinemia or chronic lymphatic leukemia can suppress antibody formation. Uremia and also uncontrolled diabetes mellitus inhibit host resistance by mechanisms not yet fully understood. It is a clinical fact that the uncontrolled or poorly controlled diabetic patient commonly has more bacterial infections that respond more slowly to therapy than those without the disorder.

The patient's defense mechanisms may be severely depressed not only by certain diseases but also by certain drugs. For example, the patient on long-term corticosteroid treatment may have his usual response to infection completely masked, inasmuch as fever, local tenderness, malaise, edema, purulence, lymphadenopathy, increase in leukocytes, or even radiological findings may be changed by these drugs. Other immunosuppressant agents and antineoplastic agents may produce a similar impairment of the host defenses. In these instances a more vigorous antibiotic treatment regimen with the bactericidal antibiotics is required; and, indeed, most practitioners agree it is wise to employ chemoprophylaxis for such dental or dental hygiene patients.

## Selected Problems in Antibiotic Use

In the clinical use of antibiotics, several well-defined problems are to be encountered. These problems may be divided into a minimum of two groups, the development of bacterial resistance to the effects of the antibiotic and the toxicities associated with the antibiotic use.

BACTERIAL RESISTANCE. A specific strain of bacteria may be intrinsically resistant to the bactericidal or bacteriostatic action of a certain antibiotic, or, it may be said, this strain of bacteria possesses natural resistance. Many resistant staphylococci produce an enzyme that inactivates penicillin G. Bacteria have a number of ways for inactivating various antibiotics.

Bacteria may also uncommonly develop acquired resistance to antibiotic action during exposure to the drug. Erythromycin possesses the unfortunate property of having rapid, one-step high resistance develop to its effects by certain bacteria. Greater attention is now being given to the phenomenon of transferred or infectious drug resistance, in which the antibiotic-resistant bacterium transfers the drug-resistant determinant or factor to another bacterium which heretofore was sensitive to the antibiotic. This confers resistance on the "infected" bacterium.

There is little doubt, however, that the continuing alarming increase in the clinical appearance of resistant strains of microorganisms is directly related to current patterns of clinical antibiotic therapy. It is important to use the antibiotics in as discriminate a manner as possible. It really makes little difference whether the resistance is natural or acquired; the indiscriminate use of antibiotics is responsible for the selecting out of drug-resistant strains.

In any culture each generation of bacteria produces a certain number of mutants with some being less sensitive to the specific antibiotic. In this situation a certain lower concentration of the antibiotic would exert its bactericidal action upon the majority of the organisms present, but the first generation mutants that are less sensitive would survive. The next generation would also produce progeny a little less sensitive to the antibiotic, and now that these organisms do not have around all the other organisms that were sensitive, these more resistant organisms flourish. Knowing these facts regarding the development of bacterial resistance will prompt the clinician to be sure the patient not only receives a sufficiently high dose to affect adversely the first and second step mutants but also takes the antibiotic over a sufficiently long enough period (usually 5 days for common acute orodental infections) and does not stop at the first sign of clinical improvement.

ANTIBIOTIC TOXICITY. Another serious problem in the use of the antibiotics is the toxicity of these drugs. To speak of toxicity to man's cells after all previous comments regarding the selective toxicity of antibiotics would appear to be a paradox.

Generally grouped, there are three types of antibiotic toxicity to consider: hypersensitivity reactions, direct toxic effects of the drug on man's cells, and indirect toxicity due to the antibiotic's ability to promote the overgrowth of nonsusceptible organisms which results in superinfections. The first (hypersensitivity reactions) and the third types (indirect toxicity) are characteristics possessed by all antibiotics, and the drugs differ from one another in producing these effects only in a quantitative sense. However, not all antibiotics directly affect man's cells to produce a specific toxicity. Unfortunately, some antibiotics, can produce irreversible damage to human cells, such as deafness or renal injury, and such direct effects will be considered with each drug discussed.

The direct and the indirect toxic effects of the antibiotics are related to the clinical dose administered and to the duration of the exposure to the drug. Remember that hypersensitivity reactions which occur relatively frequently to some antibiotics are not related to the dose administered to the patient.

In order for an antibiotic to produce a hypersensitivity or allergic reaction, a prior sensitization contact is required, either with the same drug or with one closely related chemically. A period of time is required, usually about 7 to 10 days, for the body's synthesis of drug-specific antibodies. Then the second exposure to the drug (the eliciting contact) results in an antigen-antibody interaction, which provokes the typical manifestations of allergy. These manifestations are numerous, involve various organ systems, and range in severity from minor skin lesions to fatal anaphylaxis. In man, involvement of the skin is most frequent. Penicillin commonly causes urticaria (or giant hives) and generalized itching.

There is no doubt that some drugs are more allergenic than others and this has little to do with how widespread the drug is used. Caffeine is certainly more widely used than aspirin, and aspirin more than penicillin. Yet allergy to penicillin is fairly common, allergy to aspirin is more rare, and allergy to caffeine is unknown.

Of all types of drugs administered by the dental practitioner, the antibiotics are the most likely to produce allergic reactions. Indeed, today penicillin is the number one drug for causing anaphylactic reactions.

This information regarding hypersensitivity reactions to antibiotics should suggest another general principle concerning their clinical use. The antibiotics, especially the penicillins, are sensitizing agents, i.e., they can (on their first contact) lead to the production of antibodies that may set up the patient for a reaction that may even be fatal on his next exposure to the antibiotic. For this reason alone, the antibiotics cannot be considered innocuous substances for man because they possess such incredible, though relative, selective toxicity for invading, infecting microorganisms.

The other unwanted effect that all antibiotics can produce is an overgrowth of nonsusceptible organisms which can then produce infection, or what is called a suprainfection. This phenomenon is based upon the fact that the human body serves as a host for bacteria, fungi, and other microorganisms living in and on each of us at all times. The general composition of man's microbiota depends upon a number of factors involving the fiercely competitive environment in which the organisms live. It is reasonable that a pathogenic organism could live in man without producing infectious disease because the pathogen is held in check by the other organisms. When an antibiotic is given if the microbial relationships are sufficiently disrupted so as to allow the nonsusceptible pathogen to grow and flourish, then infectious disease can occur as a result of giving an antibiotic. This is iatrogenic or drug-induced disease.

### Antibiotics in Dentistry

The antibiotics are used in general dentistry for two basic purposes: to treat acute infections of the orodental region and to be given prophylactically either to prevent primarily subacute bacterial endocarditis or to assist the patient's defense mechanisms when they are definitely known to be impaired. These indications for antibiotic use are summarized in Table 10.1.

Many groups of antibiotics are available, and each group consists of a number of individual drugs. In fact, some 500 antibiotic substances have been isolated and evaluated.[3] For the pharmacologist it is tempting to consider each antibiotic in some detail, but such a time and space expenditure cannot be justified in terms of the purposes of this text. Therefore, only selected antibiotic groups and, furthermore, only specific antibiotics will be considered which are in widespread use today as the antibacterial agents of first, second, and third choice in the treatment of infection of the oral cavity and surrounding tissues. These are the infections the general dental practitioner would be called upon to treat. Particular antibiotics used as chemoprophylactic agents will be emphasized.

Fortunately, many bacterial infections of the oral cavity are due to gram-positive cocci, both streptococci and staphylococci. Drugs most effective in the eradication of these organisms are reviewed in detail.

### THE PENICILLINS

Approximately 90% of the infections the dentist treats and/or prevents are caused by microorganisms that are susceptible to one of the penicillins.

### Chemistry

The mold, *Penicillium notatum*, biosynthesizes benzylpenicillin G by condensing phenylalanine and two amino acids, D-valine and L-cysteine. The antibiotic, whose structure is shown in Figure 10.4, is an acid with the unusual beta-lactam ring that is readily opened by the bacterial enzyme penicillinase, a process which inactivates penicillin.

It was learned very early that the mold's production of penicillin G could be greatly enhanced if phenylacetic acid or a precursor were added to the growth medium. When other precursors were

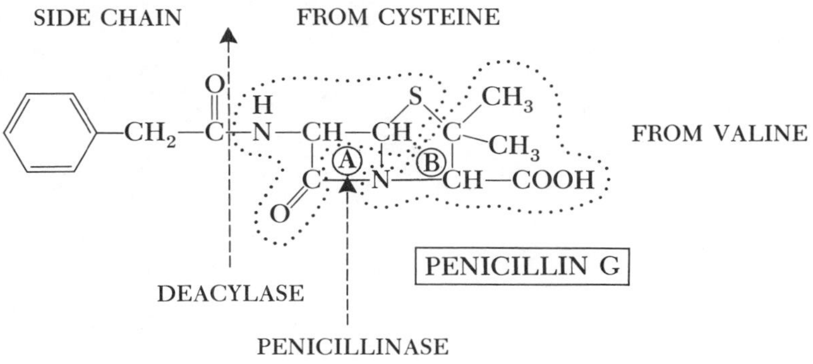

**Figure 10.4** Chemical structure of benzylpenicillin G: A = beta-lactam ring; B = thiazolidine ring.

added, the mold made different penicillins, such as phenoxymethyl penicillin (also known as penicillin V) and phenoxyethyl penicillin or phenethicillin. All the remaining penicillins available today are semisynthetic products. The mold makes benzylpenicillin G; then a bacterial producer of a deacylase enzyme is added to the growth medium. The deacylase splits the molecule to phenylacetic acid and the all-important 6-aminopenicillanic acid. The 6-aminopenicillanic acid is isolated and acylated with the various side chains necessary to produce the many other different specialized penicillins.

### Penicillin G Potassium (Pentids)

Penicillin G is not water soluble, but it does form water-soluble potassium or sodium salts. A U.S.P. unit for penicillin G is that activity, measured by bacteriological assay, which is present in 0.6 micrograms of the standard crystalline sodium salt of penicillin G. Therefore, one milligram of standard crystalline sodium penicillin G contains 1667 U.S.P. units. One milligram of potassium penicillin G contains approximately 1.5 million U.S.P. units. Thus the usual 300,000 U.S.P. unit dose is equivalent to about 0.2 grams of the salt. Penicillin G is the only one of the penicillins whose dosage is still expressed in U.S.P. units. The dosage of the other penicillins is usually expressed in the range of 250 to 500 milligrams.

ANTIMICROBIAL SPECTRUM. If a comparison were made between the range of bacteria that most often causes dental infections with the range of bacteria that is susceptible to penicillin G, it would be observed that almost the same organisms were involved. The rough approximation today indicates that penicillin is effective in 90 to

# Table 10.1. Dental Applications of Antibiotics

| Orodental Indication | Antibiotic of Choice | | |
| --- | --- | --- | --- |
| | First | Second | Third |
| I. ACUTE INFECTIONS | | | |
| A. Usual Causative Organisms | | | |
|   1. Acute dentoalveolar abscess | | | |
|   2. Toxic cellulitis | | | |
|   3. Infections following surgery or trauma | | | |
|   4. Suppurative infections of major salivary glands | Penicillin | Erythromycin | Tetracycline |
|   5. Ludwig's angina | | | |
|   6. Oral antral fistulae with sinusitis | | | |
|   7. Mucous membrane infections | | | |
|     a. If patient has agranulocytosis or agammaglobulinemia | | | |
|     b. Involved with pemphigus | | | |
|   8. Pericoronitis with cellulitis; toxic systemic manifestations | | | Cephalosporin |
|   9. Osteitis (dry socket), especially purulent osteitis or if patient is febrile | | | |
|  10. Osteomyelitis | | | |
| B. Others (Specific Organisms) | | | |
|   1. Vincent's infection (Spirochetes) | Penicillin | Tetracycline | Erythromycin |
|   2. Penicillinase-producing staphylococci | Dicloxacillin | Erythromycin | Cephalosporin |
|   3. Gram-positive penicillin resistant organisms (not penicillinase producer) | Erythromycin | Cephalosporin | Tetracycline |
|   4. Mixed infection, gram-positive and gram-negative, not sensitive to penicillin G, known etiology and testing | Ampicillin | Tetracycline | Sulfonamide |
|   5. Oral moniliasis | Nystatin | — | — |

**Table 10.1.** Continued

| | Antibiotic of Choice | | |
|---|---|---|---|
| Orodental Indication | First | Second | Third |
| II. PROPHYLACTIC INDICATIONS | | | |
| A. Protection against subacute bacterial endocarditis | Penicillin | Erythromycin | (Tetracyclines are not recommended because of possible presence of β-hemolytic streptococci) |
|   1. History of rheumatic fever | | | |
|   2. Heart valve prosthesis | | | |
|   3. Congenital heart disease | | | |
|   4. Arteriosclerotic heart disease | | | |
|   5. Hypertensive heart disease | | | |
|   6. Syphilitic heart disease | | | |
| B. Impaired host defense mechanisms | Penicillin | Erythromycin | Tetracyclines |
|   1. Agranulocytosis | | | |
|   2. Aplastic anemia | | | |
|   3. Agammaglobulinemia | | | |
|   4. Diabetes mellitus | | | |
|   5. Addison's disease | | | |
|   6. Lupus erythromatosus | | | |
|   7. Drugs | | | |
|     a. Corticosteroids (large doses) | | | |
|     b. Anticancer agents | | | |
|   8. Generalized systemic disease | | | |
|   9. Geriatric patient with senility (arteriosclerotic disease) | | | |
|   10. Extraction in X-ray treated area | | | |

94% of the cases. Penicillin G is effective in treating infections caused by penicillin G-susceptible streptococci, including *Streptococcus viridans*, as well as infections caused by pneumococci. In addition, penicillin G will cure infections caused by nonpenicillinase-producing staphylococci, including both coagulase-negative and coagulase-positive strains. Furthermore, this antibiotic will inhibit *Actinomyces israelii* and such gram-positive anaerobes as clostridia and corynebacteria. The gram-negative neisseria are inhibited by penicillin G. The causative agent for syphillis, *Treponema pallidum*, and the fusiform organisms of Vincent's disease are susceptible to penicillin G.

MECHANISM OF ACTION. The volume of printed articles on the mechanism of penicillin action is practically beyond the imagination. The evidence is now well confirmed that the site of penicillin's action in susceptible bacteria is an enzyme, a cross-linking transpeptidase, which catalyzes one of the final steps in the biosynthesis of the cell wall component called murein. The similarity between the D-alanyl-D-alanine end group, which is the substrate for the transpeptidase, and the penicillin structure is striking.

Much more important for the dental hygienist than knowing the details of the mechanism is that penicillin acts only upon susceptible bacteria when they are rapidly and actively dividing. It is at this time that new cell wall structure is made. The drug has no effect upon resting bacteria, even if the bacteria are sensitive to penicillin when they are rapidly dividing. Of course, if a bacterium does not synthesize its own cell wall component called murein, penicillin has no effect on the organism. It is of interest perhaps that from this general description of penicillin's site and mechanism of action it can be understood that the drug is not directly bactericidal but indirectly so. Penicillin causes the susceptible bacteria's progeny to have a hole in their cell walls. The susceptible gram-positive bacteria possess an enormous internal osmotic pressure which requires the rigid cell wall to keep them from lysing in the normal osmotic environment of man. When the cell wall fails, the organisms lyse and die. Thus penicillin really alters the susceptible bacteria in such a way that they kill themselves.

ABSORPTION. When penicillin G potassium is administered orally about one fifth to one third of the dose is absorbed from the upper small intestine. This is the case if the dose is given either up to 30 minutes before a meal or no sooner than 2 or 3 hours after a meal. Otherwise, the fraction is smaller. The other two thirds of the dose is destroyed by the acidity of the gastrointestinal tract or passes on to the colon where bacteria usually inactivate it. Penicillin G is rapidly transformed to an inactive product by the acid of gastric juice (pH 2). Therefore it is necessary to give orally a dose four to five times the size of the intramuscular dose in order to get comparable blood levels and durations of action. Following oral administration maximum blood levels occur in 30 to 60 minutes. In contrast with the oral route, the peak blood level following the intramuscular injection of penicillin G is reached in about 15 to 30 minutes. Unfortunately with this form of penicillin the blood level falls quickly; one-half peak level is reached in about 1 hour and virtually all drug is out of the circulation in 3 to 4 hours.

A penicillin G blood serum level of 0.2 to 0.3 $\mu$g/ml is required for successful combat of most susceptible invaders. A single oral dose of 500 mg given to the fasting patient will produce an average peak blood serum level of 0.5 $\mu$g/ml with a serum half-life of 4 hours. A single intramuscular dose of 600 mg will produce an average peak blood serum level of 12.0 $\mu$g/ml with a serum half-life of 30 minutes.

DISTRIBUTION. Penicillin G is widely distributed throughout the body once it reaches the circulation. It appears to be bound to plasma protein to the extent of approximately 65%. There may be a considerable variation in the concentration of penicillin G from one site to another in the body. Penicillin G does not enter easily into the cerebrospinal fluid under normal conditions of the meninges, nor does the drug distribute in significant amounts to bone (although with high dosage the agent will reach effective concentrations in bone). The poor vascularity of abscesses also reduces the distribution of penicillin G in these tissue states.

EXCRETION. Penicillin G is excreted with remarkable speed from the body by the kidneys. The rapid renal excretion accounts for the short half-life of penicillin G in the blood. Much of the drug can be recovered in active form from the bladder urine. Of that found, approximately 10% came by glomerular filtration; the remaining 90% was secreted by the renal tubules. This same tubular secretory mechanism handles the elimination of a number of organic acids from the body and serves as the basis for several drug-drug interactions. Since the adult human male renal tubular mechanisms can secrete up to 1.8 gm of penicillin G per hour, it can be difficult to maintain steady blood levels of the drug. One of the means used to maintain higher and longer blood levels of penicillin G is to give simultaneously a drug that inhibits renal tubular secretion of penicillin. An example of such a drug is probenecid.

UNDESIRABLE PROPERTIES. The major undesirable features of penicillin G potassium are its instability in acid, its rapid renal excretion, and its increasing inability to inhibit certain strains of gonococci and staphylococci, both of which were originally sensitive to it. Initially over 95% of the strains of gonococci could be inhibited by as little as $0.1\,\mu g/ml$ of penicillin G; it now requires at least $1.0\,\mu g/ml$. Approximately 15% of the *Staphylococcus aureus* strains in outpatients are resistant to penicillin G, and upwards of 90% of the *S. aureus* strains in hospitals are now resistant and not susceptible to any dose of penicillin G. These staphylococci produce the enzyme, penicillinase, which inactivates penicillin before it can reach its site of action.

Perhaps the most undesirable property of penicillin G is its allergenicity. Indeed, penicillin is the most allergenic of all antibiotics and holds the record for producing more instances of anaphylactic reactions than any other drug. A cross-sensitivity exists between all penicillins, which means that if the dental patient has a history of allergic reactions to one penicillin, the patient will probably be allergic to all penicillins and must not be given any type of penicillin.

### Penicillin G Procaine (Wycillin)

The procaine salt of penicillin G possesses such a low water solubility that the drug may be injected deeply within skeletal muscle and thereby becomes a tissue depot from which the drug is slowly absorbed over a period of 12 hours to several days. Penicillin G procaine is a repository form of penicillin G. The drug has the same antibacterial spectrum as penicillin G. This drug provides lower blood levels of penicillin G and gives much longer duration of action of blood levels than does an equivalent intramuscular dose of penicillin G potassium. Peak blood levels occur in about 2 hours and persist for usually 18 to 24 hours. The usual adult dose is 600,000 U.S.P. units intramuscularly every 24 hours.

It must be kept in mind that procaine occurs mole for mole with the penicillin G. If a patient has a history of allergic reaction to either penicillin or procaine, the drug cannot be given. The drug is never administered intravenously or subcutaneously.

This repository form of penicillin G may be used in dentistry as part of the procedure for chemoprophylaxis against subacute bacterial endocarditis.

### The Acid-Stable Penicillins

The acid-stable penicillins resulted from the search for a penicillin which would not be inactivated by gastric acid to the same extent as penicillin G. Two penicillins possess this characteristic as their primary reason for existence: phenoxymethyl penicillin potassium or penicillin V potassium (V-Cillin K) and phenethicillin potassium (Darcil). By far the more popular of the two is penicillin

V potassium, and the properties described for an acid-stable penicillin are those specifically for penicillin V potassium.

The antibacterial spectrum for penicillin V potassium is, for the purposes of this textbook, identical to that of penicillin G potassium.

The acid-stable penicillins are better absorbed from the gastrointestinal tract, but the absorption is not complete. Penicillin V potassium is only available in oral dosage forms, and when given in a single oral dose of 500 mg to a fasting patient, penicillin V reaches a peak serum level of 2.9 $\mu$g/ml in about 1 hour with an average serum half-life of 2 hours.

Oral dosage forms for children include drops or suspensions. In order to make the preparations palatable, high concentrations of carbohydrates are added. Therefore, following administration, parents should be certain that good oral hygiene is maintained to prevent the undesirable cariogenic effect of this additional sugar.

The body handles penicillin V potassium in the same manner as reported for penicillin G potassium. If the patient is allergic to one penicillin preparation, he is probably hypersensitive to all penicillins.

### The Penicillinase-Resistant Penicillins

There are five penicillins in this category on the market in the United States, and at least one more is about to be introduced. These penicillins are reserved for one specific situation. When microbiological tests indicate the infecting organism is a strain of penicillinase-producing *Staphylcoccus aureus* which is resistant to penicillin G, then one of these penicillinase-resistant penicillins is the drug of choice. For our purposes only a prototype of this group will be described, i.e., dicloxacillin sodium (Dynapen).

The primary characteristic of these penicillins is their resistance to the enzymatic effects of penicillinase. Although dicloxacillin has a similar antibacterial spectrum to that of penicillin G plus being effective against penicillinase-producing organisms, it must be remembered that dicloxacillin is much less effective than penicillin G against all of those bacteria with the one exception of penicillinase-producing microorganisms. Therefore, dicloxacillin is not to be considered equivalent to penicillin G or to be used interchangeably for it.

Dicloxacillin is only available in oral dosage forms. When it is administered orally in a single 500 mg dose to a fasting patient, the average peak serum level reaches 11.5 $\mu$g/ml with an average serum half-life of 3 hours. The distribution in the body is similar to that of penicillin G with the exception that dicloxacillin is much more highly bound to plasma protein (90 to 95%) than is penicillin G (about 65%). Dicloxacillin is eliminated from the body to a much larger extent via the hepatic-bile route. Table 10.2 shows a comparison between the penicillins regarding their relative degree of acid resistance and penicillinase resistance.

## The Extended-Spectrum Penicillins

The extended-spectrum penicillins are the most rapidly growing group of penicillins and understandably so. The extended-spectrum penicillins are semisynthetic drugs that possess a wider or broader spectrum of antibacterial effects than penicillin G. Whereas penicillin G is extremely effective against the gram-positive cocci (nonpenicillinase-producing) and rods and also against the gram-negative neisseria, it is ineffective against the remaining gram-negative bacteria that infect man. In an attempt to broaden penicillin's range of antibacterial action, ampicillin (Polycillin) was deliberately synthesized and has become the prototype of the extended-spectrum penicillins.

Ampicillin is more effective than penicillin G against enterococci such as *Streptococcus faecalis*. Ampicillin is a drug of first choice in treating infections caused by *Hemophilus influenzae, Escherichia coli, Proteus mirabilis, Salmonella* species, and *Shigella* species. However, when it comes to organisms susceptible to both penicillin G and ampicillin, penicillin G is shown to be more effective in realizing a cure, and therefore penicillin G is still the drug of first choice in these particular situations.

#### Table 10.2.   Resistance of the
#### Penicillins to Destruction by Acid and Penicillinase

|  | Acid Resistance (pH 2) | Penicillinase Resistance |
| --- | --- | --- |
| Penicillin G | + | 0 |
| Penicillin V | + + | 0 |
| Phenethicillin | + + + | + |
| Methicillin | 0 | + + + |
| Nafcillin | + + | + + + |
| Oxacillin | + + | + + + |
| Cloxacillin | + + + | + + + |
| Dicloxacillin | + + + | + + + |
| Ampicillin | + + + | 0 |
| Carbenicillin | 0 | 0 |

Relative degree of resistance: 0 = no resistance; + + + = most resistant

Ampicillin is bactericidal and has the same mechanism of action on cell wall biosynthesis as penicillin G. Ampicillin is well absorbed following oral administrations. A single oral dose in the fasting patient will give an average peak serum level of 3.0 $\mu$g/ml with an average serum half-life of 5 hours. A single intramuscular dose of 500 mg yields an average peak serum level of 4.3 $\mu$g/ml.

Ampicillin is widely used by the oral route, since it is acid-resistant, but unfortunately ampicillin is inactivated by staphylococcal penicillinase as quickly as is penicillin G.

In general dentistry ampicillin is considered the antibiotic of first choice (see Table 10.1) in the treatment of a mixed infection of both gram-positive and gram-negative infecting bacteria that are not sensitive to penicillin G but which microbiological tests show to be sensitive to ampicillin. Remember a patient allergic to one penicillin is allergic to all penicillins. Other extended-spectrum penicillins include amoxicillin, hetacillin, and pivampicillin.

### Specific Purpose Penicillins

The specific purpose penicillins are the latest in penicillin therapy. These penicillins are highly specialized agents used only in selected cases of resistant infections due to especially *Pseudomonas* species and some indole-positive *Proteus* species. These penicillins, exemplified by carbenicillin (Geopen) and its indanyl ester (Geocillin), are not likely to be used in outpatient dentistry. Carbenicillin has an antibacterial spectrum similar to that of ampicillin. The dose required varies greatly from species to species of infecting organism and may range from a few grams to 40 grams for a course of therapy. The drug is very expensive.

### Use of Penicillins in Dentistry

The dental practitioner must treat a variety of acute infections. In the large majority of these cases penicillin is the antibiotic of first choice (see Table 10.1). When penicillin is to be used in dentistry, it is penicillin G specifically or the acid-stable penicillin V that is the penicillin of choice. Of course, if the oral route is indicated, the preparation of choice is penicillin V potassium. The other penicillins are indicated only if there is a specific infection not susceptible to penicillin G or V. Certainly the penicillinase-resistant penicillins, extended-spectrum penicillins, and specific purpose penicillins are not to be considered just "better" penicillin G compounds or as equivalent substitutes for penicillin G or V.

For the purpose of chemoprophylaxis in the dental office the American Dental Association and the American Heart Association establish and restate periodically acceptable guidelines or procedures to follow to achieve the goal of affording the dental patient the best antibiotic prophylaxis possible. There are circumstances that require the dental hygienist to take a specific course of action in this regard. Table 10.1 lists a number of patient conditions that call for the patient to receive chemoprophylaxis if he is to be treated in any way that will lead to bacteremia. Bacteremia is produced by most manipulative procedures in the mouth, including those performed by the dental hygienist. Therefore, before any treatment is carried out, the dental hygienist must determine if each and every patient is in the category of those to receive chemoprophylaxis or those who do not require the procedure. There is no patient who is the exception. All patients will fall into one category or the other. Should the patient be one who requires chemoprophylaxis, then the patient must receive penicillin according to one of the procedures recommended in Table 10.3 or if the patient is allergic to penicillin or if a patient is already on continual oral penicillin for rheumatic fever prophylaxis and may harbor penicillin-resistant *Streptococcus viridans*, then erythromycin as a penicillin substitute is the drug of choice. It is to be noted carefully that the instructions for taking the antibiotics, either penicillin or erythromycin, are very specific. The first dose is to be given 1 hour before the dental procedure if penicillin is the drug of choice. The first dose of erythromycin is to be given 90 minutes to 2 hours before the procedure.

It would be less than bright to think that the penicillins, as used in dentistry, are free of problems. Although directly toxic effects of penicillin in man are rare and usually are unknown except when large doses are given over a number of days to a patient who has severe renal insufficiency, these individuals cannot excrete penicillin and the blood levels can become so high as to produce convulsions by a neural mechanism not yet understood. The most serious problem clinically with penicillin is its allergenicity. The penicillins are the most allergenic drugs available today, and no penicillin of any kind should be given to any dental patient with a positive history of allergic reactions to any one of the penicillins. The allergic reaction to penicillin may include only a mild delayed reaction of a skin rash which may not require any form of treatment. Then again the hypersensitivity reaction may be immediate and take the form of acute anaphylaxis which commands the prompt administration of epineprhine to the patient.

Under no circumstances should any penicillin be administered topically to the skin or mucous membranes, as this route is the most likely to cause sensitization. If there is ever any question in the mind of the dental hygienist or dentist regarding whether a particu-

## Table 10.3.   Suggested Prophylaxis for Dental Procedures

I. *FOR MOST PATIENTS*

Penicillin administered intramuscularly

> 600,000 units of procaine penicillin G mixed with 200,000 units of crystalline penicillin G 1 hour prior to procedure and once daily for the 2 days following the procedure (or longer in the case of delayed healing).

Penicillin administered orally

> A. 500 mg of penicillin V or phenethicillin 1 hour prior to procedure and then 250 mg every 6 hours for the remainder of that day and for the 2 days following the procedure (or longer in the case of delayed healing).
>
> B. 1,200,000 units of penicillin G 1 hour prior to procedure and then 600,000 units every 6 hours for the remainder of that day and for the 2 days following the procedure (or longer in the case of delayed healing).

II. *FOR PATIENTS SUSPECTED TO BE ALLERGIC TO PENICILLIN OR FOR THOSE ON CONTINUAL ORAL PENICILLIN FOR RHEUMATIC FEVER PROPHYLAXIS, WHO MAY HARBOR PENICILLIN-RESISTANT STREPTO-COCCI VIRIDANS*

Erythromycin administered orally

> For adults: 500 mg 1.5 to 2 hours prior to procedure and then 250 mg every 6 hours for the remainder of that day and for the 2 days following the procedure (or longer in the case of delayed healing).
>
> For children: The dose for small children is 20 mg/kg orally 1.5 to 2 hours prior to procedure and then 10 mg/kg every 6 hours for the remainder of that day and for the 2 days following the procedure (or longer in the case of delayed healing).

Source: Data from American Heart Association, 1972.[7]

lar patient may react adversely to penicillin, then the simplest and safest procedure would be to have the patient take the initial penicillin dose in the dental office where the staff may watch the patient closely and be ready to treat any acute drug reaction that may develop.

## THE ERYTHROMYCINS

The erythromycins are, for the most part, used in general dentistry only when the patient is allergic to the penicillins or when the invading organism shows resistance to the penicillins. The erythromycins are, therefore, antibiotics of second choice in general dentistry.

For many years the erythromycins have been referred to as the penicillin substitute antibiotic. The erythromycins are also members of the macrolide group of antibiotics because they contain a many-membered lactone ring to which are attached one or more deoxy sugars. Of this group the erythromycins are the most important. Whereas there are a number of erythromycin products available on the market, there is only one chemical substance known as erythromycin. Except where necessary to point out specific differences between one or more of the erythromycin esters, the following profile refers to the basic compound erythromycin (Ilotycin).

ANTIBACTERIAL SPECTRUM. Erythromycin has an antibacterial spectrum similar to that of penicillin G, but it is much weaker against the gram-negative neisseria. Erythromycin, which is not destroyed by penicillinase, may be used to treat infections caused by penicillinase-producing organisms. It may be of interest to the dental hygienist that erythromycin is the drug of first choice in treating infections caused by mycoplasma. In contrast to the penicillins, erythryomycin is also effective against certain rickettsiae. There is little evidence of sensitization with erythromycin and no cross-sensitivity with penicillins, so erythromycin may be used in safety for the dental patient allergic to the penicillins.

MECHANISM OF ACTION. Erythromycin exerts its mechanism of action by inhibiting microbial protein synthesis, especially the production of highly polymerized peptides. The drug appears to accumulate one hundred times more in gram-positive than in gram-negative bacteria, and the specific site of binding is the 50S ribosomal unit. Because erythromycin is not the only drug that binds at this particular site, there is a potential for a drug-drug interaction. It is of importance to realize that erythromycin does not bind to mammalian ribosomal units nor, therefore, inhibit mammalian protein synthesis. As used in general dentistry erythromycin is essentially bacteriostatic in its action; however, recent claims have been made for the antibiotic's bactericidal activity when it is administered in higher oral dosage.

PHARMACOKINETICS. Erythromycin is adequately absorbed from the upper duodenum to give antibacterial blood levels. The drug is, however, partly inactivated by the gastric juice acidity. Furthermore, the presence of food retards absorption of the drug. The variety of esters of erythromycin are claimed not to be as susceptible to acid destruction, and the manufacturer of the oral dosage form of the ethylsuccinate ester (E.E.S.) states the erythromycin is absorbed more completely in the presence of food. Certainly the presence of food should reduce the drug's tendency to irritate the gastric mucosa. As for many drugs the major portion of the antibiotic is absorbed from the upper duodenum. A single oral dose (500 mg) of the base or the stearate ester (Erythrocin stearate) will give average serum concentrations in the fasting person of approximately 1 $\mu$g/ml and show an average serum half-life of 4 hours. A single oral dose of the estolate ester (Ilosone) (500 mg) will yield a level of 2.5 $\mu$g/ml for an average half-life of 3.5 hours. The serum peak attained by the estolate ester is reached more slowly. Smaller doses of erythromycin can be administered intramuscularly or intravenously, but these routes of administration are rarely required in general dentistry.

Erythromycin is bound to plasma protein to the extent of about 18% and is one of the least bound of the antibiotics. Since the antibiotic cannot cross the blood-brain barrier, the drug is useless in the treatment of meningitis. The drug accumulates in the liver and is excreted in large amounts in the bile; only 2 to 5% is excreted in the urine.

TOXICITY. The estolate ester of erythromycin would appear to cause the most serious toxicity which is manifested as the hypersensitivity reaction cholestatic hepatitis. Erythromycin does not produce any significant, direct adverse reactions, and the most common complaint from the dental patient may be lower intestinal cramping when large oral doses are ingested. The drug is irritating. Suprainfections or overgrowth of nonsusceptible microorganisms can occur when erythromycin is administered orally over a long period or repeatedly. The incidence is low. Erythromycin is not cross-allergenic with the penicillins. Except for the estolate ester there is little evidence of hypersensitivity reactions.

DEVELOPMENT OF RESISTANCE. There has been a definite problem in recent years with a rapid increase in erythromycin-resistant staphylococci. Erythromycin is unusual as an antibiotic regarding the rapidity with which certain bacteria appear to develop resistance. Although this fact should not call for reduction in the use of the drug, it does clearly call for all practitioners to prescribe erythromycin with greater care than in the past so that the tremendous benefits of this antibiotic will exist for the next generations.

CLINICAL USE IN GENERAL DENTISTRY. There is little question in anyone's mind, based upon a long clinical experience, that erythromycin is one of the best antibiotics of second choice to treat or prevent susceptible infections in patients who are hypersensitive to the penicillins or who cannot take the penicillins for some other reason. The question commonly arises as to why erythromycin is a drug of second choice and not a drug of first choice. Some of the reasons for this important second choice position are given as follows: At the usual doses employed clinically in treating oral infections, erythromycin is bacteriostatic and not bactericidal. Bacterial resistance of organisms known to cause oral infections can develop rapidly. Erythromycin, in dental clinical experience, would appear to be slightly less effective than penicillin in treating the common dental infections. It should be fairly stated, however, that more definitive, comparative studies of orofacial infections using erythromycin and penicillin are needed. In erythromycin's favor is its lack of cross-resistance (of microbes) or cross-sensitivity (of hosts) with the penicillins.

At the present time erythromycin is the antibiotic of second choice for chemoprophylaxis in dentistry. Table 10.3 shows the circumstances in which erythromycin is required and the dosage procedure to follow in its administration.

### CLINDAMYCIN

Clindamycin hydrochloride hydrate (Cleocin) is an antibiotic of importance today in general dentistry and, owing to its unusual toxicity, the drug must be evaluated carefully. Clindamycin is a chemical derivative of lincomycin (Lincocin) and offers several advantages over the parent compound. Clindamycin was widely used as a penicillin substitute in dentistry and especially as a drug of first choice in the treatment of acute bone infections (e.g., osteomyelitis) until evidence for a severe lower intestinal adverse effect appeared.

ANTIBACTERIAL SPECTRUM. Clindamycin has a somewhat narrower spectrum of antibacterial activity than erythromycin, but the antibiotic is effective against *Mycoplasma hominis* infections as well as the gram-negative intestinal bacteroides. Although there is some difference of opinion, this text will consider clindamycin as a narrow spectrum antibiotic.

MECHANISM OF ACTION. Like erythromycin, clindamycin exerts its antibacterial effect by inhibiting microbial protein synthesis. Clindamycin binds to the 50S ribosomal subunit of susceptible organisms and in turn inhibits the binding of aminoacyl transfer-RNA to these ribosomes. This mechanism is proposed to be identical or similar to that observed for chloramphenicol. However, the antibacterial spectra of these two antibiotics are not similar. There would also seem to be a drug-drug interaction between clindamycin and erythromycin based upon a closely similar binding site in the microbial ribosome. Erythromycin has a greater affinity for the site than does clindamycin; therefore, erythromycin can antagonize clindamycin's antibacterial properties. If erythromycin is present in the body and the organisms in question are resistant to erythromycin and the drug is still attached to the 50S ribosomes, clindamycin's action is blocked, even though the organisms are susceptible to the clindamycin.

Clindamycin may be bacteriostatic or bactericidal. To most susceptible organisms the drug is bacteriostatic in therapeutic dosage, but there are indications that other mechanisms are involved because it would appear to affect both rapidly growing as well as resting susceptible bacteria.

PHARMACOKINETICS. Following the usual oral single dose clindamycin is absorbed to the extent of 90% from the upper duodenum, and the drug's absorption does not seem to be affected by the presence of food in the stomach, nor is the drug inactivated by gastric acidity. A single oral dose of 450 mg in the fasting individual will produce an average peak serum level of $4.5 \mu g/ml$ in approximately 45 minutes with an average half-life of 3.5 hours. Twenty five percent of circulating clindamycin is protein bound. The antibiotic is quickly and widely distributed in body fluids and tissues and especially in bone, which gives the drug one of its major advantages.

Clindamycin is metabolized in the body to N-demethylclindamycin and clindamycin sulfoxide, and only 10% of a dose is excreted unchanged. Approximately 10% of the drug is excreted in the urine, with the remainder believed to be excreted in the feces.

TOXICITY. The toxicity of clindamycin is of major concern at the present time, and the drug's future use in dentistry is in jeopardy. Until more is learned about the severe colitis clindamycin may produce, no dental practitioner can justify its use in the treatment of orofacial infections in outpatients. There may be a few, unusual instances in which the drug must be administered, but administration must be accomplished in the hospital.

The Food and Drug Administration issued the following statement in early 1975:

The incidence of pseudomembranous colitis, a serious, potentially fatal gastrointestinal disease, following lincomycin (Lincocin) and clindamycin (Cleocin) therapy, is considerably greater than has been appreciated heretofore. Estimates of incidence now range from 1 in 10,000 in a review of clinical experience to as high as 1 in 10 in a study using proctoscopy. The mortality rate is as yet undetermined. As of January 1975, a total of 28 deaths reported to the FDA appear to be related to colitis induced by one or another of the two drugs, the deaths occurring mostly in older persons with other serious illness. Additional deaths have probably not been reported. Because of this new information, FDA will order revisions in the Warning and restrict the Indications as follows:

Clindamycin (or lincomycin) can cause severe colitis which may end fatally. Therefore, it should be reserved for serious infections where less toxic antimicrobial agents are inappropriate, as described in the Indications section. It should not be used in patients with nonbacterial infections, such as most upper respiratory infections. The colitis is usually characterized by severe, persistent diarrhea and severe abdominal cramps and may be associated with the passage of blood and mucus. Endoscopic examination may reveal pseudomembranous colitis.

When significant diarrhea occurs, the drug should be discontinued or, if necessary, continued only with close observation of the patient. Large bowel endoscopy has been recommended.

Antiperistaltic agents such as opiates and diphenoxylate with atropine (Lomotil) may prolong and/or worsen the condition.

Diarrhea, colitis, and pseudomembranous colitis have been observed to begin up to several weeks following cessation of therapy with clindamycin (or lincomycin).

Clindamycin is indicated in the treatment of serious infections caused by susceptible anaerobic bacteria.

Clindamycin also (or lincomycin) is indicated in the treatment of serious infections due to susceptible strains of streptococci, pneumococci, and staphylococci. Its use should be reserved for penicillin-allergic patients or other patients for whom, in the judgment of the physician, a penicillin is inappropriate. Because of the risk of colitis, as described in the Box Warning, before selecting clindamycin (or lincomycin) the physician should consider the nature of the infection and the suitability of less toxic alternatives (e.g., erythromycin).[4]

It would be a considerable loss to dentistry to lose clindamycin forever, but under the FDA clear warning the drug cannot be used routinely in general dentistry. Clindamycin still is a fine penetrator of bone and effective in the treatment of osteomyelitis, but it must remain on the shelf until more is understood regarding pseudomembranous colitis.

## THE TETRACYCLINES

Seven antibiotics currently on the market in the United States are classified by their chemical structure as tetracyclines. Since these drugs are similar in terms of their chemistry, pharmacology, antibacterial spectrum, and therapeutic indications, only the prototype, tetracycline (Achromycin) will be discussed. The other members of this group will be mentioned only when necessary to emphasize a difference from the prototype.

The tetracyclines represent one of the early successful groups of antibacterial substances which have continued over the last 30 years to fulfill a need for a broad spectrum antimicrobial agent. Unfortunately, their widespread use is accompanied by even wider-spread misuse.

ANTIBACTERIAL SPECTRUM. The tetracyclines are the broadest of the broad spectrum antibiotics. Their antibacterial activity extends to many gram-positive and gram-negative bacteria as well as to rickettsiae, the Chlamydia, the Mycoplasma, and amebae. The only large group of pathogens not affected by the tetracyclines is the fungi. In general terms the gram-positive bacteria are more sensitive to tetracycline than the gram-negative, but since these antibiotics in usual therapeutic doses are bacteriostatic at best, other more specific, more narrow spectrum antibiotics are considered as the antibiotics of first choice. Indeed, in general dentistry there is no one single indication for which tetracycline is the antibiotic of first choice either in terms of treating an acute infection (see Table 10.1) or in terms of chemoprophylaxis. Tetracycline is usually the antibiotic of third choice after penicillin and erythromycin.

MECHANISM OF ACTION. The tetracyclines bind specifically and, for the most part, reversibly to the 30S ribosomal subunit of susceptible microorganisms. By preventing the binding of aminoacyl-tRNA, effective microbial protein synthesis is suppressed. The action is essentially bacteriostatic only.

PHARMACOKINETICS. Tetracycline is usually administered orally and readily, though incompletely, absorbed from the stomach and upper duodenum. The absorption is definitely reduced by the presence of divalent and trivalent cations such as calcium, aluminum, magnesium, and iron. These cations form insoluble tetracycline chelates that are not absorbed. A single oral dose of 500 mg to the fasting patient will give an average peak serum level of $3 \mu g/ml$ within 2 to 4 hours and show an average serum half-life of 8.5 hours if the patient has normal renal function. Tetracycline distributes widely throughout the body, and the highest concentrations may be found in bone, lymph nodes, liver, and kidneys. These antibiotics cross the placental barrier and are deposited in the fetal skeleton and calcifying teeth. Tetracyclines are excreted in both the feces and the urine. These drugs are secreted in bile and enter the enterohepatic cycle. The duration of action of the tetracyclines is greatly dependent upon proper renal function. In renal failure or in the elderly whose usual glomerular filtration rate may be one third of its normal rate at 30 years of age, these antibiotics demonstrate a prolonged serum half-life. Doxycycline (Vibramycin) would appear to be an exception to the rule, since this antibiotic does not accumulate in patients with renal failure.

TOXICITY. The tetracyclines also produce a broad spectrum of toxic effects or certainly unwanted side effects. The most commonly occurring undesirable effect involves gastrointestinal disturbances. Tetracycline may produce upset due to its directly irritating properties or, as is more often the case, suprainfections arise because of the broad spectrum of antibacterial activity. Fungi, especially *Candida albicans*, overgrow, and this overgrowth in turn may produce gastrointestinal irritation, glossitis, stomatitis and pruritus ani.

Another symptom of gastrointestinal disturbance produced by the tetracyclines is diarrhea. The watery expulsion of the bowels is not uncommon, and the practitioner must follow the patient's condition closely in order to be certain the diarrhea is not the result of colonic suprainfection caused by tetracycline-resistant staphylococci. This condition, like that which may be caused by clindamycin, may be fatal.

There is evidence to indicate that tetracycline can prolong blood-clotting time by mechanisms not yet understood.

Certainly of greater interest to the dental hygienist is the enamel hypoplasia and tooth pigmentation that may result from the use of tetracyclines. Tetracyclines may produce these unwanted effects at any time between the fourth month of gestation and the eighth year of life.[5, 6] The deposit of tetracycline in the teeth is permanent. There may be a slight variation in the color of the stain, depending upon the particular tetracycline administered, but the color is usually yellowish when the tooth erupts and then changes to a darker more brown tone. It is believed that the reaction of tetracycline to light brings about the color change. The degree of discoloration does not appear to correlate well with the total dose administered per day.

The inhibition of proper enamel and dentin mineralization may accompany the discoloring of the teeth. Therefore the best evidence would dictate the withholding of all tetracyclines during the last trimester of pregnancy and during the first 8 years of life.

Another form of toxicity involves the kidneys. Renal insufficiency leads to the profound prolongation of the biologic half-life of most tetracyclines in the body. The levels of tetracycline may reach sufficient levels to produce renal damage.

Tetracyclines at easily attainable high blood levels may produce profound metabolic disturbances (azotemia) due to a nonspecific catabolic action. By mechanisms still unknown, tetracyclines would appear to enhance the renal excretion of the B vitamin riboflavin. This enhancement is the basis for the drug interaction.

Lastly, the tetracycline, demeclocycline, has a tendency to produce photosensitization of the skin.

DENTAL USE. The tetracyclines do have a definite but not large role in clinical dentistry. The situation may arise in which the first and second antibiotics of choice (penicillin and erythromycin, respectively) cannot be given to the dental patient, and it is at this point that serious consideration must be given to tetracycline. The emergence of many resistant strains of staphylococci and group A beta hemolytic streptococci makes the tetracyclines doubtful agents for chemoprophylaxis against bacteremias from dental procedures. Certainly the effectiveness of the tetracycline should be proven with the appropriate bacterial sensitivity tests. A general rule would be to use the tetracycline only when an antibiotic with a more narrow spectrum and bactericidal activity cannot be used.

Combinations of tetracycline with antifungal agents in fixed dosage combinations have not been demonstrated to be clinically superior to each type of drug given alone when indicated. The combination of bacteriostatic tetracycline with bactericidal penicillins creates a definite drug-drug interaction. If the tetracycline inhibits the growth of bacteria susceptible to penicillin, penicillin will be unable to kill the organisms, since penicillin only acts upon rapidly growing bacteria by inhibiting synthesis of new cell wall.

## TOPICAL ANTIBACTERIAL ANTIBIOTICS

The dentist has always wanted to treat oral disorders locally and not get involved (so they would like to believe) with the rest of the body. The basis for this philosophy is historical and to some extent understandable, although unrealistic. Dentists were the first to use antibiotics topically in the oral cavity much in the same way mouthwashes (containing local antiinfectives) had always been used. The modern dentist and dental hygienist should know why topical antibiotics are a subject of special concern. There are occasions when a topically applied antibiotic is indicated, and the general rules of chemotherapy would dictate the following: (1) When an antibiotic is used topically, it may have only a superficial action and its effectiveness is limited to the superficial, susceptible microorganisms. (2) Topical antibiotics may produce severe local reactions. (3) Sensitization of the patient may occur more frequently when a drug is applied to skin and/or mucous membranes. (4) Although high concentrations of the antibiotic may be achieved locally, dilution in the oral cavity occurs readily and allows low concentrations of the drug to be swallowed. (5) A combination of systemic administration and local administration of the same antibiotic may be required in some rare instances. (6) If a topical route alone for the antibiotic is indicated in the management of dental infection, then the practitioner should use one that is not also used systemically. This would circumvent the possible problem of severe sensitization reactions and development of resistance to the systemically administered antibiotic.

Three antibiotics are essentially used only topically. These are the drugs of choice when only the topical route of administration is indicated.

POLYPEPTIDE ANTIBIOTICS. The polypeptide antibiotics are all cyclic structures produced by bacilli and possess surface-active properties. If these antibiotics are absorbed to a significant extent or are given parenterally, there is an excellent chance that nephrotoxicity will result. Fortunately when these antibiotics are applied topically to mucous membranes they are not usually absorbed.

Polymyxin-B (Aerosporin) is bactericidal by attaching to bacterial membrane lipoproteins, damaging the osmotic barrier, and producing a leakage from the bacterial cell of essential nucleotides. Polymyxin-B appears to be active against both growing and resting susceptible microorganisms. The antibacterial effect of the drug is antagonized by divalent metals such as calcium, magnesium, and ferrous iron. Its spectrum of antibacterial activity includes mainly the gram-negative bacteria. Development of bacterial resistance is slow, and toxicity by the topical route of administration is rare and involves only mild gastrointestinal disturbances. When applied topically to oral lesions, polymyxin-B is not absorbed into the systemic circulation to any significant extent. This is fortunate, since the parenteral route of administration (not used in dentistry for this agent) leads to such severe toxicities as renal damage, nerve damage (paresthesias), and curarelike neuromuscular blockade. In dentistry polymyxin-B serves as an excellent topical anti-gram-negative antibiotic.

Bacitracin (Baciguent) is bactericidal by inhibiting the biosynthesis of the bacterial cell wall, an action in which it synergizes with penicillin. Evidence would indicate that bacitracin also suppresses bacterial-induced enzyme synthesis. The antibacterial spectrum for bacitracin includes mainly gram-positive bacteria, but the antibiotic is also effective against neisseria and amebae. Bacitracin is bactericidal for virtually all staphylococci, regardless of the organisms' established resistance to other antibiotics. Development of bacterial resistance is slow. When it is applied locally in the oral cavity and then subsequently swallowed, there is insignificant absorption of the antibiotic into the systemic circulation. Bacitracin is nonsensitizing (thus far) when applied topically and is also nonirritating. In dentistry bacitracin is a good topical anti-gram-positive antibiotic.

AMINOGLYCOSIDE ANTIBIOTICS. The aminoglycoside antibiotics are important chemotherapeutic agents used to treat a wide variety of serious infectious diseases in man. Included in this group are antibiotics such as streptomycin, gentamicin, tobramycin, kanamycin, and neomycin, but for our purposes in general dentistry only the topical administration of neomycin will be considered.

Neomycin sulfate (Mycifradin) is bactericidal by acting as a detergent on bacterial cell surfaces and thereby interfering with the selective permeability of the bacterial cell membrane. Neomycin also inhibits bacterial protein synthesis. The antibacterial spectrum is broad enough to cover most gram-positive and gram-negative bacteria, including the tubercle bacilli and *Proteus* species as well. Bacterial resistance develops in a slow, stepwise manner, and cross-resistance exists between neomycin and the other amino-glycosides. When neomycin is applied topically, it produces little or no reported sensitization nor is the drug irritating. If neomycin is administered topically only in recommended amounts, the drug is not significantly absorbed into the systemic circulation. Neomycin is an example of a relatively safe antibiotic when used locally, but a very toxic agent when used parenterally. Neomycin is known to cause ototoxicity (auditory nerve damage and deafness) as well as kidney damage when administered by injection. As used in general dentistry by topical administration to oral cavity lesions, neomycin is an excellent relatively broad spectrum (both anti-gram-positive and anti-gram-negative) antibiotic.

## ANTIFUNGAL ANTIBIOTICS

The general dental practitioner must treat fungal infections of the oral cavity, and the most frequently employed means of doing so is to apply a topical antifungal antibiotic. The systemic treatment of fungal infections is complex and should be referred to a hospital and to experienced practitioners in this area of therapy. In outpatient dentistry the dental hygienist will most often observe the dentist prescribing only one topical antifungal agent, nystatin.

Nystatin (Mycostatin) can be either fungistatic or fungicidal, depending upon the concentration of the antibiotic in contact with the fungal cells. Nystatin is not absorbed from intact skin or mucous membranes. Although useful in the topical treatment of a variety of infectious fungi in man, nystatin's major use in general dentistry is in the treatment of mucocutaneous infections caused by *Candida albicans* (Monilia), such as oral thrush. Nystatin does not possess antibacterial or antiviral properties and only acts upon fungal organisms containing sterol in the cell membrane.

Nystatin produces a low incidence of adverse effects when held in the mouth or swallowed. However, the drug is slightly irritating. Oral tablets (500,000 units each) are allowed to dissolve in the oral cavity every 6 to 8 hours. The oral suspension dose is divided in half, and one half held in contact with each side of the mouth for several minutes before swallowing. If the dental patient who has oral monilial infection also has removable prosthetic devices in the mouth, these items should be treated with nystatin as well as the oral cavity.

## REFERENCES

1. Weinstein, L.: Chemotherapy of microbial diseases. *In* The Pharmacological Basis of Therapeutics. 5th Edition. Edited by L.S. Goodman and A. Gilman. New York, Macmillan, 1975.

2. Davis, B. D., Dulbecco, R., Eisen, H.N., Ginsberg, H.S., and Wood, Jr., W.B.: Microbiology. 2nd Edition. Hagerstown, Md., Harper and Row, 1973.
3. Pratt, W.B.: Fundamentals of Chemotherapy. New York, Oxford University Press, 1973.
4. Serious gastrointestinal toxicity due to clindamycin and lincomycin. FDA Drug Bulletin, 5:2, 1975.
5. Annotation. Tetracyclines and teeth. Lancet, 2:71, 1965.
6. Leading Article. Tetracyclines and teeth. Lancet, 1:917, 1966.
7. American Heart Association: Prevention of bacterial endocarditis. J. Am. Dent. Assoc., 85:1377, 1972.

## SUPPLEMENTARY REFERENCE

Hoeprich, P.D. (ed.): Infectious Diseases. Hagerstown, Md., Harper and Row, 1972.

# 11

## DENTAL SPECIALTY AGENTS

There are many types of dental specialty agents such as cavity liners and bases, pulpal protectants, desensitizing agents (see Chapter 7), fluorides (see Chapter 6), root canal sealants, and pit and fissure sealants. It is not uncommon in dentistry to find practical applications for drugs in addition to their more traditional uses in the prevention, diagnosis, and/or treatment of oral diseases. One such group of dental specialty compounds known as the gingival retraction agents serves as a good example and will be the group considered in this chapter.

### GINGIVAL RETRACTION AGENTS

When various hydrocolloid and rubber base impression materials are to be used, it is necessary to allow the impression material to creep into the gingival crevice to the cementoenamel junction in order to reproduce the negative of the marginal lines of the particular tooth preparation. In the usual situation, therefore, it is necessary to move the free marginal gingiva away from the tooth for a brief time while the impression is being taken.

In addition to the many nondrug means by which the free marginal gingiva may be temporarily (or with some procedures permanently) displaced, there are chemical substances or drugs which also enjoy widespread use because they produce a similar tissue response. As one might imagine, many drugs can accomplish the task of retracting the free marginal gingiva from the tooth. The number is much smaller when the condition is added that, once the impression-taking is completed, it is expected that the drug's effects will be reversed so that the free marginal gingiva returns to its normal size and position. Remember that any damage to the gingiva so as to prevent its return to normal position may lead to injury to the gingival attachment and thence to recession which defeats the entire procedure.

There is little pharmacology regarding the gingival retraction agents used today. Therefore there is a desperate need for well-controlled experimental as well as clinical investigations to shed light upon not only how these agents work, but also how one agent compares in safety and effectiveness with another.

What drugs can actually bring about the type of tissue response desired? Various astringents could be utilized, since their major effect on tissue when applied topically is to reduce or condense the surface area or size. Secondly, various vasoconstrictors, when properly applied topically and locally, could reduce the bulk of this highly vascular tissue by reducing the flow of blood through the localized area and thereby induce the free marginal gingiva to move away from the cementoenamel junction.

## Astringents

Astringents act, it is believed, by precipitating tissue protein, but they have so little penetrability that only the cell surfaces in direct contact with the agent are affected. The permeability of the cell is greatly reduced, but the cell still remains alive. As the surface condenses, the general effect is experienced as a puckering of the tissue. There are two classes of astringents: the aqueous solutions of heavy metal salts and the aqueous solutions of naturally occurring vegetable substances such as tannic acid.

ALUMINUM PREPARATIONS. Aqueous solutions of aluminum salts are some of the most widely used astringents and find use as gingival retracting agents. Solutions of 1 to 5% hydrated aluminum ammonium sulfate ($AlNH_4(SO_4)_2 \cdot 12H_2O$; ammonium alum) or hydrated aluminum potassium sulfate ($AlK(SO_4)_2 \cdot 12H_2O$; potassium alum) have a pH of approximately 4 and 3, respectively. The procedure for either preparation involves soaking a multistranded cotton cord in the astringent solution and then applying the cord to the gingival sulcus around the tooth. A modification would be to place the dry cord in the sulcus first and then apply the astringent solution to the cord. As the name would indicate, exsiccated alum contains no water of hydration, is extremely hygroscopic, and when applied to living tissue draws moisture from that tissue. Therefore, it must be remembered to use a lower concentration of the exsiccated product.

Aluminum acetate solution (5%), otherwise called Burrow's solution, is also used as a gingival retracting agent (pH 4.2).

Aluminum chloride solutions ranging in concentrations of 8 to 25% of the hydrated salt ($AlCl_3 \cdot 6H_2O$) are widely used as exemplified by the well-known products, Hemodent and Nephrostat, which contain 8% and 25% aluminum chloride, respectively. Hemodent is known to have a pH of approximately 1.72.

IRON PREPARATIONS. The water-soluble iron salts are noted for their unpleasant staining characteristics and their corrosive effect on living tissue (both hard and soft tissues). Perhaps they should be limited to their biggest market, styptic pencils. Ferric chloride in an aqueous solution of 8 to 10% (pH 1.12) has been employed as a gingival retracting agent but should no longer be so used because it irreversibly damages the gingival tissue (chemical burn) and is not good on the enamel either (decalcifies). Hydrated ferric subsulfate ($Fe_4(SO_4)_5(OH)_2 \cdot 10H_2O$), or Monsel's solution, offers no advantage over the ferric chloride preparations.

ZINC PREPARATIONS. Only one zinc salt, 8 to 20% aqueous solutions of zinc chloride, still shows some popularity. The higher concentrations are definitely corrosive to soft tissue.

Tannic acid, the naturally occurring astringent, has been used as a gingival retracting agent in the past, usually in 0.5 to 1% aqueous solutions (such concentrations as found in tea infusions), but it has never had many supporters.

In general, the use of one of these astringents locally (via the cotton cord procedure) will produce greater retraction of the free marginal gingiva than many of the nondrug, nonsurgical means. Their degree of desired effect, however, may not be sufficient because the concentration that must be used is really toxic locally or the time of placement (or exposure to the astringent) may become simply too unrealistic for the usual dental practice.

### Vasoconstrictors

It is not surprising that a strong vasoconstrictor, such as epinephrine, would become a gingival retracting agent. No one knows who first used epinephrine in this manner, but probably it was observed to retract the gingiva and reduce the tissue bulk while a 1:1,000 aqueous solution of epinephrine was being used to control local bleeding (certainly not an uncommon practice today in general dentistry).

The gingiva is highly vascular, and its bulk is regulated in part by the volume of blood flow which in turn stretches the tissue. When the blood flow through localized areas of the gingiva is greatly reduced, the local area fed by these vessels shrinks. There is no question but that epinephrine applied topically in the proper concentration will give the desired tissue retraction. There are no studies (to the author's knowledge) comparing epinephrine's effectiveness and safety at a number of dose levels or comparing epinephrine with other adrenergic and nonadrenergic vasoconstrictors. It is being assumed that when epinephrine is applied topically to the gingival crevice it is being absorbed to the extent of reaching at least the vascular smooth muscle. Secondly, it is being assumed that the concentration of epinephrine used will be just enough to produce a mild ischemia without causing local gingival hypoxia or necrosis.

Several epinephrine-containing products are used as gingival retracting agents. Ranephrine is an aqueous solution (pH 2.69) that contains racemic epinephrine hydrochloride in a concentration of 1:500 or 2 mg/ml. Adrenalin solution contains levo-epinephrine hydrochloride in a concentration 1:1,000 or 1 mg/ml. Perhaps the most widely used epinephrine-containing commercial gingival retraction agent is a product called Gingi-pak which, according to its labeling, is a cotton cord impregnated so as to obtain 0.5 mg of racemic epinephrine hydrochloride per inch. This cord, it is stated,

### Table 11.1. Comparison of Gingival Retraction Agents

| Agent Used | Effectiveness* | Tissue Recovery | Other Bad Qualities |
|---|---|---|---|
| 1. Alum (saturated solution) | 4.25 | Good | None |
| 2. Cocaine 10% + epinephrine 1:1,000 | 2.0 | Good | — |
| 3. Hemodent | 5.4 | Good | None |
| 4. Gingi-pak (alone) | 5.0 | Fair | None |
| 5. Gingi-pak + alum (saturated solution) | 6.0 | Fair | None |
| 6. Cord, 8% zinc chloride + 8% epinephrine racemic | 6.0 | Fair | Cauterizes |
| 7. Monsel's solution | 5.75 | Good | Messy to use |
| 8. Negatan | 6.0 | Poor | Decalcifies |
| 9. Cord, plain cotton | 1.0 | Good | None |
| 10. Tannic acid, 20% solution | 4.0 | Good | None |
| 11. Cord, 8% zinc chloride | 4.9 | Fair | Cauterizes |
| 12. Cord, 40% zinc chloride | 5.6 | Poor | Cauterizes |
| 13. Cord, 8% r-epinephrine | 4.5 | Fair | None |

Source: Data taken from Woycheshin, 1964.[2]
Note: * rating scale in arbitrary units.

### Table 11.2. Ranking of Gingival Retraction Agents According to Effectiveness Only

| Agent Used | Effectiveness Rating* |
|---|---|
| Gingi-pak + alum (saturated solution) | 6.0 |
| Cord, 8% zinc chloride + 8% r-epineph- rine | 6.0 |
| Negatan | 6.0 |
| Monsel's solution | 5.75 |
| Cord, 40% zinc chloride | 5.6 |
| Hemodent | 5.4 |
| Gingi-pak (alone) | 5.0 |
| Cord, 8% zinc chloride | 4.9 |
| Cord, 8% r-epinephrine | 4.5 |
| Alum (saturated solution) | 4.25 |
| Tannic acid, 20% solution | 4.0 |
| Cocaine 10% + epinephrine 1:1,000 | 2.0 |
| Cord, plain cotton | 1.0 |

Source: Data modified from Woycheshin, 1964.[2]
Note: * rating scale in arbitrary units.

is presoaked in a sterile 8% r-epinephrine HCl solution with 1% benzyl alcohol as preservative.[1]

When these epinephrine-containing products are applied to the gingival crevice, the epinephrine is absorbed into the circulation with the rapidity of an intramuscular injection. Hence the use of any epinephrine-containing gingival retraction agent is absolutely contraindicated in dental patients with a history of cardiovascular disease. It would also be unwise to employ such agents in patients with hyperthyroidism or in patients who are currently taking any one of the tricyclic antidepressants.

There are few comparative investigations of gingival retraction agents, but the most comprehensive thus far is that of Woycheshin reported in 1964.[2] As shown in Table 11.1, the agents tested were ranked according to what was considered to be the individual product's effectiveness in addition to the tissue's ability to recover after each agent's application and any bad qualities manifested. If the reported data are rearranged to show only the ranking by effectiveness, Table 11.2 results. However, using the same data but eliminating every agent possessing "other bad qualities" and listing the remaining agents according to their effectiveness rating

**Table 11.3.   Ranking of Gingival Retraction Agents According to Effectiveness and Ability of Tissue to Recover**

| Agent Used | Effectiveness Rating* | Tissue Recovery |
|---|---|---|
| Hemodent | 5.4 | Good |
| Alum (saturated solution) | 4.25 | Good |
| Tannic acid, 20% solution | 4.0 | Good |
| Cocaine 10% + epinephrine 1:1,000 | 2.0 | Good |
| Cord, plain cotton | 1.0 | Good |
| Gingi-pak + alum (saturated solution) | 6.0 | Fair |
| Gingi-pak (alone) | 5.0 | Fair |
| Cord, 8% r-epinephrine | 4.5 | Fair |

Source: Data modified from Woycheshin, 1964.[2]
Note: * rating scale in arbitrary units.

and the ability of the tissue to recover produces a different grouping of the possible agents of choice (see Table 11.3).

For the sake of emphasis, let it be stated clearly that many more well-controlled experimental and clinical studies need to be carried out to serve as a rational basis for the existence of gingival retraction agents.

## REFERENCES

1. Gingi-pak labeling. Surgident, Ltd. Los Angeles, California.
2. Woycheshin, F.F.: An evaluation of drugs used in gingival retraction. J. Prosthet. Dent., *14*:769, 1964.

# 12

## VITAMINS

A vitamin may be defined broadly as a chemical substance that is essential for the maintenance of normal metabolic functions but is not synthesized by the body and, therefore, must be furnished from an exogenous source. As the definition implies, the vitamins are involved in a wide number of metabolic reactions that are necessary for the proper utilization of other nutrients such as fats, proteins, and carbohydrates and are, thus, necessary for growth, maintenance, and repair of the body. This chapter is not intended to be a complete discussion of the vitamins. The dental hygienist is referred to a comprehensive text for a detailed discussion of vitamin pharmacology[1] as well as to *Accepted Dental Therapeutics* for a discussion of the oral manifestations of disorders related to the vitamins.[2] The following is a brief consideration of the unique aspects of the vitamins when used as drugs.

### VITAMINS AS DRUGS

The healthy adult who eats a well-balanced diet will usually get amounts of vitamins adequate to meet basic body requirements through his food intake. Most authorities agree that administration of purified vitamins in amounts in excess of those needed to supply the basic body requirements provides no further beneficial effects, although this is an area of intense controversy. One reason for the controversy is the difficulty in defining the dietary vitamin intake required to maintain optimal body levels. The most widely accepted standard of adequate vitamin intake in this country is the Recommended Dietary Allowances (RDA) of the National Academy of Science's Food and Nutrition Board. The RDA are intended to serve only as a guide to the dietary amounts of vitamins needed to maintain good health in healthy adults in the United States under normal living conditions.

There are several situations, however, when the dietary intake of vitamins may result in suboptimal body levels. In these situations it may be necessary to administer chemically pure vitamin preparations as drugs. The most obvious situation leading to suboptimal body levels of one or more vitamins is an inadequate dietary intake resulting from such causes as decreased food consumption associated with alcoholism or prolonged reducing diets, improperly balanced diets (e.g., fat diets, prevalence in the diet of one particular food), or poverty. Suboptimal vitamin body levels may result, however, even though dietary intake conforms to the RDA, for it is not only the amount of vitamin ingested but also the amount absorbed into the blood stream that determines the body level. Hence, diseases that compromise gastrointestinal function (e.g., prolonged diarrhea, diseases of the liver or biliary tract, lack of vitamin-synthesizing intestinal flora) may prevent adequate absorption of vitamins, even with adequate ingestion. It is also known that tissue requirements for vitamins may increase under certain conditions so that normal body levels become suboptimal. This may occur in chronic diseases accompanied by fever, tissue wasting, and increased metabolism (e.g., hyperthyroidism). Tissue vitamin requirements may also be elevated in healthy individuals during periods of severe emotional or traumatic stress, rapid growth, hard physical work, and pregnancy.

In any of the aforementioned situations, the dentist may consider prescribing vitamins for his patient. If this is deemed necessary, two types of vitamin preparations are available:

(1) SUPPLEMENTAL PREPARATIONS. The United States Food and Drug Administration (FDA) has proposed that these preparations contain from 50 to 150% of the RDA (maximum of 100% of RDA for preparations containing vitamins A and D and folic acid). They are intended to provide amounts of vitamins necessary to prevent the occurrence of vitamin deficiency disorders.

(2) THERAPEUTIC PREPARATIONS. The FDA has proposed that preparations containing more than 150% of the RDA be reserved for the treatment of existing specific vitamin deficiencies or some other medical purpose.

Rationally, supplemental vitamin preparations prescribed as adjuncts to the daily diet should contain only the vitamin or group of vitamins for which evidence indicates that the diet provides inadequate intake. This limitation is often impractical, since vitamin deficiencies usually involve more than one vitamin, and multiple vitamin preparations are customarily prescribed. A case may also be made for the prophylactic administration of vitamins during periods of increased need. For example, preoperative administration of vitamin K may be advisable in patients whose intestinal flora (which synthesizes most of the human vitamin K requirement) has been disrupted by chemotherapeutic agents. The dosage ranges for prophylactic use differs according to the individual situation but usually involves therapeutic concentrations.

## CLASSIFICATION, PHARMACOKINETICS, AND SUMMARY OF VITAMINS

The vitamins can be classified into the water- and fat-soluble vitamins. The solubility of the vitamins influences their pharmacokinetics. In general, the water-soluble vitamins are well-absorbed from the gastrointestinal tract and are distributed freely in the body tissues. They are not significantly stored in the body and are rapidly excreted by the kidney. Lack of storage and rapid renal excretion probably account for their low incidence of toxicity, as well as for the fact that signs of deficiency often occur within a few weeks when they are withdrawn from the diet. In contrast, the gastrointestinal absorption of the fat-soluble vitamins is generally linked with fat absorption (i.e., bile dependent), and these vitamins are preferentially distributed in the liver and fat where they are stored. Excretion of the fat-soluble vitamins is primarily by biliary excretion, and they may undergo enterohepatic cycling, which prolongs their stay in the body. Consequently, extended administration of high doses of at least two of the fat-soluble vitamins may result in cumulative toxicity. Tissue storage probably also accounts for the fact that relatively long periods of deprivation are required before symptoms of deficiency develop.

### Water-Soluble Vitamins

Vitamin B complex is a group of vitamins, all water-soluble, found in significant amounts in liver and yeast. A brief description follows for these well-known individual agents.

Thiamine ($B_1$) was the first member of the vitamin B complex to be identified. Physiologically, it acts as a coenzyme in carbohydrate metabolism. Thiamine deficiency results in a characteristic clinical syndrome, beriberi, characterized by neurological and circulatory disorders. Thiamine has no significant pharmacodynamic or toxic actions when administered in therapeutic doses.

Riboflavin ($B_2$) physiologically acts as an essential part of coenzymes—flavin mononucleotide (FMN) and flavin adenine dinucleotide (FAD)—in many metabolic reactions. Riboflavin deficiency results in a syndrome which includes glossitis, lesions at the corners of the mouth (cheilosis), and sore throat. Riboflavin has no significant pharmacodynamic or toxic actions when administered in therapeutic doses.

Niacin (nicotinic acid) acts physiologically as coenzymes—nicotinamide adenine dinucleotide (NAD) and nicotinamide adenine dinucleotide phosphate (NADP)—in many metabolic reactions. Niacin deficiency results in a characteristic clinical syndrome, pellagra, characterized by stomatitis with the tongue red and swollen, excessive salivation, enlarged salivary glands, central nervous system disturbances, and photosensitive dermatitis. The pharmacodynamic effects when nicotinic acid is administered in high doses include vasodilation, flushing, tingling of the skin, and decreases in plasma lipids. Niacin has also been used to treat a variety of mental disorders, but this use is controversial.

Pantothenic acid acts physiologically as part of the coenzyme A molecule. Experimentally produced deficiency in man (using an antagonist of pantothenic acid) is characterized by fatigue, malaise, gastrointestinal disturbances, neuromuscular disorders, and headache. It has no significant pharmacodynamic or toxic actions.

Pyridoxine ($B_6$) acts physiologically as a coenzyme in a number of metabolic reactions involving amino acid transformation. Deficiency of pyridoxine results in a variety of symptoms, including oral lesions, glossitis, stomatitis, as well as convulsions. Pyridoxine has no significant pharmacodynamic or toxic actions.

Choline serves as the precursor of acetycholine and also plays an important role in fat metabolism. It is synthesized by the body from serine, and deficiencies in man are difficult to demonstrate, but experimental choline deficiency in animals results in hepatic cirrhosis. Choline has the same qualitative pharmacodynamic actions as acetylcholine but is much less potent.

Biotin acts physiologically as a coenzyme in several carboxylation reactions. It is thought to be synthesized by intestinal bacteria, and deficiency is rare but may be induced by chemotherapeutic agents that destroy the intestinal flora. A deficiency may cause dermatitis, lassitude, loss of hair, and neuromuscular disorders. Biotin has no significant pharmacodynamic or toxic actions.

Folic acid acts physiologically as tetrahydrofolic acid as an acceptor for single carbon units in many metabolic reactions, including pathways involved in DNA and RNA synthesis. Deficiency of folic acid results in a megaloblastic anemia, glossitis, and diarrhea. It has no significant pharmacodynamic actions.

Cyanocobalamin ($B_{12}$) acts physiologically as coenzymes in many metabolic reactions involved in fat, carbohydrate, and protein metabolism. It is probably indirectly involved in DNA synthesis and is necessary for maintenance of myelin throughout the nervous system. Inadequate absorption results in a fatal syndrome, pernicious anemia, characterized by a megaloblastic anemia similar to that seen in folic acid deficiency but with a progressive degeneration of the nervous system as a result of inadequate synthesis of myelin. Cyanocobalamin has no significant pharmacodynamic actions.

Inositol's physiological function is unknown. It has no pharmacodynamic or toxic actions.

Paraaminobenzoic acid is historically classified as one of the vitamins of the B complex even though it does not conform to the definition of a vitamin.

Vitamin C (ascorbic acid) is thought to play an important role in oxidation-reduction reactions, although its exact physiological role is unknown. It is essential for the normal synthesis and maintenance of collagen and the intercellular ground substance. Deficiency of ascorbic acid results in a characteristic syndrome, scurvy, which among other symptoms has numerous oral manifestations, including gingival swelling, capillary fragility and bleeding, resorption of dentin, decrease in odontoblastic activity, degeneration of alveolar bone, and loss of teeth. Ascorbic acid has no significant pharmacodynamic actions.

### Fat-soluble Vitamins

Vitamin A (retinol) plays an essential role in the integrity of epithelial cells, formation of tooth enamel, and the function of the retina as well as possibly participating in the synthesis of adrenal corticosteroids. Deficiency of vitamin A results in night blindness and keratinization of epithelium throughout the body, especially that of the gingival tissue, conjunctiva, and cornea. Chronic administration of excessive doses of vitamin A results in a toxic syndrome (hypervitaminosis A) characterized by irritability, loss of appetite, headache, sloughing of the skin, fatigue, myalgia, gingivitis, fissures of the oral mucosa, increased intracranial pressure, and neurological symptoms. The Council on Dental Therapeutics of the American Dental Association does not accept preparations containing vitamin A.

Vitamin D (Calciferol) is formed from the irradiation of certain sterols. This vitamin plays an important role in the regulation of calcium and phosphate metabolism which includes increasing intestinal absorption of dietary calcium and, in high doses, mobilizing calcium and phosphate from old bone for use in the formation of new bone. Vitamin D is essential for normal development of bone, including the teeth and their supporting structures. Vitamin D deficiency results in the syndrome, rickets, a fairly common disease of children in some parts of the world manifested by gross abnormalities in the formation of the skeleton. Chronic administration of excessive doses of vitamin D result in a toxic condition characterized by weakness, fatigue, gastrointestinal disturbances, headache caused by an elevation in blood calcium, as well as impairment of renal, cardiovascular, and respiratory functions caused by precipitation and deposition of calcium salts in the soft tissues of the kidneys, heart, and lungs. The Council on Dental Therapeutics of the American Dental Association does not accept preparations containing vitamin D.

Vitamin K (phylloquinone) is essential for the normal biosynthesis of several factors required for blood coagulation. Because vitamin K is synthesized by intestinal bacteria, deficiency, characterized primarily by an increased bleeding tendency, is relatively rare, although it may be caused by drugs (antibiotics) or disease (biliary obstruction). Although the naturally occurring forms of vitamin K apparently cause no pharmacodynamic or toxic effects in normal man, synthetic forms of the vitamin (e.g., menadione) have produced hemolytic anemia, elevated serum bilirubin, and kernicterus in infants.

Vitamin E (alpha-tocopherol) needs to have its exact physiological role defined, since human deficiencies have not been reported. Experimentally produced deficiencies in animals are characterized by sterility (in male rat), spontaneous abortion (in female rat), lesions of skeletal and cardiac muscle, and anemia. Although vitamin E has been used empirically to treat many human disorders, there is little evidence to justify the rationality of any such therapeutic use. Vitamin E has no significant pharmacodynamic or toxic actions.

## DRUG INTERACTIONS INVOLVING THE VITAMINS

Table 12.1 lists several selected drug interactions involving the vitamins. Examination of the table will show that vitamin C (ascorbic acid) modifies the rate of renal excretion of many acidic and basic drugs. Daily administration of supraphysiological doses (gram quantities) of vitamin C has been advocated as a method of preventing or decreasing the severity of symptoms of the common cold. Discussion of this controversial issue is beyond the scope of this text, but it should be recognized that large quantities of this acidic vitamin may significantly decrease the pH of the renal tubular fluid and thus inhibit excretion of acidic drugs (e.g., barbiturates) and increase excretion of basic drugs (e.g., atropine).

## Table 12.1. Selected Vitamin-Drug Interactions

| Primary Agent | Interactant | Possible Interaction |
|---|---|---|
| Vitamin A | Corticosteroids | Topically applied vitamin A overcomes the antihealing effect of corticosteroids and promotes wound healing by enhancing tissue lysosomal enzyme production. |
| Vitamin $B_{12}$ (Cyanocobalamin) | Alcohol (ethyl) | Alcohol causes malabsorption of this vitamin. |
| | Neomycin | Neomycin inhibits the absorption of this vitamin. |
| | Potassium Chloride | Potassium chloride impairs absorption of this vitamin from the gut. May lead to deficiency owing to low intestinal pH. Below pH 5.5 the vitamin is not absorbed. |
| Vitamin B complex | Anticoagulants, oral | Vitamin B complex increases prothrombin time and may cause hemorrhage with anticoagulants. |
| Vitamin C (ascorbic acid) | Acidifying agents | Large doses of vitamin C (as is commonly being ingested for the common cold) enhance excretion of weak bases and inhibit excretion of weak acids. |
| | Anticoagulants, oral | Vitamin C with oral anticoagulants shortens the prothrombin time and antagonizes the anticoagulant therapy. |
| | Atropine | Vitamin C increases excretion of atropine (inhibition) and vice versa. |
| | Barbiturates | Vitamin C decreases excretion of barbiturates (potentiation of sedation). Barbiturates increase excretion of vitamin C. |
| | Ferrous iron | Vitamin C in doses of 1 gram or more enhances absorption of ferrous iron (potentiates). |
| | Quinidine | Vitamin C inhibits quinidine by increasing its renal excretion. |

**Table 12.1. Continued**

| Primary Agent | Interactant | Possible Interaction |
|---|---|---|
| Vitamin C (ascorbic acid) | Salicylates (aspirin) | Salicylates increase excretion of vitamin C. Vitamin C decreases salicylate excretion. |
| | Sulfonamides | Vitamin C decreases excretion of sulfonamides (potentiation) and sulfonamides increase excretion of vitamin C (inhibition). The vitamin-acidified urine promotes sulfonamide crystalluria. |
| Vitamin K (natural and synthetic products) | Antibiotics | Antibiotics inhibit production of the vitamin by intestinal flora. Result is potentiation of anticoagulants and decrease in liver-made prothrombin, factors VII, IX, and X. |
| | Anticoagulants oral | Vitamin K inhibits anticoagulants by enhancing formation of liver prothrombin and clotting factors. |
| Pyridoxine | Levodopa (Dopar; Larodopa) | Pyridoxine rapidly reverses the antiparkinsonian effects of levodopa. This vitamin is contraindicated in patients taking levodopa. |
| Riboflavin (vitamin $B_2$) | Tetracyclines | Riboflavin decreases the antibiotic activity by decomposing tetracycline. Tetracyclines may increase excretion of riboflavin in patients with renal disease. |

Source: Data adapted and selected from Martin, 1971.[3]

## SPECIAL PRECAUTIONS REGARDING VITAMIN $B_{12}$ AND FOLIC ACID

The serious consequences of administration of large doses of folic acid to patients who have pernicious anemia (vitamin $B_{12}$ deficiency) has led the FDA to limit the amount of folic acid permissible in dietary supplemental preparations. The deficiency syndromes of the two vitamins resemble each other, in part, since they both are characterized by a megaloblastic anemia. In addition, however, vitamin $B_{12}$ deficiency is also characterized by progressive degeneration of the nervous system which, if allowed to go unchecked, is fatal.

The biochemical actions of folic acid and vitamin $B_{12}$ are closely interrelated, especially with respect to their role in the synthesis of nucleoprotein (see Figure 12.1). This interrelationship is apparently responsible for the typical megaloblastic anemia associated with deficiencies of the two vitamins, since megaloblastic anemia is a usual consequence of inhibition of DNA synthesis, regardless of cause. Folic acid, in the active form of tetrahydrofolic acid, is involved in both purine and pyrimidine synthesis. As a result of its metabolic activity, a significant portion of the metabolic pool of folic acid is converted into $N^{5,10}$methylene tetrahydrofolic acid which is in turn irreversibly converted to $N^5$methyl tetrahydrofolic acid. The reaction resulting in regeneration of tetrahydrofolic acid from the $N^5$ derivative requires vitamin $B_{12}$ as an essential cofactor. Consequently, in the absence of vitamin $B_{12}$, a significant portion of the metabolic pool of folic acid becomes trapped in the form of $N^5$methyl tetrahydrofolic acid, reducing the amount of folic acid available for other metabolic pathways.

This functional folate deficiency, despite continued ingestion of folic acid, appears to be the mechanism by which vitamin $B_{12}$ deficiency causes megaloblastic anemia. It has been shown that lack of folic acid directly causes megaloblastic anemia; a similar direct causative role for vitamin $B_{12}$ deficiency has not been shown. High doses of folic acid will correct the megaloblastic anemia of vitamin $B_{12}$ deficiency, presumably by a mass action effect, and supply adequate tetrahydrofolic acid for DNA synthesis. Herein

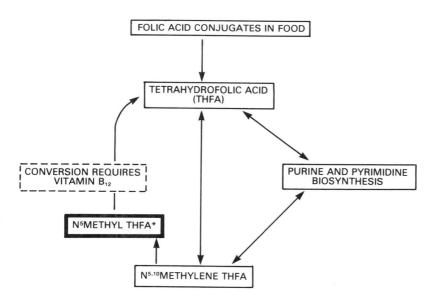

**Figure 12.1** Metabolic interrelationships of vitamin $B_{12}$ and folic acid on purine and pyrimidine biosynthesis: (*) = In the absence of adequate amounts of vitamin $B_{12}$, $N^5$methyl THFA accumulates, other folates are reduced, and there is a deficiency of metabolically active tetrahydrofolic acid. The result is a defect in nucleic acid metabolism with resultant megaloblastic anemia. (Adapted and redrawn from Herbert, 1975.[4])

lies the danger, since the neurological lesions of vitamin $B_{12}$ deficiency result from actions of vitamin $B_{12}$ unrelated to those actions involving folic acid, and large doses of folic acid do not correct these neurological lesions. Thus, large doses of folic acid in patients with pernicious anemia may correct the easily recognized megaloblastic anemia, but allow the more obscure neurological degeneration to progress to an irreversible stage.

## REFERENCES

1. Ciacco, E.I.: The vitamins. *In* Drill's Pharmacology in Medicine. 4th Edition. Edited by J.R. DiPalma. New York, McGraw-Hill, 1971.
2. Nutritional factors. *In* Accepted Dental Therapeutics. 36th Edition. Chicago, American Dental Association, 1975.
3. Martin, E.W.: Hazards of Medication. Philadelphia, Lippincott, 1971.
4. Herbert, V.: Drugs effective in megaloblastic anemias: vitamin $B_{12}$ and folic acid. *In* The Pharmacological Basis of Therapeutics. 5th Edition. Edited by L.S. Goodman and A. Gilman. New York, Macmillan, 1975.

## SUPPLEMENTARY REFERENCES

Burns, J.J.: Water-soluble vitamins: ascorbic acid (vitamin C). *In* The Pharmacological Basis of Therapeutics. 5th Edition. Edited by L.S. Goodman and A. Gilman. New York, Macmillan, 1975.

Cohn, V.H.: Fat-soluble vitamins: vitamin K and vitamin E. *In* The Pharmacological Basis of Therapeutics. 5th Edition. Edited by L.S. Goodman and A. Gilman. New York, Macmillan, 1975.

Greengard, P.: The vitamins: introduction. *In* The Pharmacological Basis of Therapeutics. 5th Edition. Edited by L.S. Goodman and A. Gilman. New York, Macmillan, 1975.

Greengard, P.: Water-soluble vitamins: the vitamin B complex. *In* The Pharmacological Basis of Therapeutics. 5th Edition. Edited by L.S. Goodman and A. Gilman, New York, Macmillan, 1975.

Mandel, H.G.: Fat-soluble vitamins: vitamin A. *In* The Pharmacological Basis of Therapeutics. 5th Edition. Edited by L.S. Goodman and A. Gilman. New York, Macmillan, 1975.

Straw, J.A.: Fat-soluble vitamins: vitamin D. *In* The Pharmacological Basis of Therapeutics. 5th Edition. Edited by L.S. Goodman and A. Gilman. New York, Macmillan, 1975.

PART IV

# DRUGS DENTAL PATIENTS ARE TAKING

# *13*

## DRUGS THE PATIENT IS TAKING

The awareness of every practitioner needs to be raised to the fact that when the patient seeks professional dental services today he may be taking one or more drugs. First the problem posed by the patient taking drugs needs to be defined so that an appropriate solution may be considered.

### CONSUMPTION OF DRUGS

A sizable number of practitioners still cannot believe that many patients are taking drugs, especially people out walking around and going to see their dentists. If the practitioner is not absolutely convinced that his patients are taking drugs, then he will see no basis for this growing clinical problem with which he must learn to cope, namely, *drug-drug interactions*. Therefore, it is essential to the effectiveness of this message that some factual information be given to support the statement that your patients *are* taking drugs.

The simplest and most direct way to prove the fact, it would seem, would be to show the results of a survey of all the people in the United States who were asked to list the names of all the drugs they were currently taking. Unfortunately no such survey exists. Without such direct evidence, consider the brief review of information to follow as indirect evidence that patients are taking drugs.

There are more drugs available today than ever before in history. In the modern world of highly sophisticated computers and information retrieval systems, there is no one—not the commissioner of the Food and Drug Administration nor the president of the Pharmaceutical Manufacturers Association—who can state accurately the number of drugs available today. A number of educated estimates may be found in literature.

Some of the more recent, authoritative, and substantiated figures to be found are shown in Table 13.1 for the year 1972 in the United States. Keep in mind there are the prescription drugs and the nonprescription or over-the-counter drugs. There were an estimated 6,780 single prescription drug entities available plus an additional 3,330 combination products of the single entities for a total of 10,110 products that were actually available in 14,250 products in different dosage forms and strengths. All of these drug products were made by only 53 drug manufacturers. There are another estimated 732 drug companies in the United States, but they are responsible for only a small percentage of the total number of prescription drug products.

Similar figures for the over-the-counter drugs are not readily available. A former commissioner of the Food and Drug Administration has estimated that in the United States more than 12,000 drug companies make approximately 200,000 drug products for over-the-counter sale. It is of interest that all of these formulations consist of only about 250 different significant active ingredients.

Another interesting statistic is that about 70% of the prescription drugs available today were not in existence in 1955. Since little more than one half of our nation's currently practicing physicians and dentists took their pharmacology courses in school, many practitioners must learn about the majority of today's drugs when they are marketed.

Although the actual number has been declining in the last several years, the number of new single entity prescription drugs introduced in the United States averaged about 10 per year over the period 1962 to 1971 as shown in Table 13.2.

#### Table 13.1.   Drugs Available in the United States (1972)

| Drug Type | Number |
|---|---|
| PRESCRIPTION DRUGS | |
| Single drug entities | 6,780 |
| Combination products | 3,330 |
| Total products | 10,110 |
| Total products in different dosage forms and strengths | 14,250 |
| NONPRESCRIPTION DRUGS | 100,000 to 200,000 |

Source: Silverman and Lee, 1974.[3]
Notes: This number of prescription drugs is made by only 53 of the estimated 785 prescription drug manufacturers. How many are made by others is unknown. This number of nonprescription drugs is made by an estimated 12,000 manufacturers. These drugs are formulations of only 250 significant active ingredients.

**Table 13.2. Drugs Introduced in the United States in Selected Categories Between 1962 and 1971**

| Category | Number |
|---|---|
| Cardiovascular drugs | 6 |
| Diuretics & related drugs | 6 |
| Respiratory drugs | 1 |
| Antibacterial & chemotherapeutic agents | 36 |
| Anticancer & immunosuppressant drugs | 13 |
| Centrally acting drugs | 26 |
| Anesthetic drugs | 5 |
| Analgesic & related drugs | 6 |
| Gastrointestinal drugs | 1 |
| Total new single drug entities = | 100 |
| Average = 10 per year | |

Source: Data from Wardell, 1973.[4]

The production figures for certain types of drugs during 1972 may be a surprise, for they too give an indication that the American public is taking drugs. As illustrated in Table 13.3 aspirin has for many years been the top drug in production; the vitamins are not too far behind. Well, just because there are a lot of drugs available does not mean people take them.

Table 8.1 shows the consumption of aspirin, one of the most popular over-the-counter drugs on the market. In 1973, it is conservatively estimated that the American public consumed approximately 35 million pounds of aspirin. That is 17,500 tons of aspirin. That is approximately 53 billion 5.0 grain tablets or about 250 tablets for every man, woman, and child in the United States. Could any dental patients have been taking aspirin when they came to the dental office? Did the patients say they were taking aspirin? Many laymen do not consider aspirin a drug.

Speaking of drugs that can be purchased over-the-counter, it may be of interest to know how much patients spent on several types of these agents. Examine Table 13.4 for the number of prescriptions dispensed in 1972. Community pharmacies, supermarket pharmacies, and dispensing physicians filled for delivery about 1.4 billion prescriptions at the patient expenditure of about $5.7 billion; hospital pharmacies filled for delivery about 938 million prescriptions at a cost to consumers of about $3.8 billion. The grand

## Table 13.3.   United States
## Production of Selected Medicinal Chemicals (1972)

| Drug Type | Production (pounds) |
|-----------|--------------------:|
| Antihistamines | 483,000 |
| Aspirin | 35,007,000 |
| Barbiturates | 567,000 |
| Vitamins | 30,030,000 |
| Antibiotics | 5,280,000 |

Source: U.S. Department of Commerce, 1974.[5]

totals are shown plus the average dollar cost per prescription. It is the last figure that is of greatest interest; i.e., the average number of new or refill prescriptions per capita in the United States in 1972 was almost 10. Each man, woman, and child obtained 10 prescription drug products. Could any of these be your patients? The figures for nonprescription drugs (Table 13.5) are for the year 1971 in the United States. The internal analgesics, some 600 in number, cost patients almost $600 million. You may note that the 200 mouthwashes and gargles were doing a brisk business in 1971. Who bought all these products?

## Table 13.4.   Prescriptions Dispensed in the United States (1972)

| Source | Number of Prescriptions | Approximate Patient Expenditure |
|--------|------------------------:|--------------------------------:|
| Community pharmacies (independents & chain stores) | 1,161,000,000 | |
| Pharmacies in supermarkets (discount stores, etc.) | 174,000,000 | |
| Dispensing physicians | 108,000,000 | |
| (Subtotal = ) | 1,443,000,000 | $ 5.7 billion |
| Hospital pharmacies | | |
| For in-patients | 752,000,000 | |
| For out-patients | 186,000,000 | |
| (Subtotal = ) | 938,000,000 | $ 3.8 billion |
| Total = | 2,381,000,000 | $ 9.5 billion |

Average prescription cost in 1972 = $4.00
Average number of new or refills per capita = 10

Source: Silverman and Lee, 1974.[3]

### Table 13.5. Selected Nonprescription Drugs United States Total Sales (1971)

| Drug Type | Approximate Number | Total Sales |
|---|---|---|
| Antacids | 575 | $108,800,000 |
| Antitussives | 500 | $270,000,000 |
| Internal analgesics | 600 | $599,900,000 |
| Laxatives | 700 | $210,000,000 |
| Mouthwashes & gargles | 200 | $411,101,000 |

Source: Data from Griffenhagen and Hawkins, 1973.[6]

Lastly, if the patient is currently seeing his physician, then the chances are three out of four that the patient is also currently taking one or more prescription drugs, as prescribed by the physician. There are many such indirect means that give every indication that the American people—dental patients—are taking drugs. The dentist deals with an unusual clientele indeed if he thinks his patients are not involved.

### DRUG INTERACTIONS

Figure 13.1 identifies in the simplest of terms four of the more important, possible interactions in the dentist-patient relationship. The patient comes to the office with diseases (both systemic and oral) and while taking drugs (both prescription drugs and/or over-

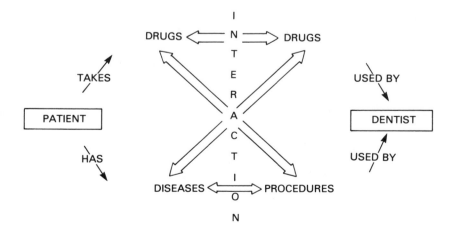

**Figure 13.1** Dentist–patient interaction possibilities.

the-counter drugs). In direct contact with the patient is the dentist, who, in his treatment of the patient, uses a variety of sophisticated procedures and who administers or prescribes a variety of drugs. The first interaction of importance, the drug-drug interaction, will be discussed last, since most of the chapter will focus on it.

### Drug-Disease Interactions

Drug-disease interaction is a factor to be considered in the treatment planning process. The dentist must determine whether a drug he plans to use will interact unfavorably with the patient's existing disease conditions. There are many examples of this type of interaction. One would be the patient who has narrow angle glaucoma; the dentist wishes to slow down the patient's salivary flow in order to take impressions. A cholinergic blocking agent, similar to atropine, is administered. If the patient's pupils dilate in response to the drug and close the normal drainage canals for intraocular fluid, intraocular pressure increases, and the patient experiences a painful glaucomatous attack.

### Procedure-Drug Interactions

Another type of interaction possibility is the procedure-drug interaction. The dentist must determine whether any of his planned procedures will interact unfavorably with a drug the patient is already taking. Once again there are many examples: extensive surgical procedures in the patient who is taking large daily doses of anticoagulants can certainly lead to an obvious unfavorable situation; the patient who is taking digitalis has a sensitive gag reflex, and the slow taking of full mouth impressions can be a messy business as well as highly stressing for the patient; or the patient who is taking one or more antihypertensive drugs usually experiences postural or orthostatic hypotension. If one of the office procedures for this patient is to return the back of the chair to its upright position rapidly, raise the chair arm, and lift the patient by his arm to a standing position, the patient may fall to the floor in syncope. Such a patient must be moved slowly from the supine position to the standing position.

### Procedure-Disease Interactions

A third type of interaction possibility is the procedure-disease interaction. An example would be the grand mal epileptic patient interacting with a procedure such as turning the light on and off in his eyes or exposing him to sudden, unannounced vibrations (e.g., the amalgam-maker). Such sensory stimulation may trigger a seizure if the patient is not well-controlled by the antiepileptic drugs he is taking. The classic example of this interaction, of course, is the stress of a dental procedure and the effect the stress will have on a patient's diseased cardiovascular system.

### Drug-Drug Interactions

The first interaction of importance is the drug-drug interaction. During the treatment planning process the dentist must determine whether the drug he plans to use will or will not interact unfavorably with a drug the patient is already taking. An example of a dental patient who may be subject to this type of interaction would be John, an older man, whom the dentist has not seen in about a year. Sitting in the office looking at John's latest roentgenograms in the viewbox and awaiting John's arrival, the dentist remembers what an unhappy patient John was. All he had talked about at his last visit over a year ago was how he was being forced to retire just because he was now 65 years old. The dentist had felt sorry for John and wondered how he had adapted to a life of retirement. John arrives, and the dentist is amazed for John's cheerfulness and adjustment to retirement. At the second appointment a couple of days later the dentist performs a routine procedure that he knows is sufficiently painful after the local anesthetic wears off that he prescribes six 100 mg tablets of meperidine (Demerol) for John to take if his pain becomes severe. Certainly there is nothing unusual about the dentist's procedure of prescribing meperidine for the patient. The dentist has done the same thing with countless other patients in the past.

When John walked out of the office that day, he never came back, because John died that same day after he had taken several tablets the dentist had prescribed. John was not allergic to meperidine. He died as a result of a drug-drug interaction.

What John did not tell the dentist was that he had been so depressed about having to retire that after moping around for a month he went to see his physician who prescribed a drug for him to take. It surely did pick him up and mask his retirement blues. The drug John was taking and about which he was too proud to tell the dentist was an antidepressant, tranylcypromine or Parnate by brand name. These two drugs, Demerol and Parnate, interact unfavorably in the body; indeed, their interaction may be rapidly fatal.

With each day that passes the chance gets better that the dentist will witness for himself an unwanted or unfavorable drug effect in one of his patients owing to a drug-drug interaction. For this discussion a drug-drug interaction will be defined as the situation in which the effects of one drug are altered by the prior or concurrent administration of another drug.

It should be understood that all possible unfavorable drug-drug interactions are not as deadly as that between meperidine and tranylcypromine. In most situations where one drug is known to intereact with another, both drugs can be used together so long as dosage adjustments are made and closer patient monitoring of drug-induced effects is carried out. Nonetheless, because dental patients are taking drugs, it becomes the dentist's responsibility to avoid or to prevent any unwanted effects from occurring as a result of a dentist's drug interacting with the drug the patient is taking. Although it cannot be stated with certainty that 100% prevention is possible, each dentist can learn how to improve greatly his ability to avoid such drug effects.

RECOGNIZING THE POSSIBILITIES. What does the practitioner do to begin working toward the ideal, namely, the ability to recognize drug-drug interaction possibilities and then to take action to prevent their occurrence? Really it comes down to just that, recognizing the drug-drug interaction possibilities, because the simplest way to prevent the situation from happening is not to give the dentist's drug.

Ideally, if a complete listing of all possible interactions existed in a computer somewhere, all the practitioner would need to do is call and ask if there is any interaction problem with giving drug A to a patient who is taking drug B. The computer would answer yes or no. Some early models of drug information systems are being created and tested now just to serve as a possible solution to this clinical problem. Without such conveniences, what can be done?

1. The practitioner must do everything possible to learn from each patient the names of the drugs he is currently taking or has taken in the past month, both prescription drugs and over-the-counter drugs. Some considerate patients know the exact names and correct spellings of the drugs they are taking. They are in the minority at the moment. Others know they are taking a prescription drug, but do not have any idea of its name. In this case, the practitioner will need to have the patient telephone when he gets home and read from the bottle's label the prescription number and the name of the pharmacy that filled it. Then a call to the pharmacy will give the name of the drug. An alternative is to contact the physician who prescribed the medication. There will be times when the only way the drug the patient is taking may be identified is by having the patient bring a tablet or capsule with him to the office and then identify it by its physical size, shape, color, and markings, using the pictorial code directory in the *Physicians' Desk Reference* (PDR).

2. Once the name of each drug the patient is taking has been obtained, then the information on the drug in the PDR should be

examined to learn to what class of drugs it belongs and to review the listing. This information may suggest possible interactions as well as give indications as to why the patient is taking the drug.

3. Next the practitioner will consult a current drug-drug interaction index to learn if any specific interaction has been reported between the drug the patient is taking and the one planned for use. The available indexes are not exhaustive, are always out of date, and this will probably continue to be the case for some time yet. The number of such indexes grows almost monthly and many are now on the market. None is directed specifically to the dental practitioner's needs; however, while learning the types of drugs that seem to interact most, as well as the ways drugs interact and how the unwanted effects can be manifested, it is helpful to have and use a good reference.[1,2]

Since no one can learn all the possible interactions and since no one index, as yet, lists all the possible interactions, what is known about general principles or concepts about all drugs that do interact must be examined. Fortunately, a number of generalities have emerged early in experience with this clinical problem.

DRUG-CONTROLLED CHRONIC DISEASES. One of the reasons why more dental patients are taking drugs these days is a direct result of medical progress. In the last 50 years, many diseases that used to kill people rather quickly are no longer doing so. Today by the proper use of drugs some of these diseases can be prevented and even cured. Many other conditions that afflict mankind may not be cured by drugs, but drugs have been found which if taken chronically—sometimes for life—can subdue or mask the debilitating symptoms and allow the individual to live a longer life than would otherwise be possible without the drug.

There are many examples of drug-controlled chronic diseases (see Figure 13.2).

Today the patient with diabetes mellitus is taking insulin or one of the oral hypoglycemic drugs; the arthritic patient takes corticosteroids; the patient with heart disease takes digitalis with or without diuretics; the patient with arterial hypertension takes one or more drugs daily to hold his blood pressure within normal limits. Note that oral contraception is also listed. This is not to say that contraception is a chronic disease that can be drug-controlled. However, it is a reason why over 20 million women in the United States each day take a drug.

In each of these cases the physician strives to establish and maintain a proper balance between the disease's effects and the drug's effects. This usually requires a number of dosage adjustments, changing to another drug or combining more than two drugs

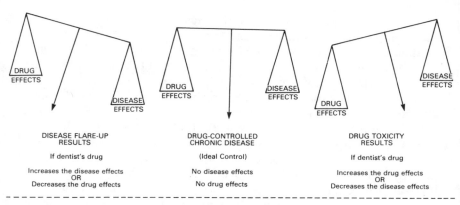

DISEASE FLARE-UP
RESULTS

If dentist's drug

Increases the disease effects
OR
Decreases the drug effects

DRUG-CONTROLLED
CHRONIC DISEASE

(Ideal Control)

No disease effects

No drug effects

DRUG TOXICITY
RESULTS

If dentist's drug

Increases the drug effects
OR
Decreases the disease effects

Selected Examples of Chronic Diseases Controlled by Drugs

| | |
|---|---|
| Allergies | Hypothyroidism and Hyperthyroidism |
| Arterial hypertension | "Oral contraception" |
| Angina pectoris | Psychoneurological disorders |
| Cardiac insufficiencies | Skin disorders (selected) |
| Postmyocardial infarction | Infections (selected) |
| Diabetes mellitus | Gastrointestinal ulcerations |
| Arthritis | |

**Figure 13.2** Drug-controlled chronically diseased patient and possible effects of dentist's drugs. Selected examples of chronic diseases that are drug-controlled today are cited.

in just the right doses. If he is successful, then the drug-controlled, chronically diseased patient will show very few if any disease effects or drug effects. This is ideal control.

In drug-controlled chronically diseased patients, it can be predicted rather accurately what effects may be expected if the dentist's drug throws the patient out of balance either one way or the other. If the dentist's drug will either increase the disease effects or decrease the controlling drug's effects, the patient can be expected to manifest a flare-up of the chronic disease. On the other hand, if the dentist's drug will add to or in any way increase the effects of the controlling drug, or if the dentist's drug will actually decrease the effects of the chronic disease, then the patient may manifest toxicity or overdosage effects of the controlling-drug. This interaction is not simple; therefore, some specific examples are in order.

Figure 13.3 illustrates how the dentist's drug actually will add to the disease effects and thereby throw the patient out of balance. The patient has angina pectoris and takes some long-term organic nitrate plus, of course, nitroglycerin when necessary. The dentist's drug is a gingival retraction agent containing epinephrine. A good impression is required. The epinephrine is absorbed, goes to the heart, and causes an increase in myocardial contractile force which

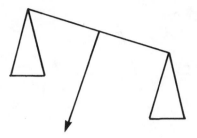

IF THE DENTIST'S DRUG INCREASES THE DISEASE EFFECTS

ANGINA PECTORIS                    GINGIVAL RETRACTION AGENT
                                   CONTAINING EPINEPHRINE

ACUTE ANGINAL ATTACK

**Figure 13.3**   Drug interaction between epinephrine and angina pectoris.

greatly increases the contracting fibers' need for oxygen. This certainly adds to the functional, diseased condition and what is seen is an acute anginal attack.

A manifestation or unmasking of the patient's drug-controlled disease symptoms is also what may be expected if the dentist's drug decreases the effects of the controlling drug. Figure 13.4 represents the congestive heart failure patient who will be taking one of the digitalis glycosides for the rest of his life. Once again the dentist needs to take impressions, but this time the patient produces such a copious flow of saliva that cotton rolls alone will not keep the area dry. The customary procedure is to administer to such a patient a single dose of an atropinelike drug which assuredly will slow down

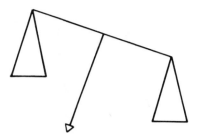

IF THE DENTIST'S DRUG DECREASES THE DRUG EFFECTS

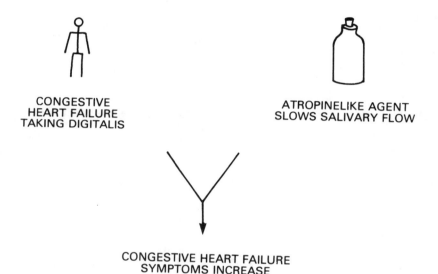

CONGESTIVE
HEART FAILURE
TAKING DIGITALIS

ATROPINELIKE AGENT
SLOWS SALIVARY FLOW

CONGESTIVE HEART FAILURE
SYMPTOMS INCREASE

**Figure 13.4**  Drug interaction between atropine and digitalis.

or even stop salivary flow for several hours. At the same time, the atropinelike drug may also be negating or opposing one of the beneficial or therapeutic effects of digitalis on the patient's heart. Part of digitalis's ability to slow the speeding, failing heart can be blocked by atropinelike drugs. What would be seen in this patient as a result of this interaction would be an unmasking of the symptoms of congestive failure.

On the other hand, the dentist's drug could throw the drug-controlled, chronically diseased patient out of balance by increasing the effects produced by the controlling drug. It would not be the heretofore drug-controlled disease symptoms that would be unmasked, but the patient would show what would appear to be an overdosage response to the controlling drug. Figure 13.5 shows what happens to the late-onset diabetic patient who is taking one of the oral hypoglycemic drugs, such as chlorpropamide (Diabinese). He takes his tablets every day, and the disease is held in balance. Following dental treatment the dentist tells him that if he needs a mild analgesic for pain lingering after the local anesthetic effect has waned, to take one or two aspirin every 3 to 4 hours. Aspirin interacts unfavorably with drugs like chlorpropamide and causes an augmentation of the antidiabetic drug's effects by a mechanism to be discussed later. The result of this drug-drug interaction is what would appear if the patient had taken an overdose of his controlling drug.

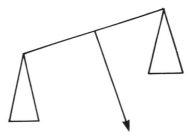

IF THE DENTIST'S DRUG INCREASES THE DRUG EFFECTS

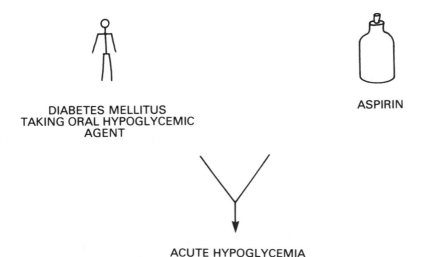

DIABETES MELLITUS
TAKING ORAL HYPOGLYCEMIC
AGENT

ASPIRIN

ACUTE HYPOGLYCEMIA

**Figure 13.5** Drug interaction between aspirin and oral hypoglycemic agent.

Lastly, one of the dentist's drugs could throw the drug-controlled, chronically diseased patient out of balance if the dentist's drug actually could decrease the effects produced by the patient's disease. It is difficult to find a straightforward example. As shown in Figure 13.6 the patient has arterial hypertension, and he is taking daily one or more antihypertensive drugs to hold down his diastolic blood pressure within what may be considered a normal range. This adult patient may be apprehensive regarding the planned dental treatment, and a secobarbital capsule will certainly allay his apprehension. The barbiturate, however, depresses the vasomotor center in the brain and thereby reduces vasoconstrictor tone, i.e., diastolic pressure. The result of the interaction is that the patient manifests a state simulating overdosage of his controlling drug.

MECHANISMS OF DRUG-DRUG INTERACTIONS. Generalities regarding how and where drugs interact in the body can now be made. It is now known that one drug can alter the effects of another drug most probably at those sites in the body where a drug reacts with the various biological systems. If all the known drug-drug interactions whose mechanisms of interaction we understand are examined, it is interesting that the majority, so far, fall into one or more of the following four general categories: (1) Drug A alters the absorption of drug B; (2) drug A alters the distribution of drug B; (3) drug A alters the metabolism of drug B; or (4) drug A alters the excretion of drug B. Consider the following few examples of known drug-drug interactions in each category which are appropriate both to the dentist's daily practice and to the goal to avoid all interactions if possible.

*Absorption.* First, there are interactions involving drug absorption. In this case the unfavorable effects produced result from one drug causing, usually, a reduction in the total amount of another drug absorbed from the gastrointestinal tract. Two common examples are tetracycline and sodium fluoride. The tetracycline antibiotics administered orally are readily absorbed, mainly from the upper small intestine. The tetracyclines, however, form insoluble complexes with both divalent and trivalent cations such as calcium ions, magnesium ions, ferrous (iron) ions, and aluminum ions. When the tetracycline is not in solution, it cannot be absorbed across the body's membranes. Therefore, it may be expected that the doses of tetracycline prescribed for the patient will not be fully absorbed *if* the patient also ingests antacids such as Tums, Rolaids, or the aluminum-containing Amphojel. Even the magnesium trisilicate in Bufferin will complex with tetracycline. Obviously, the patient must be instructed against washing down the tetracycline capsule with a glass of milk. The patient must not take

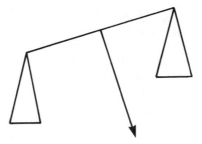

IF THE DENTIST'S DRUG DECREASES THE DISEASE EFFECTS

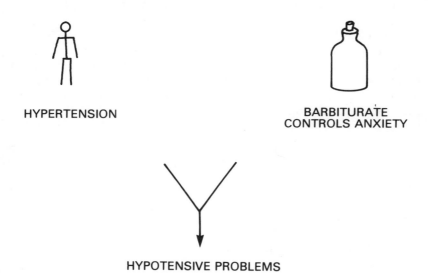

HYPERTENSION            BARBITURATE
                                 CONTROLS ANXIETY

HYPOTENSIVE PROBLEMS

**Figure 13.6**   Drug interaction between barbiturate and hypertension.

supplemental iron preparations at the same time the tetracycline is administered. The result of this drug-drug interaction is not deadly, but indeed quite misleading and frustrating when the expected-to-be-effective tetracycline is not absorbed.

Another appropriate example of this same mechanism of drug-drug interaction involves the significant reduction in absorption of fluoride from the gastrointestinal tract in the presence of divalent and trivalent cations. Here again, calcium fluoride, magnesium fluoride, ferrous fluoride, and aluminum fluoride are all insoluble in water, and if the fluoride is not in solution it cannot be absorbed across the membranes into the circulation.

Not all drug-drug interactions lead to unfavorable responses from the patient. For example, the dentist has used a drug-drug interaction to the patient's advantage for a long time, i.e., the administration together of the local anesthetic and a vasoconstrictor such as epinephrine. Epinephrine is present only to retard the absorption of the local anesthetic.

*Distribution.* Next, there are several drug interactions the mechanism of which involves the alteration of one drug's distribution in the body by the presence of another drug. Most drugs, as they circulate in the blood stream, are present in two forms: bound drug and free drug. The free drug may diffuse out of the circulation into the tissues to the drug's site of action and there may produce its effects. The free drug may also be metabolized by the liver and excreted by the kidney. The bound drug that is also circulating in the blood is linked or bound in a reversible manner usually to plasma albumin. While the drug is bound, it is unable to leave the circulation and proceed to the site of action where it would produce its effects. Therefore, bound drug is temporarily and pharmacologically inactive. If bound drug could be quickly converted to free drug, then there would be more free drug to produce immediate effects. This would be especially true for a drug that is highly bound, for example, to the extent of 90 to 95%. In this situation, the drug is producing its desired effects when only 5% of the drug is free in the circulation and able to diffuse to the site of action; 95% of the drug in the circulation is bound to plasma protein. If 5% of the bound drug was suddenly displaced and converted to free drug, there would be a doubling of the concentration of the free, active drug that can go to the site of action and produce its effects.

There are examples of this type of mechanism of interaction which involves drugs used in dental practices. Table 13.6 applies to the dental patient who is taking an oral anticoagulant, such as dicumarol, for some thromboembolic disorder. The dentist finds it necessary to allay the patient's apprehensions about the planned dental treatment and prescribes the classic agent chloral hydrate. Chloral hydrate (or one of its metabolites) has a stronger affinity for a common binding site on plasma protein to which a large percentage of the patient's circulating anticoagulant is bound. The chloral hydrate displaces the anticoagulant from the binding site, which results in a sudden increase in free anticoagulant that now goes to its site of action and produces what could be called overanticoagulation. The response seen is the same as if the patient were given two, three, four, or more times the usual dose of the anticoagulant.

The commonly prescribed drug, aspirin, is also known to be involved in drug-drug interactions resulting from this drug dis-

**Table 13.6.   Drug Interactions
Involving Drug Binding Displacements**

| Strongly Bound Drug | Bound Drug Replaced | Effect of Interaction |
|---|---|---|
| Chloral hydrate | Oral anticoagulants | Hemorrhage following "over-" inhibition of blood clotting factor synthesis |
| Salicylates, e.g., aspirin | Methotrexate | Increased methotrexate toxicity |
| Salicylates, e.g., aspirin | Tolbutamide (Orinase) | Hypoglycemia |
| | Chlorpropamide (Diabinese) | |

placement mechanism. Aspirin will remove the anticancer drug methotrexate from its plasma protein binding site. Methotrexate is a toxic substance under perfectly usual conditions, and aspirin will then greatly increase the occurrence of methotrexate toxic effects by means of this mechanism. It may be mentioned that methotrexate has become popular recently in the treatment of psoriasis; so if the dental patient has psoriasis, the practitioner might well ask if he is taking any drugs (especially methotrexate) to control the disease. By the same type of mechanism, aspirin will displace the oral hypoglycemic agents, tolbutamide and chlorpropamide, from their plasma protein binding sites and thus lead to sudden hypoglycemia. The late-onset diabetic is most often the patient who is taking one of these drugs.

*Metabolism.* It might be logically predicted that another common mechanism for drug-drug interaction is that in which one drug alters the metabolism of another drug. Certainly, this could lead to dire effects. Although not all commonly used drugs are metabolized or chemically changed in the body to other chemicals (called metabolites), the large majority of drugs is so altered to varying extents. Usually, but not always, the active drug administered is biotransformed or metabolized to a much less active substance that the kidney can more easily eliminate. The liver, which is the primary organ for metabolism of drugs, possesses the ability to biosynthesize additional amounts of various enzymes when necessary. The very presence of a particular chemical in the liver may stimulate the hepatic cells to make more of an enzyme that will then act upon the drug to metabolize it. It was learned over the last 10 years that the liver uses the same enzymes to metabolize a number of different drugs. Some drugs have been found to be especially effective in stimulating the induction of liver enzymes which in turn will then metabolize more rapidly another drug that may be present. Obviously, if that second drug is now more rapidly inactivated, then its desired effects become not only shorter in duration but also much less intense.

As shown in Table 13.7, barbiturates (especially phenobarbital) are well-established enzyme inducers. When a barbiturate is taken for 2 to 5 days, the amount of a number of liver enzymes is actually increased. As a result, drugs that are normally metabolized by these enzymes are more quickly inactivated. Some of the more important potential unwanted effects would occur as a result of too little anticoagulant, corticosteroid, digitoxin, phenytoin, testosterone, or oral contraceptive.

Another enzyme inducer is chloral hydrate. It is known to induce the synthesis of enzymes that normally metabolize the anticoagulants such as dicumarol.

Yet another example of interest is that between vitamin $B_6$ or pyridoxine and the new antiparkinsonian drug, levodopa. One of the greatest advances in therapeutics during the last 10 years has been the discovery of the phenomenal relief of the distressing symptoms of Parkinson's disease or palsy by the drug levodopa. This drug is widely used today. If a multiple vitamin preparation containing vitamin $B_6$ is prescribed, the beneficial effects of levodopa would be effectively antagonized and the patient would begin to experience the characteristic involuntary motor movements. Fortunately, most physicians treating such patients warn them not to take any vitamin preparation without the physician's

### Table 13.7. Drug Interactions Involving Increased Drug Metabolism (Hepatic Microsomal Enzyme Induction)

| Enzyme-inducing Drug | Drug Activity *Decreased* by Enhanced Metabolism |
|---|---|
| Barbiturates (requires 2–5 days) | Oral anticoagulants<br>Hydrocortisone<br>Digitoxin<br>Phenytoin (Dilantin)<br>Testosterone<br>Estrogens and progestogens (oral contraceptives) |
| Chloral hydrate | Oral anticoagulants |
| Pyridoxine ($B_6$) (in multiple vitamins) | Levodopa (Dopar; Larodopa) |

knowledge and consent. If the dentist knows this interaction, the vitamin will not be prescribed in the first place.

It could be predicted that if one drug could increase the metabolism of another drug, surely there must be drugs that could decrease or inhibit the metabolism of other drugs. Yet another known mechanism whereby one drug will interact unfavorably with another is through decreased drug metabolism. If the metabolism of a drug is reduced, then free, active drug remains around longer in the body and will show more intense effects over a longer duration of time.

As shown in Table 13.8 it is through the mechanism of hepatic microsomal inhibition that meperidine and monoamine oxidase inhibitors may lead the patient rapidly down the road to death. The monoamine oxidase inhibitors inhibit specific enzymes in the liver which normally metabolize not only the narcotic analgesics but also a number of the barbiturates. As a result of the inhibition the active drugs remain, accumulate, and produce rather promptly the effects of gross overdosage of the central nervous system depressants.

Furthermore, by this same mechanism of enzyme inhibition, aspirin depresses the enzymatic metabolism of the oral hypoglycemic agents, tolbutamide and chlorpropamide, allowing them to accumulate and produce their overdosage, toxic effects.

*Excretion.* The last general mechanism involves how one drug can alter the renal excretion of another drug. There are actually several mechanisms by which drugs may interact during their renal elimination. Only one will be mentioned, i.e., the influence of urinary pH upon drug excretion. Since many drugs are either weak organic acids or weak organic bases, it may be accurately predicted that drugs which are weak acids will be more ionized or charged in an alkaline urine than in a more acidic urine. Likewise, drugs which are weak bases will be more ionized or charged in an acidic

**Table 13.8. Drug Interactions Involving Decreased Drug Metabolism (Hepatic Microsomal Enzyme Inhibition)**

| Enzyme-inhibiting Drug | Drug Activity *Increased* by Decreased Metabolism |
|---|---|
| Monoamine oxidase inhibitors (MAOI) | Narcotic analgesics, e.g., meperidine (Demerol) |
| Aspirin | Tolbutamide (Orinase) Chlorpropamide (Diabinese) |

urine than in a more alkaline urine. When a drug is in its ionized or charged form, it will not readily cross lipid membranes and therefore will not be reabsorbed from the renal tubular urine back into the blood. It passes on into bladder urine ready for final removal from the body. It is the nonionized, noncharged form of the drug that is more lipid soluble and will diffuse across cell membranes out of urine back into the blood. Table 13.9 summarizes this mechanism of drug interaction.

Drugs such as barbiturates, salicylates, and sulfonamides are weak acids and may be expected to be more readily excreted in an alkaline urine than in an acidic urine. The opposite is true for the weak bases, such as most antihistamines and narcotic analgesics. These are more readily ionized and thereby excreted in an acidic urine than in an alkaline urine. Not only does a patient's diet determine the pH of his urine, but also the drugs he takes will influence the urinary pH. Perhaps the best known acidifying agent today is the drug, ascorbic acid or vitamin C. Since the public has widely read and accepted the purported usefulness of large oral doses of vitamin C to prevent the common cold, more Americans than ever before are consuming large amounts of this urinary acidifying agent. This agent's acidification of the urine will significantly prolong the duration of action of some barbiturates as well as aspirin and, on the other hand, significantly shorten the duration of action of drugs such as the narcotic analgesics or other weak bases, such as the amphetamines.

The most readily available urinary alkalinizing agent in the United States today is another drug that can be purchased over-the-counter or without a prescription, namely, sodium bicarbonate or baking soda. This drug will effectively alkalinize the urine rather

**Table 13.9.  Drug Interactions Involving Altered Renal Excretion Urinary Acidifers and Alkalinizers**

| Drugs | Excretion Rate in Acidic Urine | Excretion Rate in Alkaline Urine |
|---|---|---|
| WEAK ACIDS | | |
| Barbiturates Salicylates Sulfonamides | Decreased | Increased |
| WEAK BASES | | |
| Antihistamines Narcotic analgesics | Increased | Decreased |

promptly and cause a shortening of the duration of action of the salicylates and barbiturates, but prolong the duration of action of the narcotic analgesics or amphetamines.

## REFERENCES

1. Martin, E. W.: Hazards of Medication. Philadelphia, Lippincott, 1971.
2. Evaluations of Drug Interactions. 2nd Edition. Washington, D.C., American Pharmaceutical Association, 1976.
3. Silverman, M., and Lee, P. R.: Pills, Profits, and Politics. Berkeley, University of California Press, 1974.
4. Wardell, W. M.: Introduction of new therapeutic drugs in the United States and Great Britain: an international comparison. Clin. Pharmacol. Ther., 14:773, 1973.
5. Statistical Abstracts of the U.S., 1974. Washington, D.C., United States Department of Commerce, 1975.
6. Griffenhagen, G. B., and Hawkins, L. L. (eds.): Handbook of Non-Prescription Drugs. 1973 Edition. Washington, D.C., American Pharmaceutical Association, 1973.

## SUPPLEMENTARY REFERENCES

Moser, R.H. (ed): Diseases of Medical Progress: A Study of Iatrogenic Disease. 3rd Edition, Springfield, Ill., Charles C Thomas, 1969.
Physicians' Desk Reference. Oradell. New Jersey, Medical Economics, 1977.

# 14

## DRUGS IN THE TREATMENT OF CARDIOVASCULAR DISORDERS

The dental patient who has cardiovascular disease presents special concerns for the dentist and dental hygienist for several reasons: (1) Cardiovascular disease decreases the patient's ability to respond to and recover from stress. (2) The pharmacology of the drugs these patients are taking must be understood in relation to the disease processes so that the artificial physiology of these drug-controlled chronically diseased individuals may be better appreciated and potential drug-drug interactions recognized. (3) Cardiovascular disease predisposes the patient to emergency situations.

It is especially important to encourage patients with cardiovascular disease to have regular dental checkups in order that dental procedures may be kept as simple as possible. Appointments should be kept short. The extent of dental procedures that may be performed safely in these individuals varies with the individual patient and is best determined in consultation with the patient's physician who should have a reasonable idea of how much stress his patient can safely withstand.

It has been recommended that "patients with coronary, hypertensive or syphilitic heart disease or with congestive heart failure from any cause should receive preanesthetic sedation with short-acting barbiturates to allay apprehension and prevent or minimize blood pressure rises during the waiting room period as well as in the dental chair."[1] It should be appreciated that any such pretreatment must be done cautiously in patients who may be (and probably are) taking several of the drugs discussed in this chapter. As we will see, many of the cardiovascular drugs can interact dangerously with central nervous system depressants such as the barbiturates.

Probably the most important step in the dental treatment of the cardiovascular patient is the establishment of local anesthesia. Care should be taken to assure profound anesthesia as painlessly as possible. A topical local anesthetic should be applied to the site of injection, and sufficient time should be allowed for it to take effect. The question of the safety of using local anesthetic preparations with added vasoconstrictors in cardiovascular patients is still debated. Accidental intravenous injection of local anesthetics or vasoconstrictors can cause central nervous system stimulation or depression, hypertensive crises, dangerous degrees of myocardial ischemia, and even cardiovascular collapse. Nevertheless, it is generally agreed that inclusion of a vasoconstrictor insures more profound anesthesia and limits the rate of absorption of a local anesthetic agent. In addition, inadequate anesthesia may result in a reflex release of significant amounts of epinephrine from the adrenal medulla in response to pain. For these reasons the concentrations of vasoconstrictors normally used in dental local anesthetic preparations are not contraindicated in the cardiovascular patient so long as preliminary aspiration and careful administration are carried out. On the other hand, the usual concentrations and the characteristics of administration of vasoconstrictors for gingival retraction or hemostasis can lead to significant absorption; thus, such use is contraindicated in these patients.

## CARDIAC GLYCOSIDES

The cardiac glycosides are widely distributed in nature, being found in several plant species and certain toads. The prototype of this group of agents is digitalis. Official digitalis is the dried leaf of *Digitalis purpurea* or purple foxglove. Actually, the plants of the foxglove family contain several active components each possessing similar pharmacological activity. The chemical structure of the most active of these components, digitoxin, is shown in Figure 14.1 and is characteristic of the other components. The cardiac glycosides are made up of a steroid-lactone (aglycone) moiety and from one to four molecules of sugar, hence the term, *glycoside*. The aglycone moiety is responsible for the pharmacological activity, and the sugars are responsible for the pharmacokinetics (e.g., solubility and cell penetrability) of the various glycosides.

The cardiac glycosides derive their name from their major site of action—the heart. These agents increase both the speed and force with which the heart muscle contracts, not only in the normal heart but also in the failing heart. In the failing heart, digitalis causes a

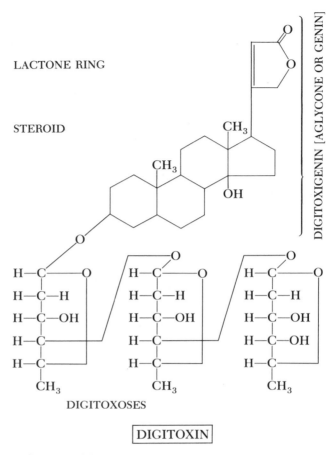

**Figure 14.1**  Structure of digitoxin.

complex combination of changes that allow it to increase the force of contraction with an accompanying net decrease in myocardial oxygen consumption, thus improving myocardial efficiency.

Digitalis also has important effects on the electrophysiological properties of the heart, both through direct actions and indirect actions that increase the activity of the vagus nerve. The effects are complex and dependent on both the dose and the particular cardiac tissue (Table 14.1). These electrophysiological effects are the basis for using digitalis to treat several types of cardiac arrhythmias and are the mechanism for its most serious toxic effects. The effects most directly related to digitalis's antiarrhythmic properties are (1) its increase in the transfer of impulses through the atrial tissue and

**Table 14.1. Electrophysiological Effects of Digitalis on the Properties of the Heart**

| | SA Node | Atrial Tissue | AV Node | Purkinje Fibers | Ventricle |
|---|---|---|---|---|---|
| Vagal effects* | ↓Automaticity (Variable) | ↑Conduction velocity  ↓Effective refractory period | ↓Conduction velocity  ↑Effective refractory period | No vagal effects | No vagal effects |
| Direct effects† | ↑Automaticity | ↓Conduction velocity  ↑Effective refractory period  ↓Excitability | ↓Conduction velocity  ↑Effective refractory period | ↑Automaticity  ↓Excitability  ↓Conduction velocity  ↓Effective refractory period | ↓Excitability  ↓Conduction velocity  ↓Effective refractory period |

Source: From Moe and Farah, 1975.[6]

Notes: Automaticity = the ability of a cell to initiate an electrical impulse.
Excitability = the ability of a cell to be stimulated electrically by an outside impulse.
Conduction velocity = the speed with which a propagated impulse is transmitted through tissue.
Effective refractory period = the time that must elapse before a previously depolarized cell may be effectively electrically stimulated.
↑ = increased; ↓ = decreased.
*In general predominate at lower doses.
†In general predominate at higher or toxic doses.

(2) its decrease in the transfer of impulses through the atrioventricular (AV) node. The effects most directly related to digitalis's toxic effects are (1) its increase in the automaticity of the "latent pacemakers" of the Purkinje system and (2) its diverse effects on excitability, effective refractory period, and conduction of ventricular tissue.

The ability of digitalis to increase the force of contraction and efficiency of the failing heart gives it a unique place in the treatment of congestive heart failure. Congestive heart failure may result from various causes, but the basic pathology is a decrease in the strength of contraction of the heart muscle. As a result cardiac output falls, and several compensatory responses are triggered. Sympathetic tone increases, causing an increase in heart rate and a decreased perfusion of the kidney. The latter, in part by increasing secretion of aldosterone from the adrenal cortex, increases water retention and expands the plasma volume. The decrease of force of myocardial contraction also leaves more residual blood in the heart, increasing its internal pressure during diastole. This, in combination with the increased sympathetic tone of the veins and the increased plasma volume, leads to a "back up" of pressure on the venous side of the vascular tree and a decrease in the reabsorption of water from the interstitial space which normally occurs in the postcapillary venules. As a result, edema forms, especially in the lungs and lower extremities.

Another important sequel to congestive heart failure is a decrease in cardiac reserve. In addition to the sympathetic nervous system, the heart has an intrinsic mechanism for increasing its force of contraction. This mechanism is a manifestation of Starling's Law of the Heart which states that, within limits, the force of contraction increases as the muscle is stretched. As a result of the increase in residual blood volume and internal cardiac pressure during diastole, the heart dilates and the myocardial fibers stretch. As long as the heart can dilate, it can increase its work and cardiac output. This is referred to as cardiac reserve (Figure 14.2). The healthy heart can maintain an adequate cardiac output at low internal pressure and dilation; it can dilate and increase its cardiac output in response to an increased demand. The patient who has congestive heart failure, but whose heart has compensated by dilation, has already used up a significant portion of his cardiac reserve and has a decreased ability to respond to stress.

Digitalis reverses the congestive processes by increasing the strength of contraction, thereby increasing the cardiac output at any given magnitude of internal pressure and dilation. This allows the heart to "de-dilate" and restores part of the cardiac reserve, as well

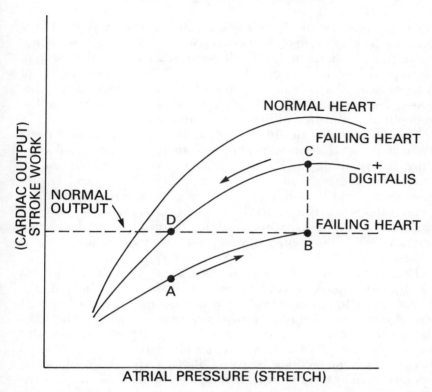

**Figure 14.2**   Effect of digitalis on cardiac reserve. (Adapted and redrawn from Mason, 1973.[5])

as decreases sympathetic tone. Heart rate is slowed, venous pressure decreases, and kidney perfusion is improved. With the increase in kidney perfusion a diuresis occurs that decreases edema and plasma volume. It is not uncommon for a patient who has congestive heart failure to be taking a diuretic in addition to digitalis to aid in this mobilization of edema fluid.

The exact mechanism of digitalis's positive inotropic effect is unknown. It is known that digitalis inhibits a $Na^+$-$K^+$-activated adenosine triphosphatase which is involved in the active transport of $Na^+$ and $K^+$ across the myocardial cell membrane. Inhibition of this enzyme results in an increase in intracellular sodium and a decrease in intracellular potassium. It appears that the toxic effects of digitalis on cardiac rhythm are closely related to this action: low serum potassium levels potentiate the arrhythmogenic effects of digitalis, whereas high serum potassium levels are sometimes effective in terminating digitalis-induced arrhythmias. Evidence linking inhibition of the triphosphatase enzyme and digitalis's positive inotropic effect is less convincing. Nevertheless, it appears that either through this, or some other action, the positive inotropic effect is a result of an increase in the availability of intracellular calcium which in turn allows greater interaction between the contractile proteins, actin and myosin, increasing the strength of contraction of the cardiac muscle fiber.

The less serious toxic effects of digitalis consist primarily of those associated with gastrointestinal upset—anorexia, nausea, and vomiting. The vomiting that occurs in patients taking digitalis is caused, at least in part, by a direct action on the chemoreceptive trigger zone located in the medulla and can be quite severe. Digitalis has other effects on the central nervous system and may cause headache, drowsiness, disorientation, confusion, and hallucinations. Vision is commonly blurred, and color vision may be disturbed.

The most severe toxic effects of digitalis are a result of its effects on the electrophysiological properties of the heart. Indeed, the cardiac arrhythmias of digitalis intoxication may take the form of almost any type of cardiac arrhythmia seen clinically. The most dangerous are of ventricular origin and include ventricular tachycardia and, of course, ventricular fibrillation.

The major interactions between digitalis and drugs of dental interest include the administration of epinephrine or atropinelike antisialagogues to patients taking digitalis. Epinephrine, through its beta adrenergic activity, may cause cardiac arrhythmias, and this effect may be synergistic with the arrhythmogenic effects of digitalis. Antisialagogues, by blocking muscarinic receptors of the AV node, may antagonize the effects of digitalis mediated by the vagus nerve, disturbing its antiarrhythmic action.

The relative characteristics of the common cardiac glycoside preparations are summarized in Table 14.2.

### Table 14.2.   Relative Characteristics of Cardiac Glycoside Preparations after Oral Administration

| Generic Name | % Absorption | Onset (hrs) | Duration (hrs) | Dosage (average adult) | | |
|---|---|---|---|---|---|---|
| | | | | Initial | Maintenance | Toxic |
| Digitalis, U.S.P. | 20 | Slow | Long | 1.2 gm | 0.1 gm | 2.25 gm |
| Digitoxin | 95 | Medium | Long | 0.2–0.6 mg | 0.05–0.3 mg | 4.0 mg |
| Digoxin | 80 | Fast | Medium | 1.0–1.5 mg | 0.125–0.5 mg | 6.0 mg |

## ANTIARRHYTHMIC AGENTS

The normal heart rate, by definition, ranges from 50 to 100 beats per minute and is regular in rhythm. Any alteration in rhythm or frequency outside of the normal range, whether regular or irregular in rhythm, is technically classified as an arrhythmia. Arrhythmias result from various causes and may range in severity from insignificant to life-threatening. An arrhythmia may originate in the sino-atrial (SA) node, in which case the rhythm is usually regular, but the heart rate is either less than 60 beats per minute (sinus bradycardia) or greater than 100 beats per minute (sinus tachycardia), or it may originate outside the SA node (ectopic arrhythmia), which usually results in an irregular rhythm and abnormal rate. Ectopic arrhythmias may originate anywhere in the heart, but regardless of the etiology, the seriousness is dependent on the ventricular rate and rhythm. If the ventricle is beating so rapidly or so erratically that adequate diastolic filling does not occur, then cardiac output will be adversely affected.

Clinically the more important drugs used to suppress or prevent arrhythmias can be loosely classified as follows:

1. Cardiac glycosides
2. Myocardial depressants
   a. Quinidine (prototype)
   b. Procainamide
   c. Propranolol (part of its action)
3. Agents having less effect on myocardium
   a. Lidocaine
   b. Phenytoin
4. Beta-adrenergic blocking agents
   a. Propranolol (prototype)

Digitalis is one of the most useful of the antiarrhythmic agents in treating arrhythmias of atrial origin. Its most important action in this regard is its action on transmission of impulses through the AV node. The AV node can be thought of as a gate regulating the number of impulses reaching the ventricle from the atrial tissue. Through both its direct and vagal actions, digitalis acts to "shut the gate," thus slowing the ventricle, even in the face of a rapid atrial rate. As a result, the ventricle has more time to fill adequately. This, in combination with digitalis's positive inotropic effect, improves cardiac output. A decrease in sympathetic tone on the heart is an added beneficial effect that results from the improved cardiac output.

Digitalis may increase the danger of ventricular fibrillation in patients who have ventricular arrhythmias and is, therefore, contraindicated in such patients.

The exact mechanisms of action of the diverse antiarrhythmic agents in various types of arrhythmias are still being investigated. However, Table 14.3 summarizes their effects on the electrophysiological properties of the heart. Although the classic antiarrhythmic agents differ in many ways, two important common characteristics are (1) the decrease in automaticity and (2) the increase in the effective refractory period relative to the action potential duration. Both of these effects are theoretically advantageous properties of an antiarrhythmic agent. The differences in the effects of the agents on cardiac electrophysiological properties may account for some of the differences in their antiarrhythmic actions, but these possibilities will not be discussed here.

### Myocardial Depressants

The pharmacological properties of quinidine and procainamide are qualitatively similar. Both drugs depress myocardial contractility and dilate peripheral blood vessels. They also both have a vagolytic action that may interfere with their effectiveness in slowing ventricular rate in patients with atrial arrhythmias. Both drugs are effective in controlling most types of ectopic arrhythmias, whether of atrial or ventricular origin.

Both quinidine and procainamide are well absorbed after oral administration and are most often given by this route. After oral administration, their onset of action is from 1.5 to 2.5 hours and their duration of action is from 6 to 8 hours. Quinidine is highly bound to plasma protein. Both drugs can be given by intramuscular injection, but intravenous administration is dangerous because severe hypotension may result from direct vasodilation and decreased force of myocardial contraction. These drugs are metabolized by the liver, and a significant percentage of the administered dose is excreted by the kidney.

### Agents Having Less Effect on the Myocardium

Phenytoin (Dilantin) is most widely used as an antiepileptic agent but also has antiarrhythmic activity. In contrast to quinidine, it has no vagolytic action and less effect on myocardial contractility and peripheral blood vessels, although rapid intravenous administration can cause significant hypotension. Phenytoin is significantly bound to plasma protein and is selectively distributed to the liver, where it is metabolized by the hepatic microsomal enzymes, and to the fat. Phenytoin is most often administered intravenously to suppress arrhythmias, but since the drug has a long duration of

## Table 14.3. Characteristic Electrophysiological Actions of Antiarrhythmic Agents

| | Procainamide Quinidine | Propranolol | Phenytoin Lidocaine |
|---|---|---|---|
| **Electrophysiologic properties, Purkinje fibers:** | | | |
| Automaticity | ↓ | ↓ | ↓ |
| Responsiveness | ↓ | ↓ | ↑ |
| Conduction velocity | ↓ | ↓ | ↑ |
| Effective refractory period | ↑ | ↓ | ↓ |
| Action potential duration | ↑ | ↓ | ↓ |
| Change in effective refractory period relative to action potential duration | ↑ | ↑ | ↑ |
| Excitability | ↓ | ↓ | ↑ → |
| Atrioventricular conduction time | ↑ | ↑ | → |

Source: Modified from Hoffman and Bigger, 1971.[3]
↑ = increased; ↓ = decreased; → = no change; Arrows indicate the direction and not the magnitude of change.

action (its half-life is approximately 24 hours), adequate maintenance can usually be accomplished with oral administration. It is ineffective against most atrial arrhythmias but is highly effective in controlling arrhythmias of ventricular origin. This is especially true for ventricular arrhythmias associated with digitalis intoxication for which the drug has an almost selective antiarrhythmic action.

The local anesthetic, lidocaine (Xylocaine), is also a well-accepted antiarrhythmic agent within relatively restricted usage. Like phenytoin, lidocaine lacks the vagolytic action of quinidine and has been reported to cause less cardiovascular depression at therapeutic concentrations. After intravenous administration, lidocaine has a quick onset and short duration of action (10 to 20 minutes after a single intravenous bolus injection). These characteristics contribute to its primary use—the emergency treatment of ventricular arrhythmias resulting from myocardial infarction and cardiac surgery. The drug is ineffective in terminating arrhythmias of atrial origin. It should be noted that lidocaine's short duration of action after a single intravenous bolus injection is due to a rapid redistribution of the drug away from the heart rather than rapid metabolism. Although lidocaine is metabolized by the liver, its metabolic half-life is about 2 hours. Prolonged infusion or repeated administration may therefore result in saturation of tissue depots and cumulative toxicity.

### Beta-Adrenergic Blocking Agents

Propranolol (Inderal), as well as other beta-adrenergic blocking agents, is effective in terminating arrhythmias caused by high circulating levels of catecholamines (e.g., pheochromocytoma) or increased sympathetic activity (e.g., thyrotoxicosis). In addition to its beta-adrenergic blocking activity, however, propranolol also has direct quinidinelike effects on the heart at higher doses. Although rarely the first drug of choice, propranolol has been used in treating various types of arrhythmias, including those of atrial origin. Its antiadrenergic action can prolong conduction through the AV node and thus slow the ventricular rate. This effect is synergistic with the effects of digitalis on the AV node, and for this reason propranolol has been administered in combination with digitalis to patients with certain atrial arrhythmias in an attempt to decrease the dose of digitalis necessary for ventricular slowing.

### Adverse Effects

The adverse effects of the antiarrhythmic agents discussed are summarized in Table 14.4. As a group, patients undergoing antiarrhythmic therapy may have episodes of dizziness, nausea, and

**Table 14.4. Characteristic Toxic Effects of Antiarrhythmic Agents**

| | Cardiac | | | CNS | Other |
|---|---|---|---|---|---|
| | Rhythm | BP | CO | | |
| Quinidine | Arrhythmias Asystole | ↓ | ↓ | Cinchonism (tinnitus, headache, impaired hearing, blurred vision) | G-I disturbances; thrombocytopenia |
| Procainamide | Arrhythmias Asystole | ↓ | ↓ | — | G-I disturbances; agranulocytosis |
| Propranolol | Pacemaker suppression Asystole | ↓ | ↓ | Mood changes; potentiation of depression caused by CNS depressants | Bronchospasm (asthmatics); hypoglycemia in predisposed individuals; potentiation of hypotensive effects of nitrates and nitrites |
| Phenytoin | Arrhythmias Asystole | ↓ | ↓ | Cerebellar signs (nystagmus, vertigo) | — |
| Lidocaine | Arrhythmias Asystole | ↓ | ↓ | Convulsions; respiratory depression; behavioral disturbances | — |

Source: Modified from Hoffman and Bigger, 1971.[3]

BP = blood pressure; CO = cardiac output; G-I = gastrointestinal; CNS = central nervous system.
Size of arrows indicates magnitude of change.

317

vomiting. They also may suffer rapid and severe falls in blood pressure; this is especially true in patients taking quinidine, procainamide, and propranolol.

Drugs that predispose the patient to hypotension, either by depressing the hypothalamic vasomotor center (central nervous system depressants) or by a direct action on the vascular smooth muscle (nitroglycerin), may precipitate a sharp fall in blood pressure in patients taking quinidine, procainamide, or propranolol. Cholinergic blocking agents such as atropine may antagonize the antiarrhythmic effects of drugs that are slowing AV conduction in patients with atrial arrhythmias. Quinidine has been reported to potentiate the neuromuscular blocking effects of skeletal muscle relaxants. Drugs that induce the enzymes of the hepatic microsomal drug metabolizing system, such as the barbiturates and some of the antihistamines, may increase the rate of metabolism of phenytoin and thus antagonize its antiarrhythmic action; on the other hand, diazepam (Valium) and chlordiazepoxide (Librium) may inhibit the metabolism of phenytoin and thus increase its toxic effects. In addition, salicylates may, theoretically, increase the toxic effects of phenytoin and quinidine by displacing them from their plasma protein-binding sites. Propranolol and phenytoin may potentiate the depression caused by the barbiturates, morphine, and other central nervous system depressants.

## DIURETICS

Diuretics are drugs that promote the net renal excretion of water and sodium ions. They are useful in many clinical situations, including cardiovascular disorders where mobilization of edema fluid and reduction of plasma volume may decrease the stress upon the cardiovascular system.

Sodium is the major extracellular cation of the body and is the primary determinant of the extracellular volume. A majority of clinically useful diuretics act on the nephron at various sites involved in the reabsorption of renal tubular sodium to promote its net excretion. Normally excretion of extracellular water follows, resulting in a decrease in the extracellular volume. Since the reabsorption of sodium is closely linked to renal regulation of other body electrolytes, the diuretics also cause modifications in these substances.

The following is a brief summary of the pertinent steps in the renal excretion of sodium and water (Figure 14.3); the reader is referred to other textbooks for a more detailed discussion.[2]

1. The fluid entering the proximal tubule from the glomerulus is an ultrafiltrate which is isosmotic with the plasma.

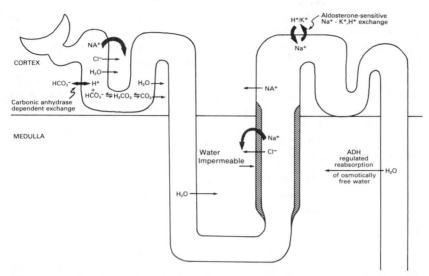

**Figure 14.3** Renal excretion of water and solutes: ADH = antidiuretic hormone; dark arrows represent enzyme- or carrier-mediated processes. (Adapted and redrawn from Thier and Sharp, 1972.[7])

2. In the proximal convoluted tubule, sodium is actively reabsorbed from the tubular fluid; water and chloride follow. Osmotic activity of the tubular fluid remains the same as the renal interstitial fluid and plasma. Within the tubular cell, carbon dioxide and water are converted to hydrogen and bicarbonate by the enzyme carbonic anhydrase. The resulting bicarbonate diffuses into the interstitial fluid while the hydrogen diffuses into the tubular lumen. Here the hydrogen associates with tubular bicarbonate to form carbonic acid and ultimately water and carbon dioxide, which passively diffuse through the tubular cell into the renal interstitial fluid. The net result is an inward movement of bicarbonate.

3. Dilution of the tubular fluid occurs in the ascending limb of the loop of Henle which is impermeable to water, but which continues the reabsorption of sodium and chloride. The active transport of sodium out of the ascending limb into the renal medullary interstitium plays an important role in the urine concentrating function of the distal portion of the nephron by maintaining hypertonicity of the interstitium.

4. In the distal tubule, sodium in the tubular fluid is exchanged for potassium from intracellular organic phosphate and hydrogen ions generated by carbonic anhydrase. The exchange of sodium for potassium and hydrogen is stimulated by the adrenal hormone aldosterone.

5. Final adjustment in tonicity of the urine occurs in the collecting ducts whose water permeability is regulated by antidiuretic hormone (ADH). In the presence of ADH, the water permeability of the cells of the collecting ducts is increased and the hypertonicity of the renal medullary interstitium promotes passive reabsorption of water (urine concentration). Absence of ADH decreases the water permeability of the cells of the collecting ducts and, hence, water reabsorption.

Among the clinically more useful diuretic agents that increase renal solute excretion are the following:

1. Agents inhibiting active transport of sodium
    a. Mercurials (e.g., mercaptomerin, Thiomerin)
    b. Benzothiadiazides (e.g., chlorothiazide, Diuril)
    c. Furosemide (Lasix)
    d. Ethacrynic acid (Edecrin)
2. Agents inhibiting the exchange of hydrogen for sodium
    a. Carbonic anhydrase inhibitors (e.g., acetazolamide, Diamox)
3. Agents inhibiting potassium excretion
    a. Spironolactone (Aldactone)
    b. Triamterene (Dyazide)

## Agents Inhibiting Active Transport of Sodium

MECURIALS. Mecurial diuretics appear to inhibit the active transport of sodium at all parts of the nephron responsible for sodium reabsorption; they do not interfere with the exchange of hydrogen for sodium. In addition, excretion of chloride is increased even more than that of sodium. These characteristics result in self-limitation of the diuretic action of these agents, since the net loss of chloride, coupled with a net increase in plasma bicarbonate generated by the still functional sodium-hydrogen exchange leads to hypochloremic alkalosis. The exact mechanism of the inverse relationship between alkalosis and diuretic action remains to be defined. The effects of these agents on potassium are complex and variable, but they generally cause less potasssium excretion than other diuretics. The major route of administration of the mercurial diuretics is intramuscular. This and the availability of more reliable oral diuretics have limited their use. The mercurial compounds are selectively distributed to the kidney and the liver, and these organs are usually the ones most often involved in the toxic effects of these agents. Toxic doses may also produce cardiac arrhythmias.

BENZOTHIADIAZIDES. The benzothiadiazides or thiazides are among the most widely used diuretics. They are effective when given orally and produce relatively moderate diuresis, including increased excretion of sodium, chloride, and potassium. Their major site of action is the distal diluting portion of the nephron where they block the reabsorption of sodium and chloride. Unlike the mercurials, the diuretic action of the thiazides is uninfluenced by body pH. Although many of the thiazides weakly inhibit carbonic anhydrase, this action does not appear to play a significant role in their diuretic action. The inhibition of sodium reabsorption in the early portion of the distal nephron presents increased sodium concentrations to the later portion where sodium-potassium exchange occurs, resulting in an increased exchange and excretion of potassium. Consequently, hypokalemia (with attendant skeletal muscle weakness, tetany, and paralysis; cardiac arrhythmias; and ileus) is one of the more common adverse effects of the thiazide diuretics. Concurrent administration of potassium-sparing agents such as spironolactone and triamterene may counteract this effect. Other adverse effects include precipitation of acute attacks of gout, as well as hyperglycemia, in predisposed individuals.

FUROSEMIDE (LASIX) AND ETHACRYNIC ACID (EDECRIN). These drugs are the most effective oral diuretics available for clinical use. Although differing chemically, their diuretic effects are similar. Both drugs cause an increased excretion of sodium, chloride, potassium, and hydrogen. Chloride excretion is increased even more than sodium excretion. A metabolic alkalosis may result, but in contrast to the mercurials this does not limit the diuretic action of furosemide and ethacrynic acid. These agents appear to block the active transport of sodium, and possibly chloride, at all levels of the ascending loop of Henle. This action not only decreases the amount of water in the distal tubule relative to the amount of solute, but the decrease in sodium transport into the medullary interstitium also reduces the osmotic gradient promoting the reabsorption of this osmotically free water from the collecting duct. Consequently, the loss of water caused by these agents may be profound and accounts for one of their more common adverse effects—hypovolemia (dehydration). This and other common adverse effects, such as potassium depletion and alkalosis, are, in fact, extensions of their therapeutic effects. Both furosemide and ethacrynic acid also cause direct toxic effects on the auditory system which result in hearing loss. These effects include destruction of the cochlear cells of the inner ear and are potentiated by the aminoglycoside antibiotics, i.e., streptomycin, kanamycin, neomycin, tobramycin, and gentamicin.

## Agents Inhibiting the Exchange of Hydrogen for Sodium (Carbonic Anhydrase Inhibitors)

The enzyme carbonic anhydrase is essential for the normal reabsorption of bicarbonate in the proximal tubule and the production of hydrogen ions for exchange with sodium in the distal tubule. Certain diuretics, such as acetazolamide (Diamox), inhibit this enzyme and thus interfere with reabsorption of sodium and bicarbonate at these sites. The resulting water diuresis is usually moderate, but these agents cause changes in the electrolyte composition and pH. For example, the decrease in bicarbonate reabsorption is associated with increased absorption of chloride; both of these actions raise urinary pH. Also a result of competition between potassium and hydrogen ions for exchange with sodium in the distal tubule, the decreased availability of hydrogen ions evokes an increased exchange of potassium for sodium which may significantly deplete body potassium. The diuretic effect of the carbonic anhydrase inhibitors is self-limiting, since the increased excretion of sodium bicarbonate, decreased net plasma bicarbonate, and increased plasma chloride produce a metabolic acidosis and enough excess hydrogen ions to restore sodium-hydrogen exchange. This metabolic acidosis can be avoided somewhat by administration of the diuretic on alternate days. Acetazolamide produces a wide range of minor adverse effects, including headache, dizziness, irritability, and gastrointestinal disturbances. It may also produce serious blood dyscrasias such as agranulocytosis and aplastic anemia.

## Agents Inhibiting Potassium Excretion

Spironolactone (Aldactone), which is a chemical homologue of the salt-retaining adrenal hormone, aldosterone, competitively antagonizes aldosterone's facilitory effect on sodium-potassium exchange in the distal tubule. The drug is most effective when aldosterone plasma levels are high, but with oral administration the diuretic effect is cumulative and several days are required for it to become maximal. At best, spironolactone causes only a mild diuresis when given alone. Its most significant effect is to decrease the excretion of potassium, and this is the basis for its most effective clinical use, i.e., concurrent administration with potasssium-depleting diuretics such as thiazides. In many patients taking these more potent, potassium-depleting diuretics, spironolactone can prevent the frequent complication of hypokalemia.

Triamterene (Dyazide) differs structurally from aldosterone and spironolactone, but its diuretic effects are similar to those of the latter agent. Triamterene interferes with the excretion of potassium in the distal tubule, but in contrast to spironolactone, it appears to act directly on the transport process involved in sodium-potasssium exchange rather than by antagonizing aldosterone's facilitory effect on this process.

## ANTIANGINAL AGENTS

Angina pectoris appears to result from a relative deficiency of myocardial oxygen supply with respect to myocardial metabolic demands. Normally there is about a 50% reserve in coronary flow, and the heart can respond to increased demands for oxygen and other nutrients with an increased coronary flow. If this reserve is reduced by disease, then factors (e.g., effort, eating, cold, and emotional stress) that increase the demand of the heart for oxygen may lead to relative ischemia and hypoxia. The result is an acute anginal attack characterized by a severe, crushing substernal pain that may radiate down either arm and, in some cases, even into the mandible. Acute anginal attacks usually last from 2 to 7 minutes; if the attack lasts for more than 30 minutes, it is likely that the patient is experiencing a myocardial infarction (heart attack).

The drugs used to prevent or terminate attacks of angina pectoris fall into two general categories. The first, and most important, are the negative myotropic agents. These agents have one thing in common—they all relax smooth muscle by a direct action on the smooth muscle cell. These agents are nonselective in that they relax smooth muscle throughout the body. This effect has led to the assumption that the negative myotropic agents relieve anginal attacks simply by dilating the coronary arteries and thus increasing total coronary flow. It now appears that the clinically successful antianginal agents act by a more complex mechanism.

The most reliable of the negative myotropic agents in treating angina pectoris are the nitrites and organic nitrates. These agents, referred to collectively as the nitrites, are discussed in more detail. Other negative myotropic agents include (1) aminophylline, a methyl xanthine, which has been shown to dilate coronary arteries but which has the disadvantage of also increasing myocardial force of contraction and oxygen consumption; (2) papaverine, an alkaloid derived from opium, which has some weak coronary vasodilator effect but which is limited in antianginal effectiveness; and (3) dypyridamole (Persantine), a synthetic coronary vasodilator, which in some experimental situations is a more potent vasodilator than the nitrites but clinically does not appear to be superior to placebo treatment in angina. Dypyridamole is thought to act by increasing the level of the metabolic by-product, adenosine, which is a potent vasodilator.

In addition to the negative myotropic agents, other agents are sometimes used to control anginal attacks. These include sedatives employed in an attempt to alleviate emotional precipitants of some types of angina. Propranolol, which prevents the increase in myocardial oxygen requirements induced by the increase in activity of the cardiac sympathetic nerves during exertion, has also been used in the treatment of angina and appears to be effective for long-term prophylaxis. In essence, beta-adrenergic blockade exchanges a decrease in force of myocardial contraction for a reduction in oxygen requirements of the heart. Since propranolol opposes the reflex sympathetic activation that may accompany administration of the nitrites, it may act synergistically with the latter agents; this too may be found to be a practical value in angina.

The nitrites are the most effective of the currently available antianginal agents. Although these agents produce vasodilation of the small coronary arteries, their beneficial effects in angina appear to be due, at least in part, to their peripheral effects. The postcapillary venules and veins are sensitive to the vasodilating effects of these agents. This venous dilation results in pooling of blood in the periphery and a decrease in venous return and load on the heart. In addition, vasodilation of arterioles decreases the arterial blood pressure and the resistance against which the heart must pump. All of these effects decrease myocardial oxygen consumption.

The most important characteristics of the nitrites and organic nitrates are summarized in Table 14.5. Amyl nitrite is a highly volatile liquid with an odor like banana oil. This drug is inactivated when administered orally and is therefore administered by inhalation. Nitroglycerin is also a volatile liquid which is adsorbed to a tablet for convenience of administration. It is the drug of choice in most dental situations related to angina. Nitroglycerin tablets quickly lose their pharmacological activity upon exposure to air. Shelf-life is about 6 months when kept in unopened *glass* bottles at room temperature; shelf-life drops to about one week after opening. Erythrityl tetranitrate, isosorbide dinitrate, and pentaerythritol tetranitrate are longer acting vasodilators promoted for prophylactic control of anginal attacks. Their effectiveness in preventing anginal attacks has been questioned, and they have no advantage over nitroglycerin in terminating an attack once it has begun.

Administration of the nitrites produces a flushing of the face, neck, and clavicular areas as a result of cutaneous vasodilation. A transient, throbbing headache occurs in many individuals as a result of vasodilation of the cerebral blood vessels. Acute toxicity due to overdosage includes postural hypotension which in turn may cause dizziness, fainting, nausea, and reflex tachycardia. If the dose is large enough, cardiovascular collapse can occur as a result of profound and widespread vasodilation of all blood vessels as well as inadequate coronary perfusion resulting from extremely low diastolic blood pressures. The nitrite ion can readily oxidize hemoglobin to methemoglobin which lowers the oxygen-carrying

## Table 14.5. Antianginal Agents

| Drug Name | Route of Administration | Average Onset | Average Duration | Purpose |
|---|---|---|---|---|
| Amyl Nitrite | Inhalation | 10–15 sec | 5–7 min | Treatment of acute attack |
| Nitroglycerin | Sublingually | 1–3 min | 10–30 min | Treatment of acute attack; prophylaxis just prior to procedure |
| Erythrityl tetranitrate | Sublingually | 5 min | 2 hr | Only for prophylaxis |
| Isosorbide dinitrate | Sublingually | 2–3 min | 1–2 hr | Only for prophylaxis |
| Pentaerythritol tetranitrate (Peritrate) | Orally | 15–20 min | 3–4 hr | Only for prophylaxis |

capacity of the blood, although this rarely causes a clinically significant problem in adults taking these agents for angina.

Repeated administration of the nitrites leads to the development of tolerance to their effects. The mechanism is unknown, but tolerance to the headache develops more rapidly than to the dilation of the coronary and peripheral blood vessels. Because this phenomenon exists, however, the smallest effective dose of these agents should be used.

The dentist will have occasion to administer nitroglycerin or some other nitrite under two different circumstances. The most usual case is that of the dental patient who has a history of angina pectoris. In such patients the dentist must administer one of the short-acting nitrites (usually nitroglycerin) before injection of the local anesthetic in order to prevent an acute anginal attack (short-term prophylaxis). The second case, which fortunately is rare, is that of the dental patient who has no history of angina, but who experiences his first anginal attack while undergoing dental treatment.

In patients who have a history of angina, visits should be kept short, fatiguing dental procedures should be minimized, and profound local anesthesia should be maintained. Premedication with sedatives, if deemed necessary, should be done in consultation with the patient's physician. For prophylaxis, the patient's own dose of his own nitroglycerin preparation should be used if at all possible. The patient should be advised to bring his own preparation to the dental office, and during treatment it should be placed within easy reach of both the dentist and the patient. Nitroglycerin should be administered 2 minutes prior to injection of local anesthetic. Whether the patient's own preparation is used or one is furnished by the dentist, it must be fresh. Reassurance of the patient and confidence of the dentist and dental hygienist are important, since studies have shown that the frequency of anginal attacks can be decreased by placebo administration when given by enthusiastic practitioners. If the dentist must determine the dose of nitroglycerin to be administered, then he should give no more than 0.3 mg sublingually. This dose may be repeated once if necessary. If the first dose does not relieve the pain, then angina may not be the problem. It should be understood that too large a dose of nitroglycerin may actually precipitate an anginal attack, since a fall in arterial blood pressure may decrease coronary flow, which will decrease myocardial oxygen supply, while at the same time increasing myocardial oxygen demands by reflexly increasing sympathetic tone on the heart.

Selected drug-drug interactions involving the nitrates and nitrites are summarized in Table 14.6.

## ANTICOAGULANTS

There are two aspects to the effects produced by the anticoagulants: (1) effects on hemostasis (the normal, extravascular clotting of shed blood) and (2) effects on thrombus formation (the potentially fatal, abnormal, intravascular clotting of blood). Their use in cardiovascular surgery involving extracorporeal circulation (e.g., through a heart-lung machine) is based on their effect on normal hemostasis. Their use in treatment of various chronic diseases (such as thrombophebitis, myocardial infarction, or cerebrovascular disease) which predispose the individual to thrombus development probably involves both effects. In such disease, the formation of an intravascular clot, or thrombus, may shut off the blood supply to vital tissues and organs causing necrosis and cellular death. In

**Table 14.6.   Drug Interactions with**
***Nitrates and Nitrites* (Antianginal Agents)**

It is assumed the dental patient is taking the usual therapeutic dose or the dentist is planning to administer the usual prophylactic dose of either a nitrate or a nitrite antianginal agent. The first column lists the drug (Interactant) the patient may already be taking and/or a drug the dentist may wish to administer. The second column lists the possible interaction that could occur.

| Interactant | Possible Interaction |
|---|---|
| Anticholinergics (Antisialagogues) | Nitrates and nitrites dilate retinal blood vessels and increase intraocular pressure. This may potentiate the anticholinergic effects of these agents in the eye and precipitate a glaucoma attack in predisposed individuals. |
| Antihistamines, e.g., Diphenhydramine (Benadryl) | Nitrates and nitrites may potentiate the anticholinergic side effects of these agents in the eye (see above). |
| Antihypertensives | Severe hypotension may occur with this combination. |
| Epinephrine | Nitrates and nitrites are antagonistic physiologically to epinephrine and can counteract epinephrine's vascular effects. |
| Meperidine (Demerol) | Nitrates and nitrites may potentiate the hypotensive effects of this and related analgesics. |

Source: Data modified from Martin, 1971.[4]

addition, portions of the thrombus may become dislodged (emboli) and travel through the vasculature until they lodge in small, but vital, blood vessels, with similar results. The goal of anticoagulant therapy in such cases is to prevent the further extension of an existing thrombus or to prevent the formation of new thrombi; these agents do not cause an existing clot to disappear. Thrombus formation is complex and poorly understood, and there is even some question as to whether anticoagulants can actually prevent thrombus development.

Although the cause of abnormal blood clotting within unbroken blood vessels is unknown, the normal clotting of blood extravascularly is better understood. The latter is a normal, homeostatic mechanism that acts to minimize blood loss when the integrity of the vasculature is breached. The major processes involved in blood coagulation are summarized in Figure 14.4.

The blood, tissue cells, and platelets contain several inactive substances or factors that are designated numerically in Figure 14.4. Contact of the blood with a foreign surface (such as broken endothelial cells) or tissue damage activates a chain reaction of these clotting factors.

The culmination of this chain reaction is the formation of thromboplastin activity (active prothrombin converting material). In the presence of thromboplastin, prothrombin is converted into throm-

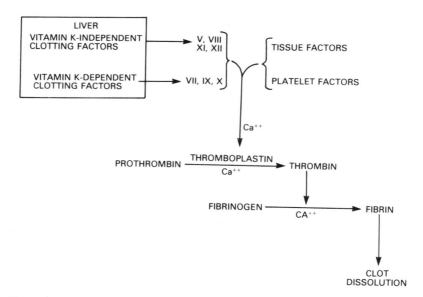

**Figure 14.4** Blood-clotting mechanism. (Adapted and redrawn from Levine, 1975.[8])

bin. Thrombin then acts catalytically to cleave soluble fibrin monomers from the protein fibrinogen. The fibrin monomers subsequently polymerize to form insoluble fibrin filaments which act as the matrix of the clot. Calcium ions are required for proper completion of each of these steps. Normally, the blood is maintained in a fluid state by a balance between these endogenous substances and substances opposing their actions. Among the apparently more important of these natural antagonists are antithrombins. These are proteins that inactivate or otherwise prevent thrombin from converting fibrinogen to fibrin.

The common anticoagulants can be divided into two groups:

1. Those acting both in vivo and in vitro
   a. Heparin
   b. Calcium-combining agents (oxalates, citrates, and chelating agents such as ethylenediamine tetraacetic acid, EDTA)
2. Those acting only in vivo
   a. Coumarin derivatives (e.g., dicumarol)
   b. Indandione derivatives (e.g., diphenadione)

## In Vivo and in Vitro Agents

Heparin is clinically the most important agent of the first group. Although calcium-combining agents are effective in vivo, they are rarely so used because of their toxicity. Their most important use is in preventing drawn blood from clotting in test tubes during laboratory tests.

Heparin, a mucopolysaccharide polymer, is the strongest naturally occurring organic acid in the body and possesses a strong electronegative charge. In the body it is stored in mast cells and has been postulated to aid in maintaining the fluidity of the blood by exerting an anticoagulant action. Such an action remains to be proven.

Although the exact mechanism of heparin's action is unknown, it is generally believed that its strong electronegative charge directly inactivates several of the enzyme systems participating in the coagulation process. Heparin's clinically most significant anticoagulant effect is its interference with the thromboplastin-mediated conversion of prothrombin to thrombin. In contrast to the oral anticoagulants, heparin does not interfere with the synthesis of prothrombin by the liver. At higher doses heparin also inactivates formed thrombin. This action requires a plasma cofactor and is related in a yet undefined way to a naturally occurring antithrombin. Heparin also interferes with the agglutination of platelets.

The drug is obtained from the intestinal mucosa of domestic animals. There is significant variation from batch to batch so that each preparation must be standardized according to its biological activity, i.e., its ability to prolong the blood clotting time. Heparin is inactivated when given orally and therefore must be given parenterally. After intravenous administration, its anticoagulant action begins within minutes, but lasts only for about 2 to 4 hours. Consequently, heparin is most often administered in the hospital to establish prompt anticoagulation. If long-term anticoagulation is required, oral anticoagulants are usually given, and heparin administration is stopped after these agents take effect (about 2 days).

The anticoagulant effects of heparin can be antagonized by basic substances having strong electropositive charges which combine with this strong acid to form a stable, inactive complex. Protamine sulfate, a low molecular weight protein, is such an agent and is sometimes used to treat severe overdosage of heparin.

## In Vivo Only Agents

The major anticoagulant agents with which the dentist and dental hygienist must contend are the orally effective agents of the coumarin and indandione classes (oral anticoagulants). These are the agents most often used for chronic control of thromboembolic diseases and, hence, are the anticoagulant agents that the dental patient will most likely be taking. The pharmacology of these agents does not differ significantly, and references to the prototype for this group, dicumarol, in the following discussion may be applied to the other coumarin and indandione derivatives.

The chemical structure of dicumarol as well as its similarity to the structures of vitamin K and aspirin, is shown in Figure 14.5. Dicumarol causes anticoagulation only when taken internally and has no effect on the coagulaton of blood in vitro. In contrast to heparin, dicumarol prolongs prothrombin time by suppressing the synthesis of prothrombin and clotting factors VII, IX, and X by the liver; it has no effect on these substances once they are synthesized. Dicumarol is thought to act as an antimetabolite of vitamin K which serves as an essential cofactor in the hepatic synthesis of these substances. This hypothesis is supported by the close chemical structural similarity between dicumarol and vitamin K, as well as the similarities between the depression of these factors as caused by dicumarol and as seen in experimentally produced vitamin K deficiency.

Dicumarol is adequately absorbed from the gastrointestinal tract. Within the circulation it is almost entirely bound to plasma protein, and this binding accounts, in part, for its slow rate of metabolism

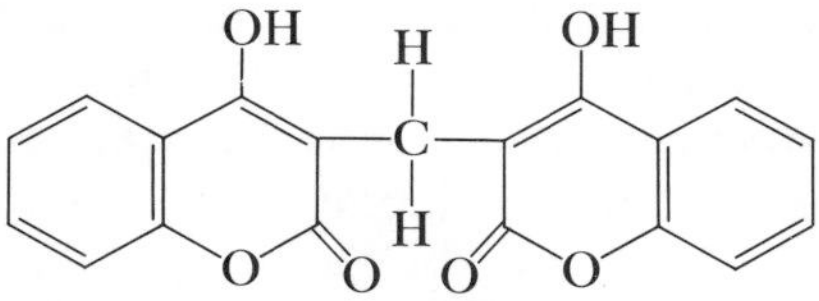

BISHYDROXYCOUMARIN (DICOUMAROL)

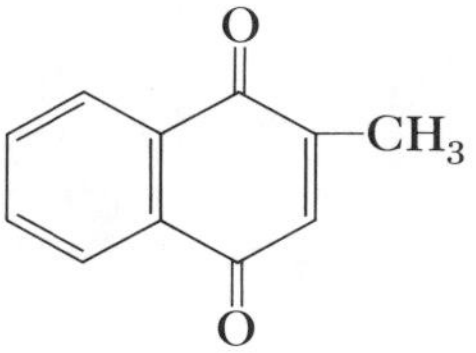

VITAMIN K (MENADIONE)

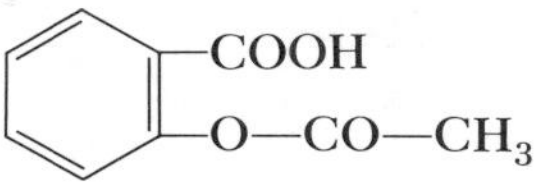

ACETYLSALICYLIC ACID (ASPIRIN)

**Figure 14.5** Comparison of chemical structure of bishydroxycoumarin (dicumarol) with that of vitamin K and aspirin.

and limited renal excretion. There is a definite lag in the onset of action of the oral anticoagulants, since time is required for the circulating clotting factors to be metabolized and their blood concentrations to fall below critical levels. In the case of dicumarol, maximum anticoagulation usually occurs within 36 to 48 hours. After administration is stopped, the duration of action is quite long (5 to 6 days) because the drug is slowly metabolized and the liver must renew its synthesis of the clotting factors.

Vitamin K antagonizes the anticoagulant effects of dicumarol. In cases of severe hemorrhage resulting from dicumarol administration, large intravenous doses of vitamin $K_1$ will reverse the anticoagulant effect. Similarly, administration of preparations containing vitamin K to patients who are adequately controlled with dicumarol is contraindicated, since this may interfere with anticoagulant therapy.

The most serious toxic effect of both heparin and the oral anticoagulants is hemorrhage. Bleeding most often occurs in the gastrointestinal tract, mucous membranes, gingiva, and urinary tract. Unless the bleeding is severe, cessation of administration is usually all that is required for control.

In times past, the patient on anticoagulant therapy was not considered a candidate for dental procedures that might result in bleeding and, indeed, every effort should be made to avoid such procedures by stressing effective preventive care. However, even though it should be appreciated that such patients are fragile patients, always on the edge of a hemorrhagic state, dental surgical procedures and exodontia can usually be performed safely, provided the patient is within the normal therapeutic dosage range and adequate preoperative and postoperative observation and care are carried out. Although clotting time of the blood is prolonged with both heparin and the oral anticoagulants, bleeding time is usually not altered significantly. The dentist should never abruptly withdraw the patient's anticoagulant therapy or administer an antagonist without approval of the physician, since this treatment may sometimes lead to a rebound hypercoagulation.

Adequate postoperative care of the dental patient on anticoagulant therapy implies the use of local hemostatic measures. These include application of pressure packs, sutures, and absorbable hemostatic agents. The latter agents act to aid the formation of artificial blood clots. Oxidized cellulose (Novocell) and oxidized regenerated cellulose (Surgicel) are chemically modified forms of surgical gauze whose hemostatic action depends upon the formation of an artificial clot by cellulosic acid. When left for prolonged periods on a surface wound, these substances have the disadvantage of delaying wound healing by inhibiting epithelization. Absorbable gelatin sponge (Gelfoam) acts as a matrix to aid clot formation. Its efficacy may be increased by wetting it with a thrombin solution. Thrombin, U.S.P., acts directly on fibrinogen to produce clotting, thus bypassing the other steps in the coagulation process. It should be administered only topically. In some cases, topical application of vasoconstrictors may provide adequate hemostasis.

It is essential in patients taking oral anticoagulants that care be taken to avoid the numerous unfavorable drug interactions possible with these agents. The more important dental drug-drug interactions are summarized in Table 14.7.

## ANTIHYPERTENSIVE AGENTS

Normal systemic arterial blood pressure is generally considered to be in order of 140 mmHg systolic and 90 mmHg diastolic (140/90). In actual fact, normal blood pressure varies and is dependent on several factors (e.g., age). Nevertheless, when the systemic arterial blood pressure persists above 160/95, it is considered abnormally elevated or hypertensive. Although systolic pressure is usually increased more than diastolic pressure in hypertension, it is the diastolic pressure which receives the most attention from the

## Table 14.7.   Drug Interactions with Coumarin Anticoagulants

It is assumed that the dental patient is taking the usual therapeutic dose of one of the coumarin oral anticoagulants when he seeks dental service. The column on the left lists drugs (Interactants) which the dentist may wish to administer in the course of dental treatment. The column on the right lists the possible interactions that could occur.

| Interactant | Possible Interaction |
|---|---|
| 1. Chloral hydrate (Noctec)<br>Mefenamic acid (Ponstel)<br>Phenylbutazone (Butazolidin)<br>Oxyphenbutazone (Tandearil) | Potentiates action of coumarin anticoagulant in man; acts by displacing anticoagulant from its plasma protein binding site |
| 2. Salicylates<br>(Aspirin) | Decrease hepatic clotting factor synthesis; potentiate coumarin anticoagulant effect |
| 3. Acetaminophen<br>(Tylenol) | *May* potentiate anticoagulant effect as seen with salicylates *but* far less in degree and *not well* shown yet in man. *If mild analgesic is needed, prescribe Tylenol rather than salicylate* |
| 4. Barbiturates and also non-barbiturates, ethchlorvynol (Placidyl), glutethimide (Doriden) | Accelerate coumarin metabolism; inhibit anticoagulant effect |
| 5. Meprobamate (Equanil) | *May* inhibit coumarin anticoagulant effect in man by same mechanism as seen with barbiturates, but more evidence is needed |
| 6. Broad spectrum antibiotics | Decrease synthesis of vitamin K by intestinal flora; potentiate coumarin anticoagulant effect |

Source: Data modified from Martin, 1972.[4]

physician, since this pressure represents the minimal level of constant mechanical strain on the cardiovascular system.

Hypertension may result from many causes, including the following: tumors of the adrenal medulla (pheochromocytoma), disease of the renal arteries, intracranial lesions, compression of the aorta, and aldosterone-producing tumors of the adrenal cortex. Most of these forms of hypertension can be treated directly by correction of the underlying cause. In a majority of hypertensive patients, however, the underlying cause cannot be identified, and the condition is given the name of primary or essential hypertension. Unless stated otherwise, the following discussion will deal with agents administered for the chronic control of essential hypertension.

As the name implies, the etiology of essential hypertension is unknown. It is commonly agreed, however, that although varying with such factors as severity, duration, rate of progression, and age, the prognosis of essential hypertension is generally poor if the diastolic pressure remains elevated and uncontrolled. Death usually results from accelerated vascular disease of the kidney, heart, or brain. The chronic elevated pressure increases the mechanical trauma to which the arterioles are exposed and hastens the onset and progression of arteriosclerosis. The arteries and arterioles of the kidney, exposed as they are to high perfusion pressures, are usually the first vessels involved, and uremia is a common cause of death in such patients. Another common complication of essential hypertension is congestive heart failure resulting from the increased work load placed on the heart by high aortic pressures as well as arteriosclerosis of the coronary arteries. Cerebrovascular hemorrhage (stroke) is also a frequent complication.

Since the pathogenesis of essential hypertension is unknown, pharmacological treatment is entirely empirical and is directed toward lowering and maintaining the diastolic blood pressure within the normal range. The rationale for this approach is based on the known dangers of uncontrolled hypertension mentioned, as well as on studies that have shown that if the diastolic blood pressure can be lowered and controlled early enough, the incidence of hypertensive complications can be decreased and life expectancy can be increased. Recognition of the importance of lowering the diastolic blood pressure, even though empirical, has led to the employment of a wide variety of drugs in controlling essential hypertension. Mechanisms of action vary, but these drugs can be loosely classified into three groups as follows: (1) agents interfering with the sympathetic nervous system; (2) agents promoting sodium excretion and decreasing blood volume; and (3) agents directly relaxing arterioles.

## Agents Interfering with the Sympathetic Nervous System

Present evidence suggests that in contrast to earlier beliefs, hyperactivity of the sympathetic nervous system is not primarily responsible for the characteristic increases in peripheral vascular resistance associated with essential hypertension. However, the sympathetic nervous system does contribute to vascular tone in hypertensive individuals just as it does in normotensive individuals. Apparently, the pressure-sensitive cells of the carotid sinus and aortic arch have the ability to adapt in the hypertensive individual in such a way as to function in relation to some new basal blood pressure far above the normal, thus adjusting sympathetic tone within a new, elevated range. Consequently, interference with sympathetic function in a hypertensive individual results in a lowering of the blood pressure. The major sites of action of antihypertensive agents that interfere with the sympathetic nervous system are as follows: hypothalamic and medullary sympathetic cardiovascular centers, autonomic sympathetic ganglia, the adrenergic nerve terminal, and the adrenergic receptors.

DRUGS ACTING ON HYPOTHALAMIC AND MEDULLARY SYMPATHETIC CARDIOVASCULAR CENTERS. Methyldopa (Aldomet) is an effective antihypertensive agent which causes a significant depletion of tissue norepinephrine, both peripherally and in the central nervous system. Methyldopa inhibits one of the enzymes (dopa decarboxylase) involved in the synthesis of norepinephrine. It has also been shown to enter the norepinephrine synthetic pathway resulting in the synthesis of alphamethyl-norepinephrine. The alphamethyl-norepinephrine formed displaces naturally occurring norepinephrine from its granular storage sites within the adrenergic nerve, depleting the nerve of its norepinephrine. When the nerve is stimulated by the action potential, alphamethyl-norepinephrine is thus released in place of norepinephrine. The preceding sequence of events is a classic example of a false transmitter. Originally the hypotensive effect of methyldopa was thought to result from actions on the peripheral adrenergic nerve terminal, either from inhibition of dopa decarboxylase or by acting as a false transmitter. It is now generally accepted, although the exact mechanism is still unknown, that the primary hypotensive effect of methyldopa is due to an action on central sympathetic cardiovascular centers, possibly involving alphamethyl-norepinephrine.

After a single dose, methyldopa evokes a progressive decrease in blood pressure and the heart rate which reaches a maximum in about 4 to 6 hours and lasts for about 24 hours. When given chronically, the hypotensive effect appears to be due to a decrease in peripheral resistance, a decrease in cardiac output, or a combination of both. The fall in blood pressure is usually greater in the hypertensive than in the normotensive individual. Most of the normal cardiovascular reflexes are not significantly reduced by methyldopa.

Methyldopa can produce several side effects related to actions on the central nervous system. The most frequent and important of these is sedation. It may also produce dry mouth, various gastrointestinal disturbances, and allergiclike reactions. Although blood pressure is lower in the erect than supine position, methyldopa evokes less frequent and less severe postural hypotension than the adrenergic neuron blocking agents (e.g., guanethidine).

Clonidine (Catapres), one of the newer antihypertensive agents, also appears to exert its hypotensive effects through an action on central sympathetic cardiovascular centers. Clonidine has many diverse actions, including alpha-adrenergic agonist activity, alpha-adrenergic blocking activity, and inhibition of norepinephrine release from adrenergic nerve terminals. Centrally, clonidine causes a decrease in sympathetic tone and an increase in vagal tone.

Chronic administration of clonidine causes a relatively mild reduction in blood pressure accompanied by bradycardia. Tolerance to the antihypertensive effect is not uncommon when the drug is given alone. Postural hypotension, if it develops, is usually not severe, and the normal cardiovascular reflexes are not significantly reduced. Sedation and dry mouth are the most frequent and severe side effects caused by clonidine.

DRUGS BLOCKING AUTONOMIC GANGLIA. Mecamylamine (Inversine) is a ganglionic blocking agent. These agents have become less important as antihypertensive agents because of their many adverse effects. They make no distinction between sympathetic and parasympathetic ganglia. Interruption of sympathetic transmission results in potentially severe postural hypotension and inhibition of heat loss through the sweating mechanism. Interruption of parasympathetic transmission results in dry mouth, blurred vision, urinary retention, and constipation. The present use of ganglionic blocking agents is limited to the acute control of severe hypertensive crises. In contrast to most of the agents effective in chronic control of essential hypertension, mecamylamine has a short onset and duration of action, allowing more flexibility in control of the hypotensive response.

ADRENERGIC NEURON BLOCKING AGENTS. The mechanisms of action of the two most important agents of this group, reserpine and guanethidine, were discussed in Chapter 3, and the present discussion will deal only with their use as antihypertensive agents.

Reserpine (Serpasil) was originally used as an early antipsychotic agent. It was noted that in addition to its antipsychotic effects, reserpine depleted peripheral and central nervous system tissues of catecholamines and serotonin, inhibited sympathetic reflexes, and lowered the systemic blood pressure. Because of these observations, reserpine became one of the first modern antihypertensive agents.

In addition to suppression of sympathetic activity the chronic administration of reserpine enhances peripheral parasympathetic activity to produce miosis, bradycardia, and increased gastrointestinal activity. The drug acts centrally to produce sedation. When administered orally in relatively small doses, reserpine produces a slowly developing fall in blood pressure that is more marked in the hypertensive than in the normotensive individual. Although reserpine is capable of suppressing all responses to peripheral sympathetic nerve activity at higher doses, in the usual chronic oral doses many sympathetic reflexes remain functional.

The mild sedation caused by antihypertensive doses of reserpine, although of importance in potential interactions with other drugs, of itself usually presents no clinical problem and may even be advantageous. However, these same doses may cause suicidal tendencies and psychic depression in a significant number of patients. The increased gastrointestinal activity caused by reserpine commonly results in cramps, diarrhea, and other gastrointestinal disturbances. Nasal stuffiness, although not serious, is an annoying complication. Reserpine, like guanethidine and mecamylamine, elicits a supersensitivity to catecholamines which may result in potentiation of the effects of injected norepinephrine and epinephrine.

Guanethidine (Ismelin) is one of the most effective of the antihypertensives available for chronic treatment of essential hypertension. However, its use is limited to more severe cases because of its adverse effects. This drug has several actions on adrenergic nerve function, and, hence, its pharmacological effects are complex. Guanethidine causes a decrease in peripheral tissue concentrations of norepinephrine which may last for several days after administration is stopped. However, responses to peripheral adrenergic nerve activity are almost completely abolished before significant depletion of tissue norepinephrine occurs. Guanethidine produces a profound fall in blood pressure. Several days may be required to establish the maximum hypotension effect, but once established, the effects are long lasting (7 to 14 days). In therapeutic doses, cardiovascular reflexes may not be completely abolished, but they are usually significantly depressed. As a result, guanethidine characteristically produces the most severe postural hypotension of the commonly used antihypertensive agents. In addition to postural hypotension, other adverse effects include gastrointestinal disturbances (primarily diarrhea), salt and water retention, and a potentially dangerous potentiation to the effects of administered catecholamines.

Pargyline (Eutonyl) is a monoamine oxidase inhibitor specifically introduced as an antihypertensive agent in response to the observation that postural hypotension was a frequent side effect accompanying administration of monoamine oxidase inhibitors for their central antidepressive effects. The mechanism of the hypotensive action of these agents remains to be elucidated, but inhibition of monoamine oxidase appears to play only a partial role, if any. The decrease in blood pressure occurs slowly (3 weeks for maximum effect) and occurs primarily in the erect position. The wide range and severity of its toxic effects limit pargyline's usefulness as an antihypertensive agent. Numerous drug-drug interactions may occur in patients taking monoamine oxidase inhibitors, and the reader is referred to Chapter 15 for a more detailed discussion of the adverse effects of these agents. It should be reemphasized, however, that residual effects of these agents may remain for weeks after administration has been stopped.

ADRENERGIC RECEPTOR BLOCKING AGENTS. Phenoxybenzamine (Dibenzyline) and phentolamine (Regitine) are alpha-adrenergic receptor blocking agents whose effectiveness in treating hypertension is limited primarily to acute control of hypertensive crises resulting from various causes, including pheochromocytoma, sympathomimetics, and drug interactions in the presence of inhibition of monoamine oxidase.

Propranolol (Inderal), a beta-adrenergic receptor blocking agent, is finding greater acceptance in the chronic control of essential hypertension. Its mechanism of hypotensive action remains to be defined but probably involves a reduction in cardiac output and plasma renin activity. Used alone, propranolol produces only a moderate reduction in blood pressure in a small number of patients. Its greatest potential lies in its use in combination with other agents. It is much more effective when used in combination with a diuretic, and it prevents the reflex increase in heart rate and cardiac output that accompanies the directly acting vasodilator antihypertensive agents. The adverse effects of propranolol are summarized in Table 14.4.

## Agents Promoting Sodium Excretion and Decreasing Blood Volume

Although many diuretics may be used in the control of essential hypertension, the present discussion will be limited to the widely used benzothiadiazide (thiazide) group of diuretics and specifically to the prototype chlorothiazide (Diuril). Although the antihypertensive effect of chlorothiazide is limited, it has become important in hypertensive therapy primarily because of its ability to potentiate the hypotensive action of other drugs.

The fall in blood pressure evoked by chlorothiazide is initially associated with the decreases in extracellular fluid, plasma volume, cardiac output, and total body sodium caused by its diuretic action on the kidney. However, after daily administration for several months the antihypertensive effect persists even though plasma volume and total body sodium return to near normal values. The exact mechanisms of this long-term antihypertensive action is not known but is associated with a significant decrease in peripheral resistance. The decreased peripheral resistance appears to be due to relaxation of arterial smooth muscle.

Chlorothiazide generally produces little or no postural hypotension. Its most frequent complication is a loss of body potassium leading to hypokalemia. This is usually not clinically significant except in patients receiving chlorothiazide and digitalis concurrently, since hypokalemia pctentiates the toxic effects of digitalis.

### Agents Directly Relaxing Arterioles

With respect to the chronic control of essential hypertension, hydralazine (Apresoline) is the most important of the antihypertensive agents that directly relax vascular smooth muscle. Others of this group (i.e., nitrites, nitroprusside) are limited to hypertensive emergencies requiring short-term, rapid reduction in blood pressure. The smooth muscle of the arterioles is more sensitive to the relaxant effects of hydralazine than is that of the veins. Since the capacitance vessels are less affected, venous return to the heart remains adequate, and cardiac output may be elevated. In addition, the fall in arterial blood pressure evoked by hydralazine reflexly stimulates the heart. Both of these effects minimize postural hypotension and limit the fall in blood pressure obtainable. The drug may also promote sodium retention and edema formation. For these reasons, hydralazine's antihypertensive effects are more apparent when it is given in combination with a diuretic or a drug (e.g., propranolol) that blocks the sympathetic nervous system and prevents the associated compensatory tachycardia and increased cardiac output.

Hydralazine causes a high incidence of adverse effects, including headache, palpitations, anorexia, nausea, vomiting, tremors, and muscle cramps. Chronic administration of hydralazine has been reported to produce an acute rheumatoid state in a small percentage of patients. It may also provoke anginal attacks as a result of the associated reflex myocardial stimulation. The frequency of adverse effects is closely related to the dose administered, and such effects occur less frequently if the dose is increased gradually.

Although closely related to the thiazide diuretics in chemical structure, diazoxide (Hyperstat) does not possess diuretic activity. However, its antihypertensive effect appears to be similar to that seen after administration of chlorothiazide for several months but is much more rapid and profound. Like hydralazine, it appears to have more effect on the arterioles than on the veins. Its clinical application is limited to short-term use by its adverse effects—salt

## Table 14.8.   Drug Interactions
## with Antihypertensive Agent Prototypes

In this listing of drug interactions it will be assumed that the dental patient is currently being treated by the physician for chronic primary hypertension with one or more of the prototype antihypertensive agents. Other antihypertensive agents that are in the same classification (i.e., possess the same mechanism of action) as one of the prototype agents may be expected to produce the same interactions as the prototype. The dentist's drug is represented by the Interactant.

| Interactant | Possible Interaction |
| --- | --- |
| PROTOTYPE 1: Reserpine (Serpasil)—norepinephrine depleting agent | |
| 1. Anesthetics, general | Anesthetics potentiate the hypotensive effect of reserpine and its derivatives, resulting in severe bradycardia. Hypotension may occur up to 2 weeks after drug is stopped. Contraindicated in surgery. |
| 2. Anticholinergics (e.g., atropine) | Reserpine antagonizes the antisecretory effects of anticholinergics. Anticholinergics counteract abdominal cramps and diarrhea resulting from increased G.I. motility and tone if given along with reserpine. |
| 3. Antihistamines | Increased central nervous system depression. |
| 4. Barbiturates | Reserpine potentiates the central nervous system depressant action of the barbiturates (bradycardia and hypotension). |
| 5. Morphine | Reserpine antagonizes the analgesic activity of morphine. |
| 6. Salicylates | Reserpine inhibits the analgesic actions of salicylates. |
| 7. Sympathomimetics | Theoretically, sympathomimetics tend to inhibit the hypotensive and sedative effects of reserpine. However, timing and the specific drug are important. Directly acting adrenergics such as norepinephrine are potentiated by reserpine. Indirectly acting adrenergics such as amphetamine have their effects inhibited or abolished by reserpine because reserpine has depleted the norepinephrine which these stimulants require for their action. |

## Table 14.8.　Continued

| Interactant | Possible Interaction |
|---|---|
| **PROTOTYPE 2: Guanethidine (Ismelin)—nonrepinephrine release blocker** | |
| 1. Anesthetics, general | Anesthetics potentiate the hypotensive effect of guanethidine which may lead to cardiovascular collapse. |
| 2. Anticholinergics (e.g., atropine) | Guanethidine antagonizes the hyposecretory effect of anticholinergics. |
| 3. Antihistamines | Antihistamines antagonize the adrenergic blocking (hypotensive) action of guanethidine. |
| 4. Catecholamines (epinephrine, norepinephrine, isoproterenol) | Guanethidine augments responses to catecholamines. Cardiovascular effects are intensified; guanethidine increases the sensitivity of the adrenergic receptor system to these amines. |
| **PROTOTYPE 3: Methyldopa (Aldomet)—norepinephrine synthesis inhibitor** | |
| 1. Anesthetics, general | The combined hypotensive effects of these two agents or methyldopa and any central nervous system depressant may be hazardous. Cardiovascular collapse and/or cardiac arrest have been reported. |
| 2. Levarterenol (Levophed) | Methyldopa potentiates levarterenol (norepinephrine) two to three times. |
| **PROTOTYPE 4: Mecamylamine (Inversine)—ganglionic blocking agent** | |
| 1. Anesthetic, general | The combined effects of mecamylamine and any general anesthetic leads to profound hypotension and in many cases cardiovascular collapse. |
| 2. Levarterenol (Levophed) | Mecamylamine potentiates the effects of all catecholamines. |
| 3. Sympathomimetics | These agents may antagonize the antihypertensive effects of mecamylamine. |
| **PROTOTYPE 5: Pargyline (Eutonyl)—monoamine oxidase inhibitor** | |
| Refer to index | |

Source: Data modified from Martin, 1971.[4]

and water retention, hyperuricemia, and hyperglycemia. At present, the drug is available in this country only for intravenous administration.

## The Hypertensive Dental Patient

If the dental patient has a history of hypertension, the person recording the medical history should be careful to note all drugs being taken, since it is not unusual for such patients to be taking a combination of antihypertensive agents. Usually chlorothiazide, or some similar diuretic, is the first drug of choice. This will produce adequate control in about 50% of patients with mild hypertension (90 to 110 mmHg, diastolic pressure). In the remainder of these patients or in patients with more severe hypertension, the diuretic is usually continued and reserpine, hydralazine, methyldopa, or propranolol added. Some physicians may combine both hydralazine and propranolol with the diuretic for the reasons already discussed. Guanethidine is usually reserved for the most severe cases of essential hypertension (> 130 mmHg, diastolic pressure).

It should be appreciated from the preceding discussion that dental patients being treated for essential hypertension have a labile blood pressure: the balance between disease and antihypertensive drug effect is usually delicate. These patients are predisposed to postural hypotension with associated nausea, dizziness, and fainting. Changes in body position from supine to erect should be gradual. Stress may precipitate a hypertensive crisis and should be avoided. For this reason, the dentist may decide to sedate the patient prior to induction of local anesthesia, but sedatives may act synergistically with the antihypertensive agent to cause dangerous hypotensive episodes. Thus, presedation must be approached cautiously with close observation of the patient. The use of epinephrine in the form of gingival retraction or local hemostatic agents is contraindicated in patients taking guanethidine, reserpine, mecamylamine, and methyldopa which potentiate the pressor effects of the catecholamines. Selected drug-drug interactions involving the antihypertensive agents are summarized in Table 14.8.

## REFERENCES

1. Anderson, T.O., et al.: Management of dental problems in patients with cardiovascular disease. J.A.M.A. *187*:848, 1964.
2. Hutcheon, D.E.: Diuretics. *In* Drill's Pharmacology in Medicine. 4th Edition. Edited by J.R. Di Palma. New York, McGraw-Hill, 1971.
3. Hoffman, B.R., and Bigger, J.T.: Antiarrhythmic drugs. *In* Drill's Pharmacology in Medicine. 4th Edition. Edited by J.R. Di Palma. New York, McGraw-Hill, 1971.
4. Martin, E.W.: Hazards of Medication. Philadelphia, Lippincott, 1971.
5. Mason, D.T.: Regulation of cardiac performance in clinical heart disease: interactions between contractile state, mechanical abnormalities, and ventricular compensatory mechanisms. Am. J. Cardiol. 32:437, 1973.

6. Moe, G.K., and Farah, A.E.: Digitalis and allied cardiac glycosides. *In* The Pharmacological Basis of Therapeutics. 5th Edition. Edited by L.S. Goodman and A. Gilman. New York, Macmillan, 1975.
7. Thier, S.O., and Sharp, W.G.: Renal disorders. *In* Clinical Pharmacology: Basic Principles in Therapeutics. Edited by K.L. Melmon and H.F. Morrelli. New York, Macmillan, 1972.
8. Levine, W.G.: Anticoagulant, antithrombotic, and thrombolytic drugs. *In* The Pharmacological Basis of Therapeutics. 5th Edition. Edited by L.S. Goodman and A. Gilman. New York, Macmillan, 1975.

## SUPPLEMENTARY REFERENCES

Angelakos, E.T.: Coronary vasodilators. *In* Drill's Pharmacology in Medicine. 4th Edition. Edited by J.R. Di Palma. New York, McGraw-Hill, 1971.
Aviado, D.M.: Diuretics. *In* Krantz and Carr's Pharmacologic Principles of Medical Practice. 8th Edition. Edited by D.M. Aviado. Baltimore, Williams & Wilkins, 1972.
Briggs, A.H., and Holland, W.C.: Antihypertensive drugs. *In* Drill's Pharmacology in Medicine. 4th Edition. Edited by J.R. Di Palma. New York, McGraw-Hill, 1971.
Lomax, P.: Diuretics. *In* Essentials of Pharmacology: Introduction to the Principles of Drug Action. 2nd Edition. Edited by J.A. Bevan. New York, Harper and Row, 1976.
Loomis, T.A.: Anticoagulant and coagulant drugs. *In* Drill's Pharmacology in Medicine. 4th Edition. Edited by J.R. Di Palma. New York, McGraw-Hill, 1971.
Moe, G.K., and Abildskov, J.A.: Antiarrhythmic drugs. *In* The Pharmacological Basis of Therapeutics. 5th Edition. Edited by L.S. Goodman and A. Gilman. New York, Macmillan, 1975.
Nickerson, M.: Vasodilator drugs. *In* The Pharmacological Basis of Therapeutics. 5th Edition. Edited by L.S. Goodman and A. Gilman. New York, Macmillan, 1975.
Nickerson, M., and Ruedy, J.: Antihypertensive agents and the drug therapy of hypertension. *In* The Pharmacological Basis of Therapeutics. 5th Edition. Edited by L.S. Goodman and A. Gilman. New York, Macmillan, 1975.
Walton, R.P., and Gazes, P.C.: Cardiac glycosides II. Pharmacology and clinical use. *In* Drill's Pharmacology in Medicine. 4th Edition. Edited by J.R. Di Palma. New York, McGraw-Hill, 1971.

# 15

## DRUGS IN THE TREATMENT OF NEUROLOGICAL DISORDERS

The patient may be taking one of the many drugs used in the treatment of the neurological disorders when he seeks the professional services of the dentist or dental hygienist. A large group of these agents, the sedatives, is presented in Chapter 9. In this chapter three additional drug groups will be considered, since each is high on the list of the drugs the patient is apt to be taking; i.e., the antiepileptic agents, the antipsychotic agents, and the antidepressant agents.

### THE ANTIEPILEPTIC AGENTS

Anticonvulsive activity is shared by a large number of drugs, e.g., the general anesthetics and the sedative-hypnotics. Administered in appropriate doses, these agents are capable of suppressing an existing convulsion or preventing the appearance of convulsions. These anticonvulsants are general or nonselective depressants of the central nervous system.

Another smaller group of drugs are both anticonvulsants and selective central nervous system depressants. These are known as the antiepileptic agents. Whereas the general term, *anticonvulsant*, refers to a drug which depresses the activity of both the motor and sensory cortex, the antiepileptic agents depress mainly the motor functions, and leave the sensorium intact. As their name indicates, the antiepileptic drugs are used specifically in the symptomatic treatment of the most prominent of all convulsive disorders, epilepsy. In particular, these drugs are employed to prevent the appearance of seizures and allow the patient to live a useful, seizure-free life.

There is as yet no complete agreement regarding the definitions of terms such as anticonvulsant or antiepileptic, convulsions and seizures, or, indeed, the disease epilepsy itself. The actual choice of drug or drugs to be used clinically is based primarily upon the patient's clinical seizure pattern type. Therefore, before the pharmacology of these drugs is presented, it is important for the practitioner to have an awareness of epilepsy and consider a brief classification of the different types of major epileptic seizures.

For our purposes, epilepsy is a symptom of malfunctioning in the central nervous system and may be defined as an intermittent cerebral dysrhythmia caused by occasional, sudden, excessive, rapid, and local discharges of gray matter. Epilepsy is characterized, electroencephalographically, by abnormal and excessive discharges of neurons and, clinically, most often by a disturbance of consciousness with or without convulsive movements.

In broad terms there are two major forms of epileptic seizures: generalized and partial. In generalized seizures, epileptiform discharges may be recorded (EEG) from anywhere on the cortex from the outset of the seizure. The discharges are bilaterally synchronous and are subcortical in origin, more specifically from what Penfield terms the centrencephalic system which includes the thalamic nuclei and the rostral portion of the ascending reticular formation of the midbrain.[2] Under this category of generalized seizures are the various forms of grand mal and petit mal epilepsy. The clinical manifestations include an immediate loss of consciousness at the seizure outset and the presence or absence of skeletal muscle movement.

In partial seizures, epileptiform discharges may be recorded (EEG) from only certain areas (the epileptogenic focus) of the cortex at the outset of the seizure. These discharges are of cortical origin. If the seizure discharge is sufficiently strong, it can spread over corticothalamic pathways to the centrencephalic system whereupon consciousness is lost and a generalized seizure ensues. In this category the most common type of all forms of epilepsy is found, namely, psychomotor epilepsy. Usually the epileptogenic focus in psychomotor epilepsy is found in the anterior region of the temporal lobe of the cortex.[3]

Regardless of the form epilepsy takes in terms of seizure patterns, there is involved in each a group of hyperexcitable neurons, referred to as the epileptogenic focus. These neuron's lowered threshold of excitability can be caused by many factors (all of which are certainly not yet known) and includes such different causes as massive tissue damage owing to traumatic injury of an anatomically invisible inherited discrepancy in cellular metabolism of one or more critically located neurons. It is conceivable that a stable supersensitive area of a few neurons could be situated so that a normal inflow of afferent sensory impulses of a particular set of characteristics may upset the delicate balance between the complex excitatory and inhibitory systems in the brain.

A second general characteristic, in addition to the presence of an epileptogenic focus, is the spread of the seizure discharge. The usual result of excessive, abnormal firing of the neurons of the focus is the spreading of these functionally abnormal impulses over normal neuronal pathways to bombard and involve other functional areas.

Based upon extensive investigations three general mechanisms of action have been proposed by which a drug with anticonvulsive or antiepileptic properties might produce its effects: (1) a depressant action directly on the hyperexcitable neurons which make up the epileptogenic focus; (2) a stabilizing action on the normal neurons of the central nervous system in order to prevent the spreading of the abnormal activity from the discharging primary focus; and (3) an action on various nonneural systems which are known to influence the appearance of seizure activity.[4]

The crucial test for the efficacy of any potential antiepileptic agent is its effects following administration to patients with various forms of epilepsy under controlled conditions by an experienced investigator. Long before the crucial test can take place, the drug must be identified as having antiepileptic properties. A battery of laboratory tests using animals has been devised in which seizures are experimentally induced by electroshock, chemoshock, and other techniques.

In this chapter the following pertinent pharmacology of three prototype antiepileptic drugs—phenobarbital, phenytoin, and trimethadione—will be presented: (1) their action as observed in laboratory tests; (2) their possible mechanism of action; (3) their relative clinical effectiveness in the major forms of epilepsy; and (4) their important side effects. Many other drugs are used specifically in the treatment of the various forms of epilepsy. Table 15.1 lists these agents in terms of their chemical structure, the form of epilepsy in which each is most commonly prescribed, and their typical total adult daily dose.

### Barbiturates

In addition to their sedative-hypnotic properties, the barbiturates also possess anticonvulsant activity (see Chapter 9). Owing to their general, nonselective depressant action on all neurons, it might be expected that in appropriate doses any one of the barbiturates could

# Table 15.1. Selected Antiepileptic Agents, Their Structures, Specific Uses, and Doses

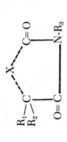

| R₁ | Substitutions R₂ | R₃ | X | Drug Names | Specific Use in Epilepsy* | Usual Oral Dose (grams)† |
|---|---|---|---|---|---|---|
| | | | | BARBITURATES | | |
| $C_6H_5$ | $C_2H_5$ | H | -CO-NH- | Phenobarbital (Luminal) | GM | 0.2 |
| $C_6H_5$ | $C_2H_5$ | $CH_3$ | -CO-NH- | Mephobarbital (Mebaral) | GM | 0.5 |
| $C_2H_5$ | $C_2H_5$ | $CH_3$ | -CO-NH- | Metharbital (Gemonil) | GM | 0.4 |
| $C_6H_5$ | $C_2H_5$ | H | -CO-NH- | Primidone (Mysoline)‡ | GM, PS | 1.5 |
| | | | | HYDANTOINS | | |
| $C_6H_5$ | $C_6H_5$ | H | -NH- | Phenytoin (Dilantin) | GM, PS | 0.5 |
| $C_6H_5$ | $C_2H_5$ | $CH_3$ | -NH- | Mephenytoin (Mesantoin) | GM, PS | 0.6 |
| | | | | OXAZOLIDINEDIONES | | |
| $CH_3$ | $CH_3$ | $CH_3$ | -O- | Trimethadione (Tridione) | PM | 0.9 |
| $C_2H_5$ | $CH_3$ | $CH_3$ | -O- | Paramethadione (Paradione) | PM | 0.9 |

Source: Modified from Toman, 1948.[4]
*= GM= grand mal; PS= psychomotor epilepsy; PM= petit mal.
†= Total daily adult oral dosage.
‡= Carbonyl oxygen of urea in barbiturate structure is replaced by two hydrogens.

abolish the overt clinical manifestations of convulsions. For the great majority of barbiturates the dosage required to show anticonvulsive effects is equivalent to the drug's anesthetic dose. However, a few barbiturates possess anticonvulsive properties at doses lower than those required to produce sedation. These barbiturates, the prototype of which is phenobarbital, are used as antiepileptic agents. The other two antiepileptic barbiturates are mephobarbital (Mebaral) and metharbital (Gemonil).

Phenobarbital is effective in elevating the minimal electroshock threshold, abolishing the tonic phase of maximal electroshock, and protecting against seizures induced by pentylenetetrazol (Metrazol) in laboratory animals. Clinically the drug is of value in both grand mal and focal epilepsies of either the tonic or clonic type, has some usefulness against petit mal, and has no effect in psychomotor epilepsy.

The most common side effect of the barbiturates used as antiepileptics is their general central nervous system depressant activity. The dose required may be so near the sedative dose for the patient that undesired drowsiness is also manifested. A major disadvantage of phenobarbital is that if it is abruptly removed from the epileptic's medication regime after a long period of use, an exacerbation of seizures occurs (abstinence syndrome?).

The two barbiturates, mephobarbital and metharbital, are N-dealkylated in the liver to phenobarbital and barbital, respectively, which exert antiepileptic activity. Although the mechanism of phenobarbital's antiepileptic action is unknown, it is believed to depress nonselectively neuronal excitation, thereby elevating the threshold of excitability of not only the cells of the epileptogenic focus but also the threshold of normal neurons and thus decreasing the spread of electrical discharge.

### Hydantoins

Until the discovery of phenytoin (Dilantin) pharmacologists thought the sedative and antiepileptic activities of a drug were inseparable. This belief was dispelled by the introduction of the hydantoin derivatives as potent, effective agents in the treatment of epilepsy.

In laboratory tests phenytoin does not raise the normal animal's electroshock threshold. However, if the animals are pretreated so as to lower the threshold of excitability of the brain, as in sodium-depleted or hydrated animals, then phenytoin is able to raise the lowered threshold toward normal. Tests show phenytoin's most dramatic effect to be its ability to abolish the tonic phase of maximal electroshock. The drug is ineffective in protecting animals against Metrazol-induced convulsions.

Phenytoin is most useful in the treatment of grand mal epilepsy. In contrast to phenobarbital, it is also effective in the control of psychomotor epilepsy. The hydantoin is not effective in the clonic type of grand mal or focal epilepsies other than the psychomotor type. Phenytoin is not only ineffective in petit mal but actually causes an exacerbation of petit mal seizures.

Whereas phenobarbital is thought to depress the abnormally firing foci, phenytoin's action is believed to be directed solely against the spread of the seizure discharge. It has been demonstrated that phenytoin, as well as the other antiepileptic agents, does not exert its beneficial effects only at specific supraspinal loci but influences neuronal processes underlying transmission at various sites on the neural axis. The actions of the antiepileptic agents were shown to possess different activities on spinal cord transmission. Phenytoin was found to have little effect on the response to repetitive stimulation. However, if the repetitive stimuli were tetanic, i.e., delivered at the rate of over 50 per second, then the drug's major effect was observable. Phenytoin reduces the zone of postsynaptic discharge, which is so characteristically enlarged by tetanic stimulation. The enhancement of the postsynaptic response after tetani, which phenytoin inhibits, is referred to as posttetanic potentiation (PTP).

Figure 15.1 depicts posttetanic potentiation in diagram form. Phenytoin acts on presynaptic nerve endings to reduce the postsynaptic discharge zone toward normal. The drug, it will be noted, does not block the normal (nontetanic) transmission pathway. Exactly how the hydantoin derivative brings about this effect is not known.

At a cellular level, phenytoin has been shown to depress neurons by increasing the activity of the mechanism that keeps sodium ions outside the cell. Based upon these insights into the drug's mechanism of action and others, it is suggested that phenytoin acts to reduce or prevent the spread of the seizure discharge.

Although 60 to 65% of the patients with grand mal epilepsy can be maintained seizure-free by this drug, it is not without undesirable side effects. Phenytoin is administered orally usually as its sodium salt. Gastric distress that commonly follows its administration can be overcome by taking the drug after meals.

Well known to the dental practitioner is phenytoin's ability, following 2 to 3 months of administration, to cause the undesirable condition of gingival hyperplasia. With continued administration the maximal hyperplastic state is reached in 9 to 12 months. There is no question but that the drug is responsible, because if the drug's administration is halted, the hyperplastic tissue spontaneously disappears in 3 to 6 months. The incidence of this condition is

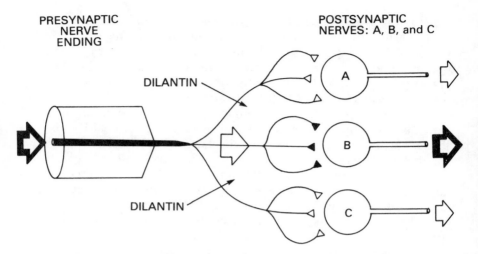

PRESYNAPTIC
NERVE
ENDING

POSTSYNAPTIC
NERVES: A, B, and C

DILANTIN

DILANTIN

A

B

C

**Figure 15.1** Phenytoin (Dilantin) inhibits the spread of seizure discharges by blocking posttetanic potentiation: ▶ = transmission path (B) during tetanic stimulation after Dilantin; ▷ = transmission paths (A, B, and C) during tetanic stimulation before Dilantin.

approximately 40%, and it occurs more often in younger patients than in adults. The mechanism by which phenytoin induces gingival hyperplasia is still not known despite the large volume of investigations on the subject.[5]

Lastly, phenytoin's metabolism by hepatic microsomal enzymes has been shown to be accelerated in experimental animals that were pretreated for several days with phenobarbital. The combination of phenytoin and phenobarbital in the treatment of grand mal epilepsy is definitely not uncommon. It was of considerable interest, therefore, when evidence was developed that phenobarbital administration in man lowers significantly the plasma levels of phenytoin. In man phenytoin has also been shown to stimulate the metabolism of cortisol to 6-hydroxycortisol through augmenting the formation of hepatic microsomal enzymes that hydroxylate cortisol.[6] It is tempting (but premature) to consider the possible interrelationship between phenytoin-induced gingival hyperplasia and the drug's ability to facilitate cortisol's metabolism. Some of phenytoin's drug interactions are shown in Table 15.2.

### Trimethadione

Trimethadione (Tridione) is the prototype of the 2,4-oxazolidinedione derivatives which possess antiepileptic activity. Its pharmacological profile differs from those of both phenytoin and phenobarbital.

Trimethadione was found to be a specific agent for the symptomatic treatment of cerebral dysrhythmias characterized by a 3 per second (EEG) pattern of spike and wave or "spike and dome." Following the administration of trimethadione, in these cases, the abnormal EEG pattern frequently reverts to more normal patterns at the same time as clinical improvement occurs. This is in contrast to the other two prototypes thus far presented which may abolish all clinical manifestation of various forms of epilepsy but which do not uniformly improve the abnormality seen in the EEG. In the laboratory tests trimethadione raises the electroshock threshold

## Table 15.2. Hydantoin Drug Interactions

It is assumed that the dental patient is taking the usual therapeutic dose of one of the hydantoin antiepileptic agents (e.g., phenytoin) when he seeks dental care. The column on the left lists drugs (Interactant) which the dentist may wish to administer in the course of dental treatment. The column on the right lists the possible interactions that could occur.

| Interactant | Possible Interactions |
| --- | --- |
| 1. Antidepressants, tricyclics | High doses of tricyclics with Dilantin may precipitate convulsions; tricyclics displace drug from secondary binding sites and also lower seizure threshold. |
| 2. Antihistamines | Antihistamines may decrease effectiveness of antiepileptic by enzyme induction. |
| 3. Aspirin | Large doses of aspirin may enhance the antiepileptic effects and toxicity of phenytoin. |
| 4. Benzodiazepines, e.g., Valium | Benzodiazepines potentiate phenytoin. |
| 5. Central nervous system depresants | CNS depressants potentiate phenytoin in general (there are some few exceptions). |
| 6. Corticosteroids | Phenytoin stimulates the metabolism of corticosteroids by enzyme induction and thus reduces steroid activity, i.e., inhibits their capacity to suppress endogenous hydrocortisone secretion. |
| 7. Phenobarbital | Additive effects of two agents initially. Phenytoin potentiates effects of barbiturate. Chronic administration of phenobarbital leads to decreased plasma levels of phenytoin. Concurrent administration of phenobarbital leads to decreased plasma levels of phenytoin. Concurrent administration, even at low doses, may decrease effectiveness of drug therapy. Doses must be adjusted carefully. |

Source: Modified from Martin, 1971.[9]

and, of the three prototypes, is the most potent antagonist of pentylenetetrazol-induced convulsions. It has little or no effect upon the seizure pattern of maximal electroshock.

In spinal cord transmission studies it has been demonstrated that trimethadione, in contrast to phenytoin, does not depress posttetanic potentiation. Its most pronounced effect is seen as a depression of the response to normal repetitive stimulation. Once the first impulse has passed the synapse, blockade ensues. More specifically, it has been demonstrated that trimethadione acts on presynaptic endings to prolong greatly the normal recovery time once the neuron has fired. This one action would explain the drug's usefulness in decreasing a self-sustained repetitively firing neuronal system. However, there must be additional actions of trimethadione that will require consideration before its action is completely understood. At the present time it is thought that trimethadione may act on the hyperexcitable epileptogenic neurons themselves to depress the origin of the seizure discharge.

Clinically trimethadione is most useful in the treatment of petit mal epilepsy. It does show some benefit in psychomotor epilepsy when administered with other antiepileptics, but it is without effect in controlling grand mal seizures.

Another unusual effect seen with trimethadione is the high incidence of hemeralopia. In 50 to 75% of the cases (especially adults) there is seen after several weeks of treatment varying degrees of blurring of the vision to bright light. It is thought this is due to a direct effect of trimethadione on the retina and not to an effect on the central nervous system. Adjustment of the dosage usually eliminates the problem.

Lastly, the drug of choice in the emergency treatment of status epilepticus is diazepam (Valium). It may be mentioned that diazepam is also the drug of choice for abolishing seizures owing to local anesthetics.

## ANTIPSYCHOTIC AGENTS

Psychopharmacology is a division of pharmacology dealing with the drugs that exert the major part of their action upon behavior, though processing, ideation, the mood, the emotions, or affective behavior. These are the important drugs used in the symptomatic treatment of the mentally ill. Some of the psychopharmacological agents have been used for many centuries, but our most recent interest in these drugs and the enormous multiplication of new drugs has come about since the early 1950's. The entire approach to the handling and treatment of the mentally ill before the advent of these drugs would be almost unrecognizable to most of us today.

One of the most vivid ways to show the effectiveness of the new antipsychotic drugs is to compare the steady increase in the number of mental patients in state hospitals prior to the widespread use of some of these drugs with the steady decrease in the number of mental patients in state hospitals after their introduction (see Figure 15.2).

The psychopharmacological agents are many and where they fit into the scheme of drugs acting upon the central nervous system is essential. Many drugs exert their primary action on the central nervous system as shown in Figure 15.3. These may be divided into two large groups of nonselective in action and the selective in action.

There are selective depressants such as the general anesthetics, barbiturates, and ethyl alcohol. There are also several nonselective stimulants of the central nervous system. The selective central nervous system drugs stimulate and depress various functional areas. The analgesics are drugs of this type. The psychopharmacological agents also act selectively upon the central nervous system. These drugs are further divided into at least three major

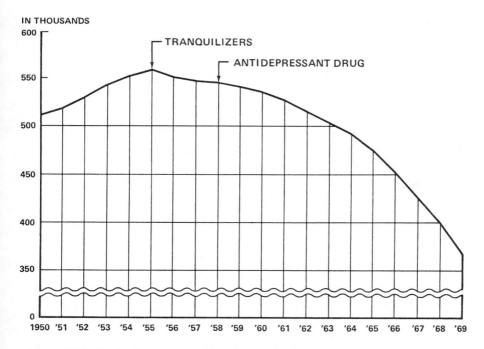

**Figure 15.2** Decline in state mental hospital population in relationship to the introduction of psychopharmacological agents. (Adapted from Facts, 1971.[7])

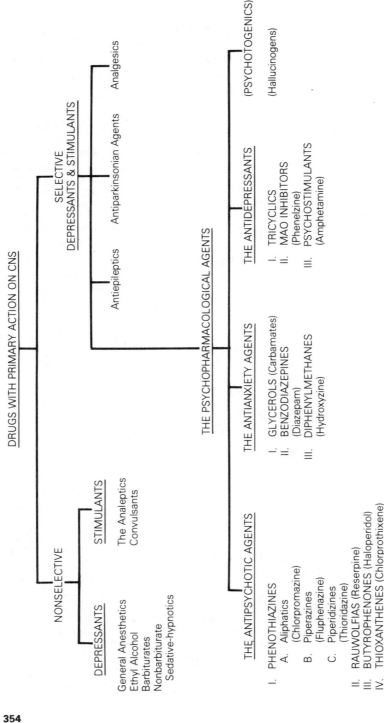

**Figure 15.3** Drugs with primary action on the central nervous system. CNS = central nervous system; MAO = monoamine oxidase.

DRUGS WITH PRIMARY ACTION ON CNS

NONSELECTIVE

DEPRESSANTS
General Anesthetics
Ethyl Alcohol
Barbiturates
Nonbarbiturate
Sedative-hypnotics

STIMULANTS
The Analeptics
Convulsants

SELECTIVE
DEPRESSANTS & STIMULANTS

Antiepileptics

Antiparkinsonian Agents

Analgesics

THE PSYCHOPHARMACOLOGICAL AGENTS

THE ANTIPSYCHOTIC AGENTS

I. PHENOTHIAZINES
   A. Aliphatics
      (Chlorpromazine)
   B. Piperazines
      (Fluphenazine)
   C. Piperidizines
      (Thioridazine)
II. RAUWOLFIAS (Reserpine)
III. BUTYROPHENONES (Haloperidol)
IV. THIOXANTHENES (Chlorprothixene)

THE ANTIANXIETY AGENTS

I. GLYCEROLS (Carbamates)
II. BENZODIAZEPINES
    (Diazepam)
III. DIPHENYLMETHANES
     (Hydroxyzine)

THE ANTIDEPRESSANTS

I. TRICYCLICS
II. MAO INHIBITORS
    (Phenelzine)
III. PSYCHOSTIMULANTS
     (Amphetamine)

(PSYCHOTOGENICS)

(Hallucinogens)

classes that are used therapeutically: the antipsychotic agents, the antianxiety agents, and the antidepressants. The psychotogenic agents are not used in therapy. The three groups are primarily based upon the general types of mental disorders the drugs best treat. There are those used in the treatment of the serious mental illness known as the psychoses, other drugs that show their greatest usefulness in the treatment of the less severe mental illnesses known as the neuroses, and, lastly, other drugs that appear to be most useful in the treatment of the abnormally depressed states.

The antipsychotic agents were formerly called by several other names which have not yet been completely purged from textbooks. One of these was the major tranquilizers. This title bore the connotation that these were the more important of the tranquilizers whereas the minor tranquilizers were insignificant. This is certainly false, and the *major-minor* semantics did not help the situation. The word *tranquilizer* is not exactly the best to use either, since the effects of the antipsychotic drugs could hardly be considered calming or pleasant as the word *tranquilizer* connotes. Among other names, these drugs have also been called neuroleptics, which is a general term meaning a drug that acts on the nervous system. These drugs also were called ataractics or ataraxics—drugs that produced a state of ataraxia or calmness and peace of mind. The official nomenclature is now antipsychotic agents.

There are four chemical classes of antipsychotic agents, and of these four there is no doubt that the phenothiazine derivatives are the most important. Indeed, the others will be mentioned only in passing. Each of these four groups, however, exerts a similar type of effect that has been referred to as the neuroleptic state. Each group may well bring about this state by a different mechanism of action and site of action. Each has its own side effects. The neuroleptic syndrome consists of two clinically observable effects: (1) the remarkable amelioration of the overt clinical picture of schizophrenia (a change is seen in the way the patient behaves and thinks); and (2) the appearance, usually simultaneously, of an unwanted side effect known as the extrapyramidal syndrome.

The proposed major site of action for these drugs is definitely subcortical. This is in strong contrast to that of the barbiturates.

Chlorpromazine (Thorazine) is the phenothiazine prototype of the antipsychotic agents, and there is no question but that thousands of persons are at home and contributing to society rather than locked away because of this one drug chlorpromazine. There are three different chemical subgroups of the phenothiazines based upon the nature of the side chain. It is important to know to which subgroup a particular phenothiazine belongs so that a better understanding of the side effects can be appreciated.

Chlorpromazine acts upon specific areas of the central nervous system, sometimes exciting, sometimes depressing, to bring about its observable effects upon behavior. The primary, desired effect is to alter the characteristically abnormal behavior of schizophrenia especially and return the patient toward more normal behavior. Chlorpromazine can do this in slightly over 75% of the cases. The withdrawn and retarded schizophrenic becomes slightly more active, and the overactive or combatant schizophrenic becomes less so. Chlorpromazine appears to bring both types back toward more normal patterns of ideation and behavior. Unfortunately, the phenothiazines produce a number of side effects, some more serious than others, but none so serious as to overshadow its remarkable antischizophrenic effects. The drug does not cure any form of mental illness.

Chlorpromazine has another effect upon general behavior which clearly contrasts it with the barbiturates. Chlorpromazine can be shown to block conditioned responses while not affecting unconditioned responses. Barbiturates are well known to block both the conditioned and unconditioned responses.

Chlorpromazine has a third general effect upon behavior. It suppresses spontaneous motor activity, especially with the higher daily doses.

There is general agreement that chlorpromazine has at least two important sites of action, both subcortical (see Figure 15.4). The drug primarily blocks the afferent collaterals to the reticular activating system. This increased filtering of all incoming sensory information definitely reduces the activity of the cortex via the thalamic diffuse projection system. Thus there is seen a reduction in general awareness without unconsciousness. The second major site of action is the hypothalamus where chlorpromazine depresses.

Chlorpromazine has many other detectable effects on the central nervous system, but they seem to be all subcortical in site. The limbic system appears depressed at low doses of the drug, but higher and higher doses are known to produce generalized seizures which have their origin in the limbic system.

Chlorpromazine has a rather specific action upon transmission in the basal ganglia. It is this action which leads to the production of unwanted extrapyramidal side effects. These motor effects closely resemble many of the symptoms of the patient with Parkinson's disease. The transmission processes at the basal ganglia level are now well-confirmed to involve (1) a cholinergic excitatory process in which one neuron releases acetylcholine to excite the next

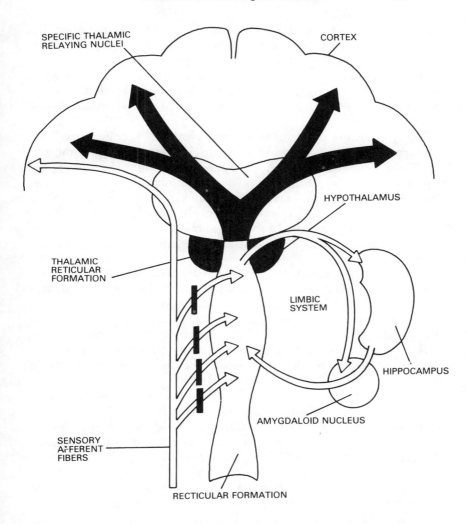

**Figure 15.4** Subcortical sites of action of chlorpromazine as shown by shaded areas. (Adapted and redrawn from Lembeck and Sewing, 1969.[8])

neuron and (2) an adrenergic inhibitory process in which acetylcholine stimulates an inhibitory neuron and in turn releases dopamine to inhibit the excitatory process. We know that chlorpromazine blocks the effects of the inhibitory transmitter dopamine. When blocking occurs, there is a release of the excitatory effects (an inhibition of an inhibitory system = disinhibition = overt excitement). These excitatory effects are seen peripherally as the extrapyramidal effects. It is of interest that we now recognize the cause of Parkinson's disease is a neuronal deficiency of dopamine.

Chlorpromazine has little effect on respiration but produces hypotension through depressing the vasomotor center. The drug is one of the most specific antiemetics available and selectively blocks the chemoreceptive trigger zone. It is of no value in treatment of motion sickness.

Chlorpromazine exerts at least three clinically significant effects upon the autonomic nervous system: (1) a strong antiadrenergic effect on both the central and peripheral autonomic receptor systems, (2) a weak peripheral anticholinergic effect, and (3) some slight degree of autonomic ganglionic blocking activity. These autonomic effects point toward such clinical problems as postural hypotension, dry mouth, and the antagonism of epinephrine's vasoconstricting effects in combination with dental local anesthetics.

The endocrinological effects of chlorpromazine are a result of inhibition of the hypothalamic-hypophyseal system and include the depression of the following: (1) gonadotropic hormone secretion, (2) antidiuretic hormone secretion, (3) ACTH secretion, and (4) somatotrophic hormone secretion. The studies on the mechanism of chlorpromazine action are legion and complex and as a result there is no one unifying theory regarding the antipsychotic action.

The phenothiazines are used to control moderate to severe anxiety, tension, and agitation associated with schizophrenia. Chlorpromazine is not to be used to control the mild neuroses as if it were an antianxiety agent or a sedative barbiturate. Chlorpromazine shows little efficacy in such cases.

Tolerance does develop to some of chlorpromazine's effects (not the antipsychotic effects), but there is no incidence of psychological or physical dependence upon the drug.

The toxic or side effects of chlorpromazine are many and the most frequent at the usual therapeutic doses include postural hypotension, chilliness, constipation, xerostomia (dry mouth), blurred vision, stuffy nose, edema, lactation, and increased appetite with subsequent weight gain. Of particular interest are the central nervous system side effects that are generally grouped together and called the extrapyramidal effects. These occur in about 40% of the cases. These include akathisia or a restlessness and constant urge to be moving; a dystonic syndrome sometimes called face, neck, tongue syndrome, which involves the trigeminal nuclei and may involve oral symptoms first seen by the dentist (especially in children on high chlorpromazine daily doses); tardive dyskinesia, which may be irreversible; parkinsonian symptoms, i.e., shaking palsy (paralysis agitans) or "pill-rolling motion."

By far the most serious effects are the direct toxicities of the phenothiazines and the hypersensitivity reactions that are known to occur. Bone marrow depression resulting in leukopenia and agranulocytosis, with an incidence of 1 in 3,000, is a direct toxic effect of the drug. The jaundice that may occur in 0.5% of the patients and skin reactions are hypersensitivity types of responses.

Chlorpromazine is well known for a number of drug-drug interactions. It potentiates almost every drug that depresses the central nervous system. Knowing that the drug suppresses the background excitability of the cortex by filtering all incoming sensory stimuli from entering the diffuse activating system should suggest other central nervous system depressants to be potentiated.

It may be of interest that chlorpromazine is able to antagonize the symptoms and behavior produced by both amphetamines and LSD. Owing to chlorpromazine's central excitatory effects, the drug should not be given to epileptics. Chlorpromazine also potentiates the *systemic* toxicity of local anesthetics, since both cause an increase in excitability of the amygdaloid nucleus in the limbic system.

It may be noted by the dental hygienist who works with a number of mental outpatients who are required to take large daily doses of chlorpromazine or one of its analogs that the dental patient has difficulty retaining his dentures (due to dry mouth and other drug-induced effects) and usually resorts to holding hard candy in his mouth continuously. Chlorpromazine is also known to produce direct chemical burn of the oral soft tissue when the drug is held in juxtaposition to the soft tissue for any length of time.

## THE ANTIDEPRESSANTS

The antidepressants make up a special group of the psychopharmacological agents and are popular drugs today. They are used to treat symptomatically the various types of depressive disorders. Whereas anxiety may be most simply defined as the behavioral response to a threat, depression may be defined as the behavioral response to a loss. It is hoped that the dental hygienist appreciates that both anxiety and depression are not always diseased states of mind to be treated by drugs. We are each daily threatened and sustain countless losses in many areas of our life experiences and yet we do not need, in fact, and should not have drugs to assist or to prevent our appropriate handling of these situations. We lose the opportunity to employ our coping mechanisms. Dental patients will be coming to you while they are taking antidepressants according to their physician's instructions. Antidepressants are potential interacting agents with the drugs used commonly in dental practice. There are two major subgroups of antidepressants: the monamine oxidase inhibitors and the tricyclics.

## Monoamine Oxidase Inhibitors

At the present time, the most dangerous of drug-drug interactions include some of the antidepressants. There are at the time of this writing only six monoamine oxidase inhibitors on the American market; these are shown in Table 15.3.

It will be recalled from Chapter 3 that the adrenergic transmitter is released from the nerve ending, interacts with the adrenergic receptor system, and then actively is taken back up into the nerve ending. Some small amount escapes and is broken down by circulating catechol-O-methyltransferase, but the majority of the norepinephrine is taken back into the nerve ending. The level of norepinephrine in the nerve is regulated by the enzyme monoamine oxidase located in the numerous mitochondria. If the activity of monoamine oxidase could be inhibited, there would be an excess of norepinephrine accumulating in adrenergic nerves. This would be more norepinephrine that could be released by the arrival of an action potential, or more that could be released by indirectly acting sympathomimetic amines. Indeed, the active norepinephrine itself can leak out of the nerve ending when too much is stored therein.

A volume of evidence, still growing, shows that adrenergic nerves with their norepinephrine, monoamine oxidase, and biosynthetic enzymes exist also in specific areas of the central nervous system. Perhaps cautious analogies can now be made between the events in the peripheral autonomic adrenergic system and those located in various areas of the central nervous system. For our purposes assume that the role of central nervous system monoamine oxidase is similar to that which it has peripherally. It is of interest that norepinephrine is found in most of the reward centers of the brain, and norepinephrine is considered to be the mediator for our coping mechanisms. Thus, a deficiency in the system might account for the two prominent symptoms of depression: the inability to cope and the inability to find enjoyment. All antidepressants thus far examined increase adrenergic transmission by various mechanisms.

What are the central effects of monoamine oxidase inhibition? It would appear that norepinephrine also accumulates in central adrenergic neural pathways so that more norepinephrine is available for release. It is believed that this excess available norepineph-

**Table 15.3.   Monoamine Oxidase Inhibitor
Products on the Market in the United States in 1977**

| Generic Name | Brand Name (Manufacturer) | Therapeutic Use |
|---|---|---|
| 1. Pargyline | Eutonyl (Abbott) | Antihypertensive agent |
|  | Eutron (Abbott) | Antihypertensive agent |
| 2. Phenelzine | Nardil (Warner-Chilcott) | Antidepressant |
| 3. Isocarboxazid | Marplan (Roche) | Antidepressant |
| 4. Tranylcypromine | Parnate (Smith Kline) | Antidepressant |
| 5. Furazolidone | Furoxone (Eaton) | Intestinal antibacterial |
| 6. Procarbazine | Matulane (Roche) | Antineoplastic agent |

rine is available for release and causes the antidepressant effects or the mood-elevating effects observed clinically. No one really knows the cellular mechanism of action, but there are some fascinating theories.

The monoamine oxidase inhibitors produce an irreversible inactivation of monoamine oxidase by forming stable complexes with the enzyme. Because the synthesis of the biogenic amines is not inhibited, there is a buildup of amines intracellularly. It takes the monoamine oxidase inhibitors about 1 to 2 weeks or longer to produce overt clinical effects, but that does not mean they are not acting. The enzyme is irreversibly inactivated right away, but the accumulation of norepinephrine and perhaps other biogenic substances takes a while. The drug is given daily to inactivate the newly formed monoamine oxidase. Once the last dose is given, it takes the body 1 to 3 weeks to resynthesize enough monoamine oxidase to get the neuronal levels of norepinephrine back to preinhibitor levels.

It is unfortunate that the monoamine oxidase inhibitors are not very specific. They also interact with hepatic enzyme systems that are responsible for the metabolic degradation of a number of drugs, such as barbiturates, the narcotic analgesics, and meperidine.

It is tempting to enumerate the known effects, both good and bad, of the monoamine oxidase inhibitors upon the various organs and tissues of man, but this interesting information will need to be obtained from the supplemental reading list so that space and effort may be given to how the monoamine oxidase inhibitors, or drugs with such a side effect, interact unfavorably with the drugs most commonly encountered in dentistry. Table 15.4 summarizes a number of established drug-drug interactions in which one of the drugs is a monoamine oxidase inhibitor. The mechanisms of each of

## Table 15.4.   Drug Interactions with MAO Inhibitors

| Drug | Reaction |
|---|---|
| A. Analgesics:<br>   morphine<br>   meperidine<br>   codeine | Potentiation of depressant effects: sedative, hypotensive, and respiratory depression may cause BP fall, cardiovascular collapse, respiratory failure, coma, and death |
| B. CNS depressants:<br>   general anesthetics<br>   local anesthetics<br>   (systemic toxicity)<br>   barbiturates<br>   nonbarbiturate sedatives<br>   phenothiazine derivatives<br>   alcohol | Depressant effects potentiated: prolonged action. Hypotension, coma |
| C. Vasopressor substances:<br>   All indirectly acting<br>   sympathomimetic amines, e.g.<br>   amphetamine, methamphetamine,<br>   ephedrine, tyramine | Central and peripheral effects potentiated. Marked rise in BP, hypertensive crises, excitement, cardiac arrhythmias, chest pain, severe headache |
|    Directly acting sympathomimetic<br>   amines, e.g., norepinephrine,<br>   epinephrine, phenylephrine | Peripheral effects not potentiated. Central effects enhanced |
| D. Antihypertensives:<br>   ganglionic blockers<br>   diuretics<br>   guanethidine (Ismelin) | Potentiates hypotensive effect; cardiovascular collapse and shock |
| E. Anticholinergics:<br>   atropine, other derivatives | Potentiates effects |
| F. Others:<br>   reserpine<br>   caffeine<br>   insulin<br>   corticosteroids<br>   thiazide diuretics | <br>Excitement, delirium, hypertension<br>Potentiated<br>Potentiated (hypoglycemia)<br>Potentiated<br>Potentiation of CNS effects of MAO inhibitor: psychomotor stimulation, postural hypotension |

CNS = central nervous system.
MAO = monoamine oxidase.
BP = blood pressure.

these interactions can be traced to (1) an alteration in monoamine storage and degradation, (2) the inhibition of drug metabolizing enzymes, or (3) unknown mechanisms.

ALTERATION IN MONOAMINE STORAGE AND DEGRADATION. The effects of the indirectly acting adrenergic agonists are profoundly augmented and the patient may succumb, if not treated, in hypertensive crisis. In the patient who is taking monoamine oxidase inhibitors there is an excess amount of norepinephrine stored and ready for release from the cytoplasmic pool by agents such as the amphetamines, ephedrine, and also the adrenergic vasoconstrictor substances in many common over-the-counter cold remedies or nasal decongestants. These indirectly acting agents are contraindicated. The dentist gets involved when he prescribes a nasal decongestant for the dental patient who is scheduled to be given nitrous oxide at a later office visit. Please note that the directly acting adrenergic agonist, phenylephrine, is a widely used nasal decongestant but it too is contraindicated, since it is inactivated by monoamine oxidase. There is no problem administering the other directly acting adrenergic agonists used in dentistry: epinephrine, levarterenol, or levonordefrin (in local anesthetic solutions), or isoproterenol (in emergency treatment of acute bronchial asthmatic attack). The peripheral effects of these latter agents do not appear to be greatly augmented in the presence of monoamine oxidase inhibitors.

INHIBITION OF DRUG METABOLIZING ENZYMES. It is more likely that the dentist will see a drug interaction with monoamine oxidase inhibitors by this particular mechanism. The monoamine oxidase inhibitors are not selective inhibitors and depress the activity of a number of drug-metabolizing enyzmes in the liver. Especially of concern to the dentist is the profound prolongation of action of not only most barbiturates but also the narcotic analgesics. The monoamine oxidase inhibitors effectively suppress the activity of the enzymes involved in side chain oxidation of barbiturates as well as oxidative deamination and the N-dealkylating enzymes; this would directly affect the inactivation of the opiates and opioids such as morphine, meperidine, propoxyphene and pentazocine. Most of the fatal drug-drug interactions of this type thus far reported have occurred between meperidine and a monoamine oxidase inhibitor. The inhibition of these enzymes lasts about one to two weeks following the last dose of the inhibitor. Therefore, it is essential to ask each patient if he had been taking any medication but now no longer is taking it.

UNKNOWN MECHANISMS. A number of other drug-drug interactions listed in Table 15.4 contraindicate the administration of a variety of seemingly unrelated drugs to patients taking monoamine oxidase inhibitors. The mechanisms for these interactions are not understood.

### Tricyclic Antidepressants

Owing mainly to the discovery of the antidepressant effects of the tricyclic agents, the monoamine oxidase inhibitor type of antide-

**Table 15.5. Differences Between MAOI and Tricyclic Type of Antidepressant Agents**

| | MAOI Antidepressants | Tricyclic Antidepressants |
|---|---|---|
| Biogenic amine stores | Increase amine stores in adrenergic nerve endings and brain; increase active amine at receptors in CNS | Block uptake of norepinephrine into nerve endings; decrease in intraneuronal stores of norepinephrine and 5-hydroxytryptamine; increase active amine (norepinephrine) at receptors |
| Autonomic nervous system | No direct effects | Potent anticholinergic activity (antimuscarinic) both centrally and peripherally |
| Antihistamine activity | None | Antihistaminic |
| Effect of tyramine (foods, wines, cheeses) | Increase pressor action of tyramine | Inhibit effects of tyramine by blocking its uptake into nerve ending |
| Effect of norepinephrine and epinephrine administered exogenously | No great alteration of peripheral effects of norepinephrine | Increased effects both centrally and peripherally of exogenously administered norepinephrine and epinephrine |
| Sedative effects | None | Sedation similar to that produced by chlorpromazine, especially prominent with imipramine and amitryptyline |

CNS = central nervous system.

pressant has grown more and more unpopular. The tricyclic antidepressants are not inhibitors of monoamine oxidase and do not possess the same types of drug-drug interaction limitations.

There are two chemical groups of tricyclic antidepressants: (1) the dibenzazepine derivatives exemplified by imipramine (Tofranil) and (2) the dibenzocycloheptadiene derivatives exemplified by amitriptyline (Elavil). The tricyclics bear a close resemblance in chemical structure to the phenothiazine antipsychotic agents with which they share a number of common effects. Tricyclic effects are compared with monoamine oxidase inhibitor effects in Table 15.5.

In the nondepressed person the tricyclics produce a calming or depressing effect, but in states of especially endogenous depression, the tricyclics elevate the mood. They have little predictable usefulness in treating situational depression, e.g., depression of usual short-term duration owing to the loss of a loved one.

The mechanism of action of the tricyclics is thought to be an inhibition of the active reuptake mechanism for norepinephrine at the ends of adrenergic fibers both in the peripheral and in the central nervous systems. This mechanism would place more norepinephrine at its receptor sites. These antidepressants also possess strong anticholinergic effects most commonly seen as a very dry mouth in the dental patient. From the point of view of the dental hygienist and the dentist these agents profoundly potentiate the effects of epinephrine, levarterenol, levonordefrin, (and isoproterenol in emergency kits); therefore, local anesthetic solutions without adrenergic vasoconstrictors should be considered or at least the amount of vasoconstrictors used should be reduced. Certainly the use of epinephrine containing gingival retracting or hemostatic agents is contraindicated. The anticholinergic effects of atropine are greatly augmented as well as those of other substances such as diazepam. The central depressant effects of barbiturates are also increased, and dosages must be reduced.

### REFERENCES

1. Taylor, J. (ed.): On epilepsy and epileptiform convulsions. Vol. 1. Selected Writings of John Hughlings Jackson. London, Hodder and Stoughton, 1931.
2. Penfield, W., and Jasper, H.: Epilepsy and the Functional Anatomy of the Human Brain. Boston, Little Brown, 1954.
3. Gastaut, H., and Fischer-Williams, M.: The Physiopathyology of epileptic seizures. In Handbook of Physiology. Vol. 1, Section 1: Nuerophysiology. Edited by J. Field. Washington, D.C., American Physiological Society, 1959.
4. Toman, J.E.P., and Goodman, L.S.: Anticonvulsants. Physiol. Rev., 28: 409, 1948.
5. Livingston, S., and Livingston, H.S.: Diphenylhydantoin gingival hyperplasia. Am. J. Dis. Child., 117:265, 1969.
6. Werk, E.E., Jr., MacGee, J., and Sholiton, L.J.: Effect of diphenylhydantoin on cortisol metabolism in man. J. Clin. Invest., 43:1824, 1964.

7.  Facts on the Major Killing and Crippling Diseases in the United States Today. New York, The National Health Eudcation Committee, Inc., 1971, p. 12.
8.  Lembeck, F., and Sewing, K-F.: Pharmacological Facts and Figures. Berlin, Springer-Verlag, 1969, p. 36.
9.  Martin, E.W.: Hazards of Medication. Philadelphia, Lippincott, 1971.

# 16

## DRUGS IN THE TREATMENT OF ENDOCRINOLOGICAL DISORDERS

Hormones that are released into the circulatory system by various glands of the endocrine system influence metabolism and other body processes. An excess or a shortage will cause malfunction that in many instances can be controlled by drug therapy. Among the patients seen by the dentist and the dental hygienist will be some being treated for adrenal insufficiency, diabetes mellitus, or thyroid deficiency.

### ADRENAL CORTICOSTEROIDS

The dentist and dental hygienist will be required to treat patients who are taking adrenal corticosteroids either for their hormonal effects or for their pharmacological antiinflammatory effects. Either situation presents special problems, both those posed by the disease for which the drug is being administered as well as those posed by the corticosteroids themselves.

The adrenal gland is actually made up of two independent parts, both involved in the stress response. The medulla, embryologically derived from neural tissue, synthesizes and secretes catecholamines. The glandular, cortical portion synthesizes and secretes two major classes of steroids—the corticosteroids and the adrenal androgens. The present discussion will deal only with the former class.

The adrenal corticosteroids are customarily classified according to their hormonal effects into mineralocorticoids and glucocorticoids. Corticosteroids whose primary effects are on electrolyte and water balance (as measured by their potency in promoting sodium retention) are referred to as mineralocorticoids; those whose primary effects are on carbohydrate and protein metabolism (as measured by their potency in promoting liver glycogen deposition) are referred to as glucocorticoids. Although many of the newer synthetic glucocorticoids have no significant mineralocorticoid activity, the naturally occurring corticosteroids have some degree of both types of activity and are classified according to their predominant activity.

In the following discussion both hormonal and pharmacological effects of the corticosteroids are considered. Although any given dose of corticosteroid may be either physiological or pharmacological depending on the external environment and internal state of the patient, it is generally agreed that an equivalent daily dose of any corticosteroid greater than 20 mg of cortisol (the average daily adrenal secretion of cortisol) is a supraphysiological dose. The pharmacological effects of the corticosteroids are generally considered to be those effects seen at supraphysiological doses. It should be appreciated that the direct hormonal effects of the corticosteroids increase in magnitude as the dose is increased so that what may be a beneficial effect, indeed a life-sustaining effect, at physiological concentrations may become a toxic effect at supraphysiological (pharmacological) concentrations.

Much has been learned about the effects of corticosteroids from so-called experiments of nature. Addison's disease, a characteristic syndrome of abnormalities caused by inadequate adrenocortical function (adrenal insufficiency), is one such experiment. Correction of the abnormalities of Addison's disease by administration of physiological doses of corticosteroids helps define their hormonal role. Similarly, Cushing's syndrome, a characteristic syndrome of abnormalities caused by hyperfunction of the adrenal cortex, resembles the toxic effects of long-term administration of supraphysiological doses of corticosteroids.

### Mineralocorticoids

Aldosterone is physiologically the most important naturally occurring mineralocorticoid (see Figure 16.1). It acts directly on the cells of the renal distal tubule to facilitate the exchange of tubular sodium for potassium and hydrogen. An excess of aldosterone consequently leads to an increase in extracellular sodium and concomitant decreases in plasma potassium and hydrogen. These electrolyte changes are associated with secondary increases in plasma chloride and bicarbonate. Metabolic alkalosis may result from the loss of hydrogen and increase in plasma bicarbonate, while the hypokalemia may cause paralysis of skeletal muscles. The most significant alterations, however, are in extracellular volume and cardiovascular function. Water is retained along with

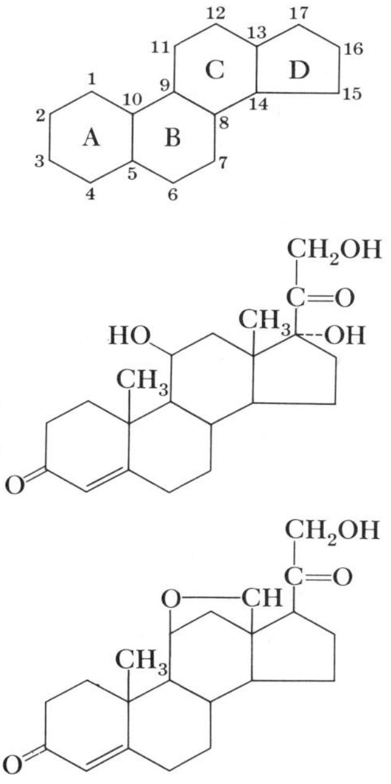

CYCLOPENTANO-
PERHYDROPHENANTHRENE RING

CORTISOL (HYDROCORTISONE)

ALDOSTERONE

**Figure 16.1**  Structures of adrenal corticosteroids.

sodium; in addition, the increased plasma electrolyte concentration usually causes thirst and a greater intake of water. This combination results in a significant increase in extracellular and plasma volumes with associated edema, as well as increased cardiac output, peripheral resistance, and blood pressure.

The exact mechanism of the regulation of aldosterone secretion by the adrenal cortex is unknown. It is known, however, that decreased plasma sodium, increased plasma potassium, decreased plasma volume, and decreased tissue perfusion (especially of the kidney) are associated with increased secretion of aldosterone. Conversely, aldosterone secretion is decreased by alterations of these parameters in the opposite direction. It has been proposed that one mechanism for regulation of aldosterone secretion by the adrenal cortex involves the renin-angiotensin system. Decreased perfusion of the kidney is believed to result in release of the enzyme, renin, which acts on proteins in the plasma to cause the formation of the polypeptide angiotensin. This polypeptide is known to increase the secretion of aldosterone by the adrenal cortex.

## Glucocorticoids

Cortisol (hydrocortisone) is physiologically the most important of the naturally occurring glucocorticoids (see Figure 16.1). The hormonal effects of cortisol are diverse but are of one of two types: (1) direct effects, varying in magnitude with the dose administered, and (2) permissive effects, those effects that are actually mediated by other substances but require some minimal level of cortisol for a normal response to the causative agent. An increase in cortisol above this permissive level does not increase the magnitude of the response.

METABOLIC EFFECTS. The most important result of cortisol's metabolic effects is an increase in available energy in the form of glucose. This is a major factor in the body's response to starvation and other types of stress. The actions of cortisol on carbohydrate, protein, and fat metabolism, although not completely understood, all contribute to this increase in synthesis of new glucose (gluconeogenesis). The major source of raw material for the increased gluconeogenesis appears to come from body protein in the form of amino acids. Cortisol increases the breakdown of body protein as well as inhibits synthesis of new protein. These effects explain the skeletal muscle wasting and loss of the protein matrix of bone which are common adverse effects of long-term administration of high doses of corticosteroids. The loss of the bone's protein matrix is followed by loss of calcium (osteoporosis) and fragility of the bone. Osteoporosis of the facial bones can sometimes be noted in dental radiographs of such patients.

Cortisol increases the rate of entry of amino acids into the liver. Several of the hepatic enzymes involved in the conversion of these amino acids into new glucose are also increased by cortisol. All of these actions result in a significant increase in the synthesis of hepatic glucose. Concurrently, cortisol inhibits peripheral utilization of glucose, apparently at some intracellular point beyond the site of insulin-induced glucose entry into the cell.

High doses of cortisol increase the total body fat and alter its distribution from the normal fat depots to other areas such as the face and behind the neck, accounting for the "moon face" and "buffalo hump," respectively, characteristic of patients with Cushing's syndrome or those receiving high doses of corticosteroids. In addition, cortisol enhances catecholamine-induced release of free fatty acids from fat depots (lipolysis) by a permissive action.

All of the above effects oppose the effects of insulin. It is not surprising, then, that corticosteroids are contraindicated in the diabetic.

EFFECTS ON GASTRIC SECRETION. Cortisol increases the secretion of both acid and pepsin by the stomach which is thought to reduce the protective mucous lining of the stomach walls. Consequently, cortisol administration is associated with a high incidence of gastrointestinal ulceration and is contraindicated in patients who are predisposed to this condition.

EFFECTS ON THE VASCULATURE. Cortisol has been shown to have a significant permissive effect on reactivity of vascular smooth muscle to catecholamines and other pressor agents. Through this action cortisol appears to play a vital role in the response of the cardiovascular system to stress. The corticosteroids may also be necessary for maintenance of the integrity of the vascular endothelium since vascular permeability is increased in their absence.

EFFECTS ON LYMPHOID TISSUE. Lymphoid tissue mass is conspicuously responsive to the glucocorticoids. The characteristic increase of the amount of lymphoid tissue in patients with Addison's disease is reduced to normal by administration of hormonal doses of cortisol. Similarly, greater than hormonal doses of cortisol greatly reduce the mass of lymphoid tissue.

EFFECTS ON BLOOD CELLS. Supraphysiological doses of cortisol decrease the number of circulating eosinophils. Normal migration of neutrophils and normal phagocytic activity of neutrophils and monocytes appear to depend upon optimal levels of corticosteroids, since these functions are depressed in patients with Addison's disease as well as in patients receiving high doses of cortisol. Supraphysiological doses of cortisol also depress the metabolism and function of lymphocytes and plasma cells.

EFFECTS ON THE CENTRAL NERVOUS SYSTEM. The glucocorticoids significantly influence the central nervous system. Patients with Addison's disease usually exhibit signs of central nervous system depression which are improved by administration of hormonal doses of cortisol. Supraphysiological doses of cortisol, however, generally produce signs of central nervous system excitation, including euphoria in some patients. Patients with Cushing's syndrome and a small percentage of patients receiving high therapeutic doses of corticosteroids may also exhibit psychotic reactions.

ANTIINFLAMMATORY EFFECTS. In pharmacological doses the glucocorticoids suppress almost all phases of the inflammatory response. Among the most obvious effects are the suppression of the local vasodilation, increased capillary permeability, and associated exudation of plasma components occurring during the early phases of the acute inflammatory response. The suppression of increased vascular permeability is probably a result of the glucocorticoid's general promotion of membrane integrity throughout the body.[1] This generalized effect on membrane integrity also probably explains the ability of these agents to prevent disruption of lysosomes and the associated release of their proteolytic enzymes. Generation of kinins, polypeptides believed to mediate portions of the acute inflammatory response, is also suppressed by high doses of the glucocorticoids. All of these effects tend to alleviate the redness, swelling, pain, and cellular destruction caused by the inflammatory response.

Pharmacological doses of the glucocorticoids also suppress many of the later manifestations of the inflammatory response. Their inhibitory effects on the migration and phagocytic activity of blood cells has already been discussed. One of their most important, and potentially dangerous, effects is their suppression of fibroblastic activity. High doses of the glucocorticoids not only decrease the number of fibroblasts but also inhibit their synthesis of collagen resulting in a thinning of the connective tissue. The danger of this effect lies in the vital role the deposition of collagen plays in walling off and localizing bacterial and viral invaders. In addition, the proliferation of capillaries into the area of insult is inhibited. Suppression of collagen synthesis and proliferation of capillaries result in a delay of wound healing.

The effects of excessive doses of glucocorticoids on the immune response are still undefined. Although the glucocorticoids do improve the clinical course of a number of diseases in which the immune response is believed to play an important role, present evidence indicates that the beneficial effects are due primarily to suppression of the accompanying inflammatory response.[2]

The rate of synthesis and release of cortisol is regulated by a polypeptide hormone, adrenocorticotropin (ACTH), secreted by the pituitary gland. In the absence of ACTH, cortisol production stops and the adrenal cortex atrophies. In turn, regulation of ACTH secretion is mediated by a balance between two opposing forces: (1) There is a positive influence from hypothalamic neural pathways activated by various stressful stimuli such as sound, emotion, pain, and anxiety. In response to these stimuli, corticotropin-releasing factor (CRF) is released from nerve endings in the median eminence into the hypophyseal-portal venous system where it travels to the pituitary and stimulates synthesis and release of ACTH. (2) There is a negative influence mediated by plasma cortisol concentrations (negative feedback). Cortisol acts directly on the median eminence to inhibit both the synthesis and release of ACTH and, hence, cortisol.

Thus, the blood concentration of cortisol is maintained within a given physiological range by a dynamic equilibrium between continual secretion of ACTH on the one hand and the negative feedback mechanism on the other. This equilibrium allows excessive plasma cortisol concentrations to shut down ACTH secretion while allowing increased output as plasma cortisol concentrations fall. This dynamic equilibrium is modulated, however, by several factors. Superimposed upon this interplay between cortisol's plasma concentration and its rate of secretion is a diurnal cyclical pattern in which an individual's plasma cortisol concentration is highest upon awakening in the morning, falls throughout the day, and reaches a minimum about midnight. The neural mechanisms responsible for this internal clock are unknown, but the cycle can be altered by changing the sleeping pattern of the individual. In addition, negative feedback mechanism can be overridden by the neural pathways activated by stressful external stimuli, allowing a greater than usual output of cortisol in periods of increased need. Consequently, the *normal* physiological range of the plasma cortisol concentration varies according to the time of day and whether the patient is under physical or emotional stress.

## Preparations

The structural core of the corticosteroids is the cyclopentanoperhydrophenanthrene (steroid) nucleus (see Figure 16.1). Other common structural features of the naturally occurring corticosteroids include a double bond between carbons 4 and 5, a ketone group at carbon 3, and a -CO-CH$_2$OH side chain at carbon 17. The structural differences among the corticosteroids, both natural and synthetic, occur in the various side groups of the steroid nucleus and account for their pharmacological differences. Studies of the structure activity relationships of the corticosteroids have resulted in significant separation of glucocorticoid activity from mineralocorticoid activity. To date, however, antiinflammatory activity and glucocorticoid activity parallel one another. Table 16.1 summarizes the relative mineralocorticoid, glucocorticoid, and antiinflammatory activity of selected corticosteroids.

Absorption of the corticosteroids is determined primarily by the water and lipid solubilities of the given preparation. Water solubility is more important after parenteral administration, and lipid solubility is more important after oral administration. The free steroids are slightly insoluble in water, whereas the acetate esters

**Table 16.1. Adrenal Corticosteroids**

| | Relative Potencies | | | |
|---|---|---|---|---|
| Generic Name (Trade name) | Glucocorticoid Activity Liver glycogen deposition | Antiinflammatory Activity | Mineralocorticoid Activity Sodium retention | Approximate Equivalent Antiinflammatory Dose (mg) |
| NATURAL PRODUCTS | | | | |
| Cortisol (Cortef) | 1 | 1 | 1 | 20 |
| Cortisone (Cortone) | 0.8 | 0.8 | 0.8 | 25 |
| Aldosterone | 0.3 | 0.3 | 3,000 | 67 |
| SYNTHETIC PRODUCTS | | | | |
| Prednisone (Delta) | 3.5 | 3.5 | 0.8 | 5 |
| Prednisolone (Hydeltra) | 4 | 4 | 0.8 | 5 |
| Triamcinolone (Kenalog) | 5 | 5 | 0 | 4 |
| Paramethasone (Haldrone) | 10 | 10 | 0 | 2 |
| Dexamethasone (Decadron) | 25 | 25 | 0 | 0.75 |
| Betamethasone (Celestone) | 25 | 25 | 0 | 0.6 |

Source: Modified from Haynes and Larner, 1975.[2]

are even more water insoluble; both are absorbed slowly after parenteral administration. On the other hand, the sodium-phosphate and succinate esters are highly water soluble and are rapidly absorbed after parenteral administration.

The appropriate form of a given corticosteroid can be chosen according to its therapeutic use. Thus, the water-insoluble esters or free steroids are employed when slow, persistent absorption or, conversely, when localization of effect is desired (e.g., topical application, pellet implantation for prolonged hormonal effect, and injection into arthritic joints). When rapid absorption and distribution are required (e.g., acute adrenal insufficiency, anaphylactic shock, and daily administration for antiinflammatory effect) the water-soluble esters are indicated. The following preparations with their respective dental uses are given as examples:

1. Hydrocortisone hemisuccinate (Solu-cortef) a water-soluble preparation given in acute adrenal insufficiency or in anaphylactic reactions to support the pressor effects of epinephrine

2. Prednisolone acetate (Meticortelone acetate), a water-insoluble preparation given by intraarticular injection for the treatment of temporomandibular joint arthritis

3. Triamcinolone acetonide (Kenalog), a water-insoluble preparation topically applied in the management of oral ulceration

### Adrenal Insufficiency

Insufficiency of secretion of the adrenal corticosteroids can result from abnormalities of the adrenal cortex itself (Addison's disease) or from inadequate secretion of ACTH by the pituitary. One example of the latter is adrenal insufficiency in patients from whom corticosteroids are withdrawn too abruptly after long-term administration of supraphysiological doses. If untreated, chronic adrenal insufficiency, as in patients with Addison's disease, results in a progression of degenerative changes over a period of weeks, including loss of appetite and gastrointestinal disturbances; hypoglycemia; muscle weakness; excessive excretion of sodium and chloride but retention of potassium; a decrease in the extracellular and plasma volumes resulting from renal excretion of water and the movement of extracellular water and potassium into the cells; hypotension and hemoconcentration; and, finally, cardiovascular collapse, renal failure, and death.

Administration of a mineralocorticoid will correct many of these alterations and maintain life as long as the individual is not placed in a stressful situation. The blood electrolyte composition, plasma volume, and cardiovascular function return toward normal. The return to more normal perfusion of muscular tissue appears to be responsible for the increased muscular strength that usually accompanies administration of the mineralocorticoids. If the individual is exposed to stress, however, acute adrenal insufficiency (adrenal crisis) may develop and the cardiovascular and renal systems rapidly collapse. Although the mineralocorticoids alone do not prevent adrenal crisis in response to stress, adequate doses of the glucocorticoids do. Although hypoglycemia undoubtedly contributes, the rapid deterioration seen in adrenal crisis appears to result primarily from an inability of the cardiovascular system to respond to the increased demands placed upon it by the stressful stimuli. The exact cause is unknown, but appears to lie, at least in part, in the permissive action of the glucocorticoids on the vascular response to epinephrine and other vasopressors. In the absence of glucocorticoids the blood vessels lose their responsiveness to these agents; administration of glucocorticoids restores this responsiveness, thus allowing control by the sympathetic nervous system of blood pressure and tissue perfusion.

Normally, the body responds to stress with an increased secretion of cortisol by the mechanisms discussed. Obviously, this cannot occur in the patient whose adrenal cortex or pituitary is compromised by disease or other factors. Normal, daily activity in such patients can be ensured by the administration of hormonal doses of exogenous corticosteroids (maintenance therapy). However, adrenal crisis may be evoked in these patients by moderate stress of any kind, including trauma, infection, and hemorrhage. In other words, the proper maintenance dose is relative to the external environment and internal state of the patient. The same dose that may adequately maintain a calm, rested individual under optimal environmental conditions may fail to do so under conditions of stress and trauma. The dentist must therefore consider increasing the dose of glucocorticoid administered to these patients prior to, during, and immediately after any stressful dental procedure in order to provide the extra glucocorticoid needed by the body. This increase should be done in consultation with the patient's physician; the proper course of action is determined primarily by the anticipated degree of stress (mild, moderate, or severe) to the specific patient.

With proper evaluation and management, patients with adrenal disorders can be treated safely. They should be watched closely for signs of adrenal crises—nausea, vomiting, and abdominal cramping; weakness; mental confusion, restlessness, or lethargy; and hypotension. If adrenal crisis does occur, its management requires parenteral administration of a water-soluble glucocorticoid, glucose, fluids (isotonic saline), and possibly, vasopressors.

### Antiinflammatory Therapy

The glucocorticoids are prescribed in a wide variety of diseases for their antiinflammatory effects. They are commonly employed in the treatment of rheumatoid conditions such as rheumatoid arthritis and rheumatic heart disease. They are also used in the treatment of severe cases of asthma, lupus erythematosus, various dermatological diseases, inflammatory diseases of the eye, and several hematological disorders. One of the most recent uses of the glucocorticoids is in combination with other drugs to suppress immunological rejection after organ transplants. Although the corticosteroids may be lifesaving, their effectiveness in all of the aforementioned diseases is entirely palliative; they do not correct the underlying cause of any disease.

The high doses of corticosteroid and prolonged treatment period required in these chronic diseases produce many adverse effects. Foremost among these is significant suppression of pituitary ACTH secretion by the negative feedback mechanism, which results in adrenal cortical atrophy and decreased cortisol synthesis and secretion. When administration of exogenous corticosteroid is stopped, the pituitary responds with an increased secretion of ACTH. Depending upon the degree of cortical atrophy, however, the adrenal cortex remains unresponsive to ACTH for significant periods. This phenomenon is referred to as suppression of the hypothalamic-pituitary-adrenal axis and is, in fact, a form of drug-induced adrenal insufficiency.

The degree of suppression depends upon several factors, most important of which are the dose and potency of the corticosteroid and the duration of treatment. In general, if the glucocorticoid is given for less than 10 days, the hypothalamic-pituitary-adrenal axis recovers rapidly and few clinical difficulties are encountered. The longer the period of administration, however, the more prolonged the recovery period—in some cases up to one year after administration has stopped.

Other adverse effects of the corticosteroids are mainly exaggerations of their hormonal effects and have been discussed.

In an attempt to avoid suppression of the hypothalamic-pituitary-adrenal axis, as well as other adverse effects, the administration of high doses of corticosteroids is advocated on alternate days.[3] With alternate day therapy one large dose of the corticosteroid is administered early in the morning, at the time of peak endogenous plasma cortisol concentration, to allow the exogenous and endogenous steroid plasma concentrations to fall together, thus mimicking the natural diurnal cycle. In a large number of patients, this regimen allows adequate antiinflammatory effects while minimizing hypothalamic-pituitary-adrenal suppression and other adverse effects.

The patient who is taking antiinflammatory doses of the glucocorticoids offers a special challenge to the dental hygienist. Not only must he or she be aware of the possible adverse effects of these agents, but the inability of the oral tissue to inflame removes one of the most obvious signs of oral disease. Thus, these patients may be practicing poor oral hygiene or have all the conditions that cause gingivitis or periodontitis without the characteristic signs of inflammation.

The inflammatory response constitutes the body's first line of defense against infection. Consequently, one of the most serious potential dangers of antiinflammatory doses of the glucocorticoids is dissemination of latent or localized infection, especially viral infection. The possibility of mobilizing oral bacteria during dental operative or surgical procedures dictates that particular attention be paid to asepsis and appropriate chemoprophylaxis. If bacterial infection develops in such patients, it may be extremely difficult to control and may require decreasing the dose of corticosteroid after consultation with the patient's physician. Such reduction of dosage, however, may exacerbate the disease for which the corticosteroid was originally prescribed, and a vicious cycle is set in motion.

## ANTIDIABETIC AGENTS

Insulin is a protein hormone synthesized and secreted by the beta cells of the pancreas primarily in response to elevated blood glucose. Whereas cortisol and epinephrine provide a readily utilizable source of energy in the form of circulating glucose and free fatty acids, insulin promotes the conservation of energy by stimulating its storage in the form of glycogen (in muscle and liver cells) and triglyceride (in fat cells).

The metabolic effects working together to produce this increased storage are varied and poorly understood. Insulin's most well-established action is its ability to increase the transport of glucose across cell membranes. In the muscle and liver cells, it also directly stimulates the enzyme system catalyzing the conversion of glucose into glycogen. At the same time there is a decrease, probably secondary, in gluconeogenesis. In the fat cell, the increase in available glucose results in its increased conversion into triglycerides. In addition, insulin directly inhibits the enzyme that catalyzes the release of fatty acids from these triglycerides.

Diabetes mellitus is a disease characterized by several signs and symptoms. The most common are increased blood glucose and increased glucose in the urine and diuresis; the most serious is a metabolic acidosis (ketoacidosis) resulting from increased production of ketone bodies (i.e., acetone, acetoacetic acid) as by-products of fat metabolism. Although other factors are probably involved, diabetes mellitus results from inadequate secretion of insulin by the pancreas. The disease may take one of two basic forms: (1) Juvenile onset diabetes usually develops before 20 years of age and is associated with a complete lack of insulin secretion, rapid development, and severity of symptoms. (2) Maturity onset diabetes usually develops after age 40, is associated with the ability of the pancreas to secrete some insulin, and involves a slower onset and less severe symptoms.

In the absence of insulin the transport of glucose into the cell is reduced, and fuel for cellular metabolism must be obtained from glycogen stores. These carbohydrate stores are quickly depleted, and the body metabolism shifts from carbohydrate to protein and fat fuel sources. Protein is broken down at an abnormally high rate, and the resulting amino acids are rapidly converted into glucose. Mobilization of free fatty acids from peripheral fat depots is increased as a result of the uninhibited lipolytic action of cortisol, catecholamines, and other hormones. These fatty acids are used as fuel by the liver with the formation of acidic ketone bodies as by-products. In response to the resulting acidosis and increased breakdown of protein, the kidney excretes increased urea and ammonia which contributes to the metabolic acidosis.

### Insulin Preparations

The solubility and, hence, the onset and duration of action of a given insulin preparation are dependent upon its physical state (whether amorphous or crystalline, and, if crystalline, the size of the crystals), its zinc content, the presence of protein modifiers, and the nature of the buffer in which the insulin is suspended. Based upon these characteristics, the available insulin preparations can be divided into three groups as shown in Table 16.2: fast, intermediate, and long-acting preparations. In general, solubility decreases and the onset and duration of action increase as the crystal size increases or if the insulin is complexed with proteins such as protamine or globin. One advantage of the lente insulins, which rely on crystal size and zinc content for prolongation of action, over

**Table 16.2  Properties of Various Preparations of Insulin**

| Type | Preparation | Protein Modifier | Approximate Time of Onset (hours) | Approximate Duration of Action (hours) |
|---|---|---|---|---|
| FAST ACTING | Insulin Injection, U.S.P. (regular insulin) | None | 1 | 6 |
| | Insulin Injection, U.S.P. "Insulin made from zinc insulin crystals" (regular insulin) | None | 1 | 8 |
| | Prompt Insulin Zinc Suspension, U.S.P. (semilente insulin) | None | 1 | 14 |
| INTERMEDIATE ACTING | Isophane Insulin Suspension, U.S.P. (NPH insulin, isophane insulin) | Protamine | 2 | 24 |
| | Insulin Zinc Suspension, U.S.P. (lente insulin) | None | 2 | 24 |
| LONG ACTING | Protamine Zinc Insulin Suspension, U.S.P. | Protamine | 7 | 36 |
| | Extended Insulin Zinc Suspension, U.S.P. (ultralente insulin) | None | 7 | 36 |

Source: Modified from Larner and Haynes, 1975.[4]

insulin preparations which rely on protein modifiers is a lower incidence of hypersensitivity reactions, since the protein modifier itself may be allergenic.

All insulin preparations must be administered parenterally, usually by subcutaneous injection. For this reason, as well as for greater control over the desired effect, it is desirable to have a preparation with a fairly rapid onset and moderately prolonged (24 hour) duration of action. This ideal can be approached by mixing compatible insulin preparations (e.g., combining regular and protamine zinc insulin).

### Oral Hypoglycemic Agents

The diabetic patient whose pancreas synthesizes and secretes no insulin must receive exogenous insulin daily. In a large number of diabetic patients, however, the basic problem is not the complete lack of insulin, but rather a subnormal rate of insulin secretion or the too rapid destruction of secreted insulin. This is often the case in the patient who has maturity onset diabetes. The diabetic condition of a large number of such patients can be effectively controlled by the oral hypoglycemic agents. These drugs act either by stimulating pancreatic secretion of insulin or by modifying its actions peripherally.

The oral hypoglycemic agents can be classified into two groups on the basis of their chemical structure (see Figure 16.2) as follows:

1. Sulfonylureas
   Tolbutamide (Orinase)
   Chlorpropamide (Diabinese)
   Acetohexamide (Dymelor)
   Tolazamide (Tolinase)
2. Biguanides
   Phenformin (DBI)

The sulfonylureas act by stimulating the secretion of insulin by the beta cells of the pancreas. The exact mechanism of this action is unknown. They are effectively absorbed from the gastrointestinal tract (hence the term, oral) and are bound to plasma protein in varying amounts. Differences in the degree of protein binding, as well as in rates of renal excretion and biotransformation, account for the differences in onset and duration of action of these agents (see Table 16.3).

The adverse effects of the sulfonylureas include gastrointestinal disturbances, hematological disorders, jaundice, and allergic skin rashes. These are usually transient and not serious. The most

SULFONYLUREA DERIVATIVES:

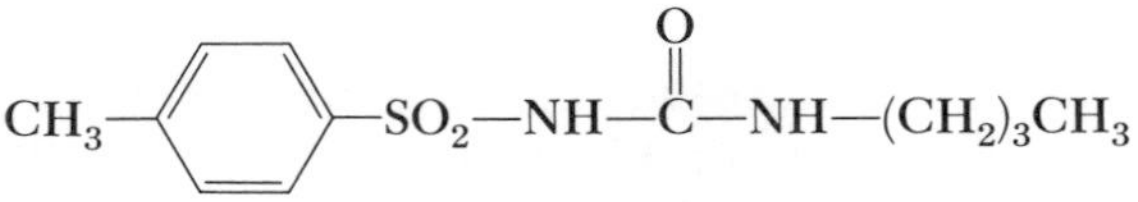

TOLBUTAMIDE

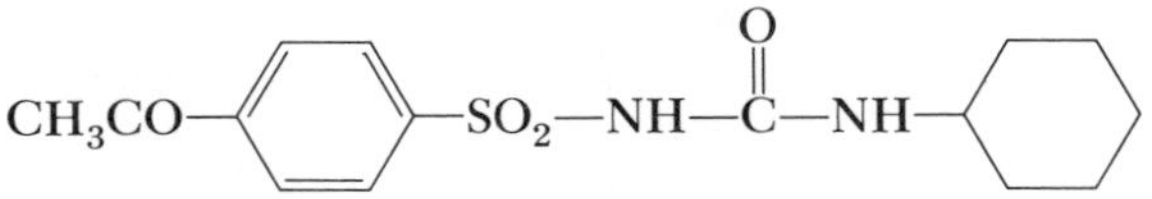

ACETOHEXAMIDE

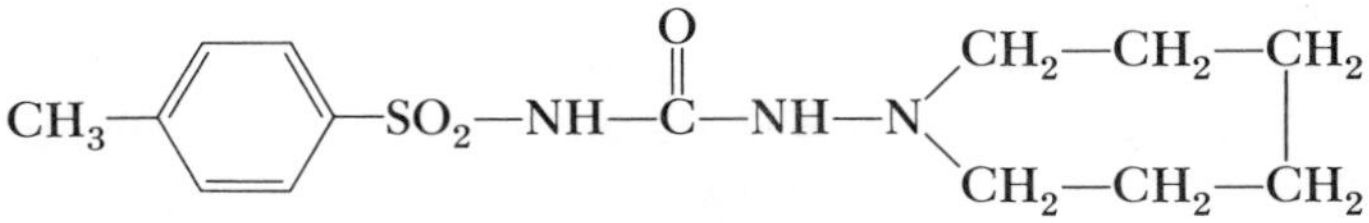

TOLAZAMIDE

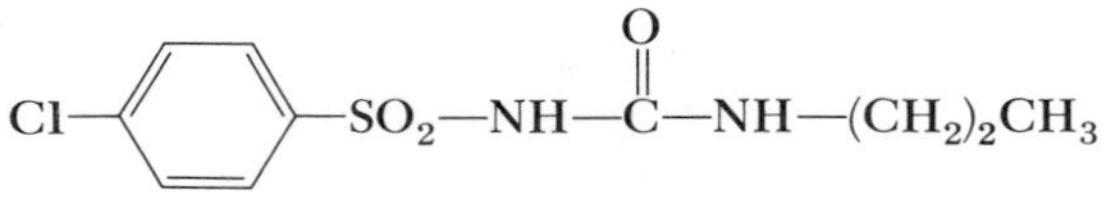

CHLORPROPAMIDE

BIGUANIDE DERIVATIVE:

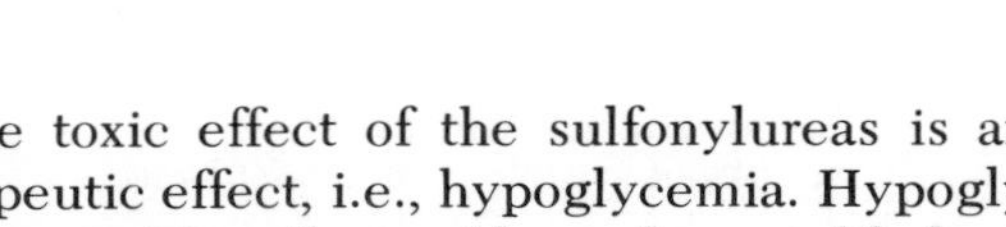

PHENFORMIN

**Figure 16.2** Structures of oral hypoglycemic agents.

severe toxic effect of the sulfonylureas is an extension of their therapeutic effect, i.e., hypoglycemia. Hypoglycemia is least likely to occur with tolbutamide and most likely to occur with chlorpropamide; it may occur as a result of overdosage, decreased excretion or metabolism, or from displacement of the hypoglycemic agent from protein binding sites by other drugs, thereby increasing the concentration of free, active agent. In the case of chlorpropamide, especially, the hypoglycemia may be severe and prolonged, lasting for days after administration has been stopped. The sulfonylureas find their greatest clinical usefulness in patients with relatively mild, maturity onset diabetes.

Many drugs have been reported to interact with the sulfonylureas, including the following: (1) Salicylates, phenylbutazone, and the sulfonamides are reported to increase the hypoglycemic effect of the sulfonylureas. Proposed mechanisms include displacement from protein binding sites, interference with renal excretion, and inhibition of metabolic inactivation. (2) Barbiturates, meperidine, and phenothiazine derivatives are reported to decrease the hypoglycemic effects of the sulfonylureas. Proposed mechanisms include induction of the liver microsomal enzyme system. (3) Under some circumstances the sulfonylureas may prolong the hypnotic and sedative effects of the barbiturates and other sedative-hypnotic agents. (4) Patients taking the sulfonylureas have been reported to have an intolerance to alcohol similar to that produced by disulfiram (i.e., nausea, vomiting).

Phenformin lowers the blood sugar concentration in the diabetic, but not in the normal individual. The mechanism of the blood glucose lowering effect in the diabetic is unknown, but it is clear that phenformin acts by a mechanism different from that of the sulfonylureas. It does not stimulate pancreatic insulin secretion, but rather appears to potentiate insulin's actions peripherally, since its actions require the presence of at least some insulin, either endogenous or exogenous.

Phenformin is adequately absorbed from the gastrointestinal tract. The onset of action after oral administration is from 3 to 5 hours. Depending upon the preparation administered, the duration of action may vary from 8 to 24 hours. Hypoglycemia can occur with phenformin administration, but high doses are required and it is less likely to occur than with the sulfonylureas. Inadvertent overdosage is limited by gastrointestinal disturbances that usually occur before hypoglycemia. These include a metallic taste, nausea, vomiting, diarrhea, and cramping. Xerostomia may also occur in patients taking phenformin. Phenformin is useful in the treatment

**Table 16.3.  Duration of Sulfonylurea Action**

| Compound | Time to Peak Effect (hours) | Usual Duration of Action (hours) |
|---|---|---|
| Tolbutamide | 5 | 8–12 |
| Acetohexamide | 3 | 12–14 |
| Tolazamide | 4–6 | 15 |
| Chlorpropamide | 6–10 | Several days |

Source: Modified from Shaw and Beaser, 1971.[5]

of relatively mild, maturity onset diabetes. It may also be effective as an adjunct to exogenous insulin in the treatment of more severe and unstable forms of diabetes, allowing better control with smaller doses of insulin by virtue of its insulin-potentiating action.

## The Diabetic Dental Patient

The severity of diabetes ranges from mild forms of maturity onset diabetes, which can be controlled by diet alone, to the brittle form of juvenile diabetes, which requires daily injections of exogenous insulin. Even with the daily insulin injections, the brittle diabetic walks a tight rope between severe hypoglycemic reactions, on the one hand, and ketoacidosis, on the other. The reasons for this unstable condition are unknown, but several possible precipitants have been suggested, including fluctuations in circulating insulin antibodies, exercise, infection, emotional factors, and changes in the diet.

As in any patient being treated pharmacologically for a chronic disease, the general health of the diabetic is a delicate balance between the disease itself and the effects of the controlling drug. Anything that augments or reduces the influence of either one of these components will throw the general health of the patient out of balance.

Many factors may increase the body's insulin requirements and thus aggravate the diabetic condition. Foremost among these is the stress response. The epinephrine and cortisol released during the body's response to stress exert antiinsulin actions. Both raise the blood glucose levels by increasing the breakdown of glycogen, stimulating the synthesis of new glucose, and promoting mobilization of free fatty acids. Cortisol also stimulates gluconeogenesis by increasing the breakdown of protein. In addition, epinephrine inhibits pancreatic release of insulin and inhibits cellular uptake of glucose. Consequently, stressful conditions such as anxiety, trauma of surgery, and infection exacerbate diabetes. The diabetic patient should be well-controlled before involved operative or surgical procedures are performed; indeed, if the patient's diabetic condition is not controlled, routine dental treatment of any kind should be delayed until control has been established by the patient's physician.

Obviously, administration of epinephrine and glucocorticoids in such a way that significant systemic absorption might occur should be avoided in the diabetic patient. Morphine and other narcotic analgesics may increase insulin requirements, and the possibility of acidosis makes general anesthesia dangerous in the diabetic patient.

In addition to avoiding factors that may exacerbate the diabetic condition, the dental practitioner must also appreciate the tenuous condition of the patient with diabetes mellitus. These patients have a higher-than-normal incidence of infection, including infections resulting from dental treatment. This lowered resistance to infection indicates that appropriate chemoprophylaxis is advised in the diabetic patient in situations in which it might not ordinarily be required. The small blood vessels of the diabetic are fragile. For this reason, procedures, such as subgingival curettage, which may injure soft tissue and bone should be avoided unless the diabetic condition is well controlled. Wound healing may also be significantly delayed.

In the majority of cases, the physician can give his diabetic patient a fairly uniform day-to-day routine by properly balancing the diet, timing of meals, and daily physical activity with the dosage schedule of insulin or oral hypoglycemic agent. Sugar tolerance is lowest in the morning, and the greatest tendency toward hyperglycemia is after breakfast. To compensate for these factors insulin is usually administered in the morning before breakfast in a carefully chosen dosage. The blood glucose concentration generally falls throughout the morning but begins to rise again in the afternoon. For these reasons it is best to schedule dental appointments for the diabetic patient about 1 to 2 hours after the patient has taken his insulin and has eaten breakfast. Under these conditions the available insulin should be enough to allow an adequate response to moderate stress. However, if the patient is controlled by oral hypoglycemic agents alone, exogenous insulin may be required before moderately stressful dental procedures are performed.

Hypoglycemia may occur in any patient treated with insulin or the oral hypoglycemic agents. This may occur through inadvertent overdosage, potentiation of the oral hypoglycemic agents by other drugs, or even failure of the patient taking insulin to eat breakfast before the dental appointment. In a few patients, the initial signs of hypoglycemia include hunger or nausea, bradycardia, and mild hypotension. In the majority of patients, hypoglycemia is characterized by lethargy and yawning; confusion and impaired mental function, hypertension, tachycardia, sweating, mydriasis, increased respiration, and other signs of increased sympathetic activity; convulsions and coma. Signs of increased sympathetic activity usually predominate when the blood glucose level falls rapidly, since a rapid fall evokes a compensatory activation of the sympathetic nervous system. Disturbances of the central nervous system usually predominate if the fall in blood glucose is moderate and occurs slowly.

The immediate need of the patient with hypoglycemia is intravenous glucose. Intramuscular injection of glucagon has also been advocated and may be beneficial, but it does not supplant the need for glucose. Glucagon is a polypeptide hormone, synthesized and secreted by the alpha cells of the pancreas. Its actions are antagonistic to insulin; it promotes the mobilization of fuel from intracellular stores. Glucagon's beneficial effects in hypoglycemia are limited by its dependence upon adequate glycogen stores. Glucagon also stimulates the release of insulin which may be a disadvantage in patients whose pancreas retains some insulin-secreting ability.

## THYROID AND ANTITHYROID DRUGS

Essentially, abnormalities of thyroid function result from iodine deficiency or from subnormal (hypothyroid) or excessive (hyperthyroid) activity of the thyroid gland. Similarly, the drugs to be discussed in this section fall into three groups: (1) agents used to correct and prevent iodine deficiency; (2) agents used as replacement therapy for the thyroid hormones in cases of hypothyroid function; and (3) agents inhibiting the biosynthesis or release of thyroid hormones and used to control excessive thyroid activity.

### Normal Thyroid Function

The thyroid gland synthesizes two hormones, thyroxine ($T_4$) and triiodothyronine ($T_3$), from iodinated tyrosine (see Figure 16.3). Normally, thyroxine is the major hormone secreted, and triiodothyronine accounts for only a small fraction of the total organically bound iodine in the blood. These hormones are essential for normal growth and development. Their absence during childhood results in a dwarfed, mentally retarded individual (cretin). Present evidence suggests that one of the thyroid hormones's most important actions in this regard is as important determinants of genetically coded developmental sequences. The activities of many enzyme systems throughout the body are also modulated by the thyroid hormones. They increase the total body metabolic rate; especially sensitive are the metabolic rates of the heart, kidney, liver, and diaphragm. These actions are largely responsible for the essential role the thyroid hormones play in the proper function of many body systems, including the nervous, cardiovascular, renal, reproductive, and temperature regulating systems in the adult.

Hyperthyroid function is characterized by excessive production of heat, increased activity of sympathetic nervous system, and increased neuromuscular excitability. The activity of the heart is especially elevated as evidenced by increased cardiac output,

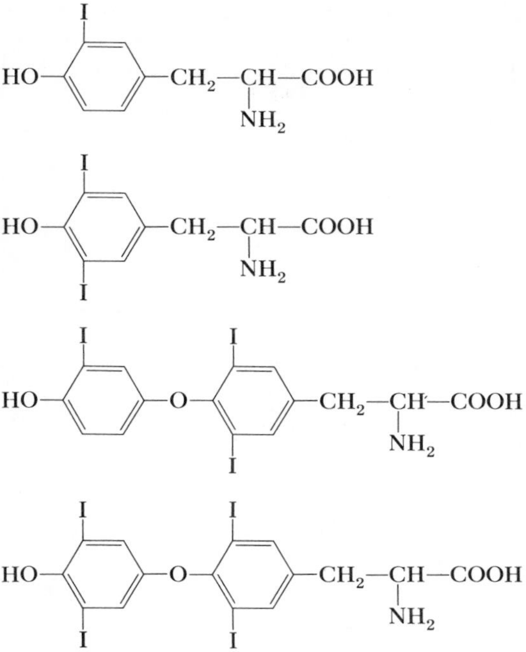

MONOIODOTYROSINE (MIT)

DIIODOTYROSINE (DIT)

TRIIODOTHYRONINE ($T_3$)

TETRAIODOTHYRONINE ($T_4$)
(Thyroxine)

**Figure 16.3** Structures of thyroid hormones and their precursors.

tachycardia, as well as possible anginal attacks and arrhythmias. Although these cardiac changes appear to be due to the thyroid hormones themselves, the similar stimulatory effects of endogenous catecholamines undoubtedly intensify the stress placed upon the myocardium in situations of thyroid hyperfunction.

The production of thyroxine and triiodothyronine can be divided into four steps—trapping of iodide, binding of iodine to tyrosine, coupling of iodotyrosines, and secretion of thyroid hormone (see Figure 16.4).

TRAPPING OF IODIDE. The thyroid gland selectively concentrates iodide, resulting in a glandular iodide concentration 20 to 50 times that of the plasma under normal circumstances. This so-called trapping involves an energy-requiring active transport process that is stimulated by thyrotropin (TSH), a polypeptide hormone secreted by the pituitary gland. In addition to the positive action of TSH, the activity of the iodide uptake mechanism is inversely related to the stores of thyroid iodine. Under normal circumstances the uptake of iodide is the rate-limiting step in hormone synthesis.

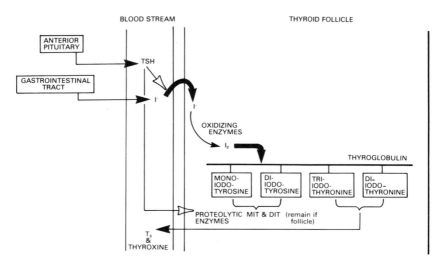

**Figure 16.4** Thyroid hormone synthesis and release. (Adapted and redrawn from Gilman and Murad, 1975.[6])

BINDING OF IODINE TO TYROSINE. Normally, the iodide taken up by the thyroid gland is rapidly oxidized by a poorly understood mechanism which appears to involve hydrogen peroxide and a peroxidase enzyme present in the thyroid gland. The resulting oxidized intermediate reacts with molecules of tyrosine at the sites shown in Figure 16.4 to form monoiodotyrosine or diiodotyrosine. The tyrosine moieties thus iodinated are constituents of thyroglobulin, the protein making up the colloid within the thyroid follicles. Normally, about four times as much diiodotyrosine as monoiodotyrosine is formed, although this ratio may be decreased significantly in iodine deficiency.

COUPLING OF IODOTYROSINES. The iodinated tyrosine moieties serve as the source for the basic constituents of thyroid hormone synthesis. Hormone synthesis occurs by coupling of two iodinated tyrosine moieties which are incorporated within the thyroglobulin molecule. This coupling is an oxidative reaction which also appears to involve a peroxidase enzyme. Thyroxine is formed by the coupling of two diiodotyrosine moieties, while triiodothyronine is formed by the coupling of one monoiodotyrosine and one diiodotyrosine moiety. The ratio of thyroxine to triiodothyronine is influenced by the relative quantities of monoiodotyrosine and diiodotyrosine available so that, normally, about four times as much thyroxine as triiodothyronine is formed. In iodine deficiency, however, the relative proportions may shift so that triiodothyronine may predominate by as much as threefold. This, and the fact that triiodothyronine is about four times as potent as thyroxine allows up to sixfold increases in hormonal activity for a given quantity of available iodine.

SECRETION OF THYROID HORMONE. The thyroid hormones, as well as monoiodotyrosine and diiodotyrosine, are cleaved from thyroglobulin by hydrolytic enzymes in the thyroid gland. Normally, however, only the hormones are secreted into the blood, whereas the monoiodotyrosine and diiodotyrosine are enzymatically deiodinated. The liberated iodide is then reused by the gland.

The activity of the thyroid gland is regulated primarily by thyrotropin (TSH). Within a few minutes after TSH makes contact with the thyroid gland, there is an increase in the secretion of thyroid hormone. This is followed by an increase in the vascularity of the gland, enlargement of the thyroid cells, and resorption of the follicular colloid. With continual TSH stimulation, uptake of iodide is enhanced. The rate of secretion of TSH by the pituitary is negatively modulated by the concentration of thyroid hormone in the blood in a manner analogous to the ACTH-glucocorticoid negative feedback mechanism. This mechanism plays an important role in the enlargement of the thyroid gland (goiter) in response to decreases in hormonal output.

## Iodine Deficiency

Chronic iodine deficiency is manifested in a characteristic clinical disorder—colloid or simple, nontoxic goiter. Since iodine is one of the basic raw materials of thyroid hormone synthesis, normal thyroid function depends on the availability of adequate amounts. Although the body has a great capacity for conserving iodine, a significant amount is excreted daily by the kidney and adequate replacement must be provided by the daily diet. Under normal circumstances, dietary intake of about 1 to 2 $\mu$g/kg/day is required to maintain proper homeostatic balance.

Iodine is not ubiquitous in most items of the human diet; seafood is the richest source. It is not surprising, then, that the most common cause of simple goiter is a lack of iodine in the daily diet and, with the exception of societies in which seafood is a major portion of the total diet, is a fairly common worldwide disorder. The introduction of iodized salt as a supplemental source of iodine has decreased the incidence of simple goiter in many countries.

Simple goiter resulting from iodine deficiency is usually not associated with decreased hormonal activity. Indeed, the enlargement of the thyroid gland (goiter) is a remarkable compensatory adaptation of this organ to the lack of iodine which allows it to make the greatest use of the iodine that is available. Although iodine deficiency initially reduces thyroid hormone synthesis and, hence, circulating hormone, removal of this negative feedback influence on the pituitary results in elevated secretion of TSH. Under the chronic influence of TSH, the thyroid glandular tissue hypertrophies, vascularity of the gland increases (10- to 100-fold), and uptake of iodide is stimulated (increasing the normal gland/plasma iodide concentration gradient up to 10-fold). As a result, the enlarged gland is extremely efficient in extracting and utilizing the reduced amounts of available iodine, allowing it to maintain normal hormonal output. In addition to hypertrophy of the thyroid gland itself, the shift in predominance from thyroxine to the more potent triiodothyronine induced by iodine deficiency aids in maintaining normal hormonal activity.

Although simple goiter resulting from iodine deficiency is of itself a relatively benign condition, with hormonal activity usually being neither subnormal or excessive (i.e., euthyroid), if the gland continues to function under these stressful conditions for prolonged periods several complications may arise. The gland may undergo so-called exhaustion atrophy and stop functioning altogether, resulting in hypothyroidism. On the other hand, the constant stimulation by TSH may convert the simple goiter into toxic nodular goiter which predisposes the patient to hyperthyroidism and thyroid carcinoma.

These complications can be prevented by early treatment which consists simply of supplying the patient with doses of iodine near his daily normal requirement (1 to 2 $\mu$g/kg/day). Iodine is usually provided by administration of the appropriate dose of either a saturated solution of potassium iodide or Lugol's solution containing 5% iodine and 10% potassium iodide. The iodide is readily absorbed from the gastrointestinal tract, and the gland usually recedes slowly back to normal size. It is important that the dosages administered in treating iodine deficiency are in the range of the normal daily iodine requirement, since large, supraphysiological doses inhibit thyroid function.

## Hypothyroidism

Deficiency of circulating thyroid hormone in the adult may range from mild (hypothyroidism) to severe (myxedema). Classic myxedema is characterized by such signs as obesity, edema, puffiness of the face, weakness of both voluntary and involuntary muscles, impaired mentality, sluggish speech, dilation of the heart, and decreased cardiac output. Thyroid hypofunction may result from many causes, including genetically determined abnormalities of the various enzymes involved in thyroid hormonal synthesis and release; the presence in the diet of foods, such as cabbage, containing chemicals (goitrogens) which inhibit thyroid hormone synthesis; inadequate TSH secretion by the pituitary; and even treatment of hyperthyroidism, either by administration of antithyroid drugs or surgery. However, inadequate circulating thyroid hormone occurs most often when the thyroid gland spontaneously stops functioning at a normal rate for unknown reasons.

Hypothyroidism is rationally and effectively treated by oral administration of exogenous thyroid hormone. The most commonly used preparations are:

1. Thyroid, U.S.P., and Thyroid Tablets, U.S.P., made from dessicated thyroid glands of domestic animals. Standardization of hormonal activity is based on the iodine content and bioassay.

2. Levothyroxine Sodium, U.S.P., the sodium salt of the L-isomer of thyroxine.

3. Liothyronine Sodium, U.S.P., the sodium salt of the L-isomer of triiodothyronine.

These thyroid preparations differ in potency, onset, and duration of action as shown in Table 16.4. Within the circulation, thyroxine is strongly bound to plasma protein, triiodothyronine less so. Protein binding protects thyroxine from hepatic metabolism, and this undoubtedly contributes to its long duration of action. It probably also plays a role in thyroxine's slow onset of action, although the magnitude of the lag time between administration and onset of action has contributed to the hypothesis that thyroxine's hormonal activity is the result of its metabolic conversion to triiodothyronine. Although it has been shown that thyroxine is metabolically transformed to triiodothyronine, the question of whether this transformation accounts for thyroxine's hormonal activity is still debated.

### Hyperthyroidism

Adverse effects from excessive levels of circulating thyroid hormones (thyrotoxicosis) may result either from administration of excessive doses of exogenous thyroid hormone or from excessive production of endogenous hormone by the thyroid gland. The latter occurs both in Graves' disease and toxic nodular goiter. Graves' disease occurs mainly in young adults and is characterized by a diffusely enlarged, highly vascular thyroid gland and a striking protrusion of the eyeballs. Toxic nodular goiter is characterized by nodules within the thyroid gland which spontaneously secrete

**Table 16.4. Thyroid Agents**

| Drug | GI Absorption Rate | Approximate Potency in Dosage-Terms | Onset of Action | Peak of Action | Duration of Action* |
|---|---|---|---|---|---|
| Dessicated thyroid | Slow | 150 mg/day | 2 days | 10 days | 21–42 days |
| Sodium levothyroxine (Synthroid) | Faster | 0.3 mg/day | 1–2 days | 10 days | 21–28 days |
| Sodium liothyronine (Cytomel) | Fastest | 0.1 mg/day | 2 hours | 2 days | 10 days |

\* = after abrupt withdrawal of drug; GI = gastrointestinal.

excessive amounts of hormone, while the rest of the glandular tissue is atrophied. It occurs primarily in older patients, often developing from a long-standing nontoxic goiter. Whatever the etiology, thyrotoxicosis is characterized by excessive production of heat, increased activity of the sympathetic nervous system, increased neuromuscular excitability, and increased sensitivity to pain.

The pharmacological agents that interfere with thyroid function are as follows: (1) inorganic anions, (2) iodine, (3) radioactive iodine, and (4) organic antithyroid agents.

INORGANIC ANIONS. Inorganic anions are found in foods, especially the thiocyanate ion, the goitrogen of cabbage. Although these agents have been used in the past to treat hyperthyroidism, their toxicity has limited their clinical use. The most important members of this group are potassium thiocyanate (KSCN) and potasssium perchlorate ($KClO_4$). Both the thiocyanate and perchlorate anions have been shown to be capable of controlling hyperthyroidism by selectively inhibiting the trapping of iodide by the thyroid gland. When these anions are administered, iodide is rapidly discharged from the thyroid gland, and the concentration gradient of glandular to plasma iodide falls until the respective concentrations are about equal. With this abrupt reduction in raw material, the synthesis of hormone significantly slows. As a result, the toxic goiter of Graves' disease takes on the appearance and activity of simple goiter, often requiring the administration of exogenous thyroid hormone.

IODINE. Iodine is the oldest remedy for disorders of the thyroid gland. The importance of daily microgram quantities to ensure normal hormone synthesis has already been discussed. In large doses (above the minimal effective dose of 6 mg/day) iodine produces a rapid reduction of circulating hormone in patients with hyperthyroidism. The mechanism of iodine's antithyroid action is not completely understood but appears to involve suppression of hormone release from the thyroid gland. Iodine also reduces the vascularity of the enlarged thyroid gland, and one of its primary clinical uses is to reduce thyroid vascularity prior to surgical thyroidectomy.

RADIOACTIVE IODINE. Radioactive iodine is another means of reducing thyroid hormone production. Concentration of the radioactive iodine by the thyroid gland results in localized destruction of thyroid tissue with negligible penetration of radiation to adjacent tissues. The patient is usually pretreated with organic antithyroid drugs to deplete the gland of hormone as well as with iodine to reduce vascularity of the gland prior to radiothyroidectomy.

ORGANIC ANTITHYROID AGENTS. Of the drugs inhibiting thyroid function, the dental practitioner is most likely to encounter patients taking organic antithyroid agents. There are numerous drugs possessing antithyroid action, but in many cases this is not their primary pharmacological action (e.g., the sulfonamides). The most important agents used clinically for their antithyroid action are derivatives of the thioamide class and include propylthiouracil (Propacil) and methimazole (Tapazole). These antithyroid agents may be used alone over a prolonged period to bring the hyperfunctioning thyroid gland to the euthyroid state. In severe thyrotoxicosis they may be given prior to surgical or radiothyroidectomy to reduce the possibility of thyroid storm, a life-threatening, acute form of thyrotoxicosis marked by high fever, tachycardia, hypertension, angina, and cardiac arrhythmias.

The mechanism of action of the antithyroid drugs is not completely understood, but much of the available evidence suggests that they inhibit hormone synthesis primarily by preventing iodination of the tyrosine moieties of thyroglobulin, probably by inhibiting the enzymatic oxidation of trapped iodide. Other evidence suggests that they may also prevent the coupling of iodotyrosines to form the thyroid hormones.

The organic antithyroid agents cause a wide range of adverse reactions, the most common of which are fever and skin rashes. The incidence of adverse effects with propylthiouracil and methimazole is lower than with other members of this group. These agents may also cause pain and stiffness of the joints. Their most serious adverse effect is agranulocytosis which occurs in less than 1% of the cases.

## Thyroid and Antithyroid Drugs and the Dental Patient

Optimally, the dental patient who is being treated for either hyperthyroidism or hypothyroidism will be euthyroid and present few problems associated with the disease during treatment. The dental practitioner, however, should be alert for signs of significant imbalance in control, i.e., either signs of the disease or signs of overdosage of the controlling drug.

Patients who are hyperthyroid, whether by virtue of a hyperfunctioning thyroid gland or by virtue of excessive administration of exogenous thyroid hormone, tend to be overactive and unusually sensitive to pain and, consequently, may require higher than normal doses of sedatives, analgesics, and local anesthetics. On the other hand, patients who are hypothyroid, whether by virtue of a hypofunctioning thyroid gland or by virtue of excessive administration of antithyroid drugs, tend to be abnormally sensitive to all central nervous system depressants, especially the narcotic analgesics.

In the dental patient who has hyperthyroidism, undue stress may precipitate thyroid storm, and medical treatment of such patients to bring them to the euthyroid state should be obtained before any elective operative or surgical procedure is performed. It should be emphasized that special precaution should be taken to avoid intravenous injection of local anesthetic solutions containing epinephrine for two reasons. First of all, epinephrine causes many of the same effects as thyroid storm, making it difficult to evaluate the problem. In addition, the combined stress placed upon the cardiovascular system by epinephrine and the thyroid hormones (the two agents tending to potentiate each other's actions) may result in severe cardiovascular problems—hypertension, angina, and arrhythmias.

## REFERENCES

1. Nocenti, M.R.: Adrenal cortex. *In* Medical Physiology. 12th Edition. Vol. 1. Edited by V.B. Mountcastle. St. Louis, Mosby, 1968.
2. Haynes, R.C., Jr., and Larner, J.: Adrenocorticotropic steroids and their synthetic analogs; inhibitors of adrenocortical steroid biosynthesis. *In* The Pharmacological Basis of Therapeutics. 5th Edition. Edited by L.S. Goodman and A. Gilman. New York, Macmillan, 1975.
3. Harter, J.G., Reddy, W.J., and Thorn, G.W.: Studies of an intermittent corticosteroid dosage regimen. N. Engl. J. Med., *269*:591, 1963.
4. Larner, J., and Haynes, R.C., Jr.: Insulin and oral hypoglycemic drugs; glucagon. *In* The Pharmacological Basis of Therapeutics. 5th Edition. Edited by L.S. Goodman and A. Gilman. New York, Macmillan, 1975.
5. Shaw, R.A., and Beaser, S.B.: The insulins and oral antidiabetic agents. *In* Drill's Pharmacology in Medicine. 4th Edition. Edited by J.R. Di Palma. New York, McGraw-Hill, 1971.
6. Gilman, A.G., and Murad, F.: Thyroid and antithyroid drugs. *In* The Pharmacological Basis of Therapeutics. 5th Edition. Edited by L.S. Goodman and A. Gilman. New York, Macmillan, 1975.

## SUPPLEMENTARY REFERENCES

Mills, L.C.: Adrenal cortex and adrenocortical hormones. *In* Drill's Pharmacology in Medicine. 4th Edition. Edited by J.R. Di Palma. New York, McGraw-Hill, 1971.
Perlmutter, M., and Levey, H.A.: Thyroid gland and antithyroid drugs. *In* Drill's Pharmacology in Medicine. 4th Edition. Edited by J.R. Di Palma. New York, McGraw-Hill, 1971.

# INDEX